T5-AFS-903

Artificial Immune Systems
and Their Applications

Springer
*Berlin*
*Heidelberg*
*New York*
*Barcelona*
*Hong Kong*
*London*
*Milan*
*Paris*
*Singapore*
*Tokyo*

Dipankar Dasgupta (Ed.)

# Artificial Immune Systems and Their Applications

With 100 Figures and 15 Tables

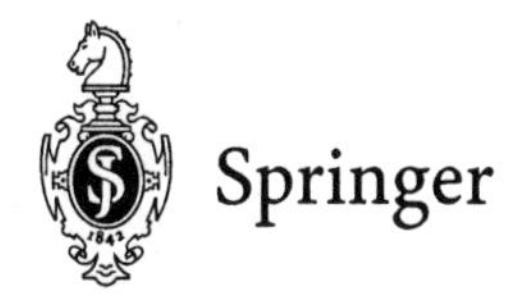

Editor:

Dipankar Dasgupta
University of Memphis
Mathematical Sciences Department
Memphis, TN 38152-6429, USA
dasgupta@msci.memphis.edu

ACM Computing Classification (1998): F.1.1, F.2.2, I.2, I.6, E.4, J.3

ISBN 3-540-64390-7 Springer-Verlag Berlin Heidelberg New York

Library of Congress Cataloging-in-Publication Data
Artificial immune systems and their applications / [edited by] Dipankar Dasgupta
p. cm.
Includes bibliographical references and index.
ISBN 3-540-64390-7 (alk. paper)
1. Immune system - Computer simulation. 2. Artificial Intelligence. I. Dasgupta, D. (Dipankar), 1958- .
QR182.2.C65A78 1998
616.07'9'0113-dc21 98-35558
CIP


Printed in Germany



Cover design: *design & production* GmbH, Heidelberg
Typesetting: Camera ready copy from the editor using a Springer TEX macro package
SPIN: 10675823 45/3142 – 5 4 3 2 1 0 – Printed on acid-free paper

# Preface

The natural immune system is a complex adaptive system which efficiently employs several mechanisms for defense against foreign pathogens. The main role of the immune system is to recognize all cells (or molecules) within the body and categorize those cells as self or non-self. The non-self cells are further categorized in order to induce an appropriate type of defensive mechanism.

From an information-processing perspective, the immune system is a highly parallel intelligent system. It uses learning, memory, and associative retrieval to solve recognition and classification tasks. In particular, it learns to recognize relevant patterns (antigenic peptide), memorize patterns that have been seen previously, and use combinatorics (within gene libraries) to construct pattern detectors (V-regions in antibody) efficiently for distinguishing between foreign antigens and the body's own cells. Moreover, the identification of antigens is not done by a single recognizing set but rather a system level mutual recognition through antigen-antibody reaction as a network. So the overall behavior of the immune system is an emergent property of many local interactions.

The natural immune system is a subject of great research interest because of its importance, complexity and poorly understood alternative mechanisms. However, its general features provide an excellent model of adaptive processes operating at the local level and of useful behavior emerging at the global level. There exist several theories (some are contradictory) to explain immunological phenomena and computer models to simulate various components of the immune system. There is also a growing number of intelligent methodologies (inspired by the immune system) toward real-world problem solving. These methods are labeled with different names – Artificial Immune Systems, Immunity-Based Systems, Immunological Computation, etc. The scope of this field includes (but is not limited to) the following:

```
* Computational methods based on Immunological Principles
* Immunity-Based Cognitive Models
* Artificial Immune Systems for Pattern Recognition
* Immunity-Based Systems for Anomaly or Fault Detection
* Immunity-Based Multi-Agent Systems
```

* Immunity-Based Systems for Self-organization
* Immunity-Based approach for Collective Intelligence
* Immunity-Based Systems for Search and Optimization
* The Immune System as Autonomous Decentralized System
* Immunity-Based approach for Artificial Life
* Immunity-Based Systems for Computer & Internet Security
* The Immune System as a metaphor for Learning System
* Immunological Computation for Data Mining
* Artificial Immune Systems for Fraud Detection
* Immunity-Based Systems in Image & Signal Processing

As the field is growing, researchers started to organize scientific meetings which can serve as a forum for presenting and disseminating current research activities in the field. The first international workshop on "Immunity-based Systems" was held in Japan on December 10, 1996. Subsequently, there was a special track on "Artificial Immune Systems and Their Applications", organized by the editor of this book, at the IEEE International Conference on Systems, Man, and Cybernetics (SMC' 97), Orlando, October 12-15, 1997. A similar event on this topics is also planned to organize at SMC' 98 to be held at San Diego, California. It seems particularly significant at this point of time, to put together important works in an edited volume in order to provide new researchers with a more thorough and systematic account of this rapidly emerging field. We feel that Artificial Immune Systems will soon receive similar attention like other biologically-motivated approaches, such as genetic algorithms, neural networks, cellular automata, etc.

This is the first book that focuses on immunological computation techniques and their applications in many areas including computer security, data mining, machine learning, fault detection, etc. Though the emphasis of the book is on the computational aspects of the immune system, biological models are also considered since they are important to understand the immunological mechanisms and derive computational algorithms. The book will be useful for academician, researchers and practitioners in any scientific discipline who are interested in the models and applications of immunity-based systems.

This volume consists of three parts: introduction, models of artificial immune systems and applications. Various chapters emphasize in-depth analysis of various immune system models and their relation to information processing and problem solving.

The chapter by Dasgupta in the introductory section covers important immunological principles and their computational aspects. It also provides an overview of immunity-based computational models and their applications in pattern recognition, fault detection and diagnosis, computer security, and others.

Bersini's chapter describes the double plasticity of the immune network that allows the system to conduct its self-assertion role while being in constant shift according to the organic's ontogenic changes and in response to the environmental coupling. The author illustrates three application areas where the endogenous double level of adaptability, weakly inspired by the double plasticity in immune networks, allows to learn rapidly a satisfactory solution.

In part II, first chapter argues that the immune system is composed of two distinct compartments, a Central Immune System (CIS) and a Peripheral Immune System (PIS). The PIS is composed of lymphocyte clones and is appropriate for reactions to immunizing antigens, whereas the CIS is appropriate for body antigens. The chapter also reviews the second generation immune network and proposes a third generation network model with an effort to establish a productive relationship between theory and experiments of the immune system.

Segal and Bar-Or view the immune system as an autonomous decentralized system. They propose three different models of such distributed systems and make some useful comparisons between the immune system and other autonomous decentralized systems.

The chapter by Chowdhury presents mathematical models for describing the population dynamics of the immunocompetent cells in a unified manner by incorporating intra-clonal as well as inter-clonal interactions in both discrete and continuous formulation.

Smith et al. argue that immunological memory belongs to the same class of associative memories as Kanerva's sparse distributed memory (SDM). They show the correspondence between B and T cells in the immune system and hard locations in a SDM. In particular, their work demonstrates that B and T cells perform a sparse coverage of all possible antigens in the same way that hard locations perform a sparse coverage of all possible addresses in a SDM.

Next two chapters in this part provide more biological insight of the human immune system. In particular, in Tan and Xiang's chapter a state space model is developed to estimate and predict the number of free HIV and T cells in HIV-infected individuals using the Kalman filter method. Their models express HIV pathogenesis in terms of stochastic differential equations. Based on observed RNA virus copies over time, their models are validated by comparing the Kalman filter estimates of the RNA virus copies with the observed ones from patient data. According to the authors, these models may be useful for monitoring the dynamic behavior of the HIV process at the cellular level in HIV-infected individuals and for assessing the efficiencies and usefulness of the anti-viral treatment.

The chapter on *Modeling the Effects of Prior Infection on Vaccine Efficacy* by Smith et al. provides computer simulations of the vertebrate humoral immune system to study the effects of prior infection on vaccine efficacy. The authors show that the effects of cross-reactive memory and original antigenic sin in the context of three antigens, and investigated how they can lead to vaccine failure. They feel that this work has applications to understanding vaccination against viruses such as influenza that are mutating continually.

In part III, the contribution by Hunt et al. describes a machine learning system based on metaphors taken from the immune system. They illustrate the current version of this Artificial Immune System (AIS), known as *Jisys*. The *Jisys* system can learn patterns in the data by incorporating existing domain knowledge explicitly within the pattern recognition and learning processes. The chapter illustrates the application of the *Jisys* system in detecting patterns in mortgage fraud data. The authors argue that the *Jisys* system is unique in nature and can address problems in a wide range of real world applications.

Watanabe et al. construct a decentralized behavior arbitration mechanism inspired by the biological immune system, and confirm the validity of the proposed system through some experiments. In particular, they experiment with a garbage-collecting problem of autonomous mobile robot that takes into account the concept of self-sufficiency.

The chapter on *parallel search for multi-modal function optimization* proposes an immune algorithm which can accommodate both diversity and learning. The proposed algorithm is shown to be effective for searching for a set of global solutions as well as local solutions.

KrishnaKumar and Neidhoefer developed immunized computational systems that combine *a priori* knowledge with the adapting capabilities of immune systems to provide a powerful alternative to currently available techniques for intelligent control. They apply this immunized adaptive critics to a flight path generator for level 2, non-linear, full-envelope, intelligent aircraft control problem.

The chapter by Kaphart et al. describe an immune system for computers that senses the presence of a previously unknown pathogen, and within minutes automatically derives and deploys a prescription for detecting and removing it. According to the authors, this system is being integrated with a commercial anti-virus product, IBM AntiVirus.

Dasgupta and Forrest develop an anomaly detection algorithm inspired by the immune system. This approach collects knowledge about the normal behavior of a system (or a process) from historical data sets, and generates a set of detectors that probabilistically notice any deviation from the normal behavior of the system. They experimented with a number of time series data and report results to illustrate the performance of the proposed detection algorithm.

The last chapter (by Fukuda et al.) describes a framework for an autonomous distributed system. This is a multi-agent management system which they applied for decision making in production line of a semiconductor plant.

Editing a book which covers interdisciplinary topics is a very difficult and time consuming project. The book could not have been successfully accomplished without support and constructive feedback from the contributors. I would like to thank all the contributors for their effort, for reviewing each others' work and for providing feedback on their own chapters. The completion of this edited volume is accompanied by a great personal tragedy, as my father died of cancer in February, 1998.

My sincere gratitude to the executive editor of Springer-Verlag, Hans Wössner, for his help throughout the project. This document has been prepared using the LATEX word processing system. I would like to thank Frank Holzwarth, Jacqueline Lenz and Gabi Fischer for their help in formatting the final manuscript of the book. I also like to thank my wife, Geeta for helping me with typing and encouraging in editing this volume.

**August 1998**

*Dipankar Dasgupta*
Memphis, USA.

# Table of Contents

**Part I. Introduction**

**An Overview of Artificial Immune Systems and Their Applications** ..... 3
*Dipankar Dasgupta*
1 Introduction ..... 3
2 Computational Aspects of the Immune System ..... 5
3 The Nervous System and the Immune System ..... 6
4 Immune System Based Models ..... 7
5 Some Applications of Artificial Immune Systems ..... 12
6 Summary ..... 17
References ..... 18

**The Endogenous Double Plasticity of the Immune Network and the Inspiration to be Drawn for Engineering Artifacts** ..... 22
*Hugues Bersini*
1 Introduction ..... 22
2 An Elementary Immune Network and the Basic Principles to be Obeyed by a Double Plastic Adaptive System ..... 28
3 The Endogenous Double Plasticity in Neural Net Classifiers ..... 30
4 The Endogenous Double Plasticity in Autonomous Agents Learning by Reinforcement ..... 34
5 The Endogenous Double Plasticity for the Control of Chaos ..... 38
6 Conclusions ..... 40
References ..... 41

**Part II. Artificial Immune Systems: Modeling & Simulation**

**The Central and the Peripheral Immune Systems: What is the Relationship?** ..... 47
*John Stewart, Jorge Carneiro*
1 Introduction ..... 47
2 Second Generation Network Models ..... 48

3 An Immune Network Incorporating B-T Cell Co-operation ........ 55
4 Concluding Remarks ........ 59
References ........ 61

**Immunology Viewed as the Study of an Autonomous Decentralized System** ........ 65
*Lee A. Segel, Ruth Lev Bar-Or*
1 Introduction ........ 65
2 A Nano-course in Immunology ........ 65
3 Overall Characterization of the Immune System ........ 67
4 Postulating a Role for Feedback ........ 67
5 Optimizing Effector Performance ........ 69
6 Optimizing Effector Choice ........ 74
7 The Importance of Geography ........ 79
8 Communication ........ 80
9 A Brief Comparison to Some Other Approaches to Decentralized Systems ........ 80
10 Overview ........ 83
References ........ 86

**Immune Network: An Example of Complex Adaptive Systems** 89
*Debashish Chowdhury*
1 Introduction ........ 89
2 A Brief Summary of Experimental Phenomena to be Modelled Theoretically ........ 90
3 Clonal Selection and Its Mathematical Modelling ........ 92
4 Beyond Clonal Selection; Immune Network ........ 98
5 Summary and Conclusion ........ 101
References ........ 102

**Immunological Memory is Associative** ........ 105
*Derek J. Smith, Stephanie Forrest, Alan S. Perelson*
1 Introduction ........ 105
2 Immunological Memory ........ 106
3 Sparse Distributed Memory (SDM) ........ 108
4 Correspondence between Immunological Memory and SDM ........ 109
5 Aspects of Associative Recall in the Immune Response ........ 111
6 Summary ........ 112
References ........ 112

**Estimating and Predicting the Number of Free HIV and T Cells by Nonlinear Kalman Filter** ........ 115
*Wai-Yuan Tan, Zhihua Xiang*
1 Introduction ........ 115
2 A Stochastic Model of the HIV Pathogenesis ........ 116
3 A State Space Model for the HIV Pathogenesis ........ 123

4 An Illustrative Example ... 130
5 Some Monte Carlo Studies ... 133
6 Conclusion and Discussion ... 135
References ... 138

**Modeling the Effects of Prior Infection on Vaccine Efficacy** ... 144
*Derek J. Smith, Stephanie Forrest, David H. Ackley, Alan S. Perelson*
1 Introduction ... 144
2 Materials and Methods ... 145
3 Results and Discussion ... 148
References ... 152

**Part III. Artificial Immune Systems: Applications**

**Jisys: The Development of an Artificial Immune System for Real World Applications** ... 157
*John Hunt, Jon Timmis, Denise Cooke, Mark Neal, Clive King*
1 Introduction ... 157
2 Research into ISYS ... 158
3 The *JISYS* System ... 163
4 Jisys System Structure ... 175
5 The Mortgage Fraud Application ... 177
6 Analysis of *JISYS* ... 179
7 Comparison with Related Work ... 180
8 Future Work ... 181
9 Conclusions ... 184
References ... 184

**Decentralized Behavior Arbitration Mechanism for Autonomous Mobile Robot Using Immune Network** ... 187
*Yuji Watanabe, Akio Ishiguro, Yoshiki Uchikawa*
1 Introduction ... 187
2 Biological Immune System ... 189
3 Proposed Behavior Arbitration Mechanism Based on the Immune System ... 191
4 Adaptation Mechanisms ... 197
5 Conclusions and Further Work ... 206
References ... 207

**Parallel Search for Multi-Modal Function Optimization with Diversity and Learning of Immune Algorithm** ... 210
*Toyoo Fukuda, Kazuyuki Mori, Makoto Tsukiyama*
1 Introduction ... 210
2 Immune Algorithm ... 211
3 Experiments and Implementation Details ... 216

4 Conclusion ..... 219
References ..... 219

**Immunized Adaptive Critic for an Autonomous Aircraft Control Application** ..... 221
*Kalmanje KrishnaKumar, James Neidhoefer*
1 Introduction ..... 221
2 Levels of Intelligent Control ..... 222
3 The Autonomous Aircraft Control Problem ..... 224
4 Immunized Computational Systems ..... 227
5 Immunized Adaptive Critics ..... 231
6 Conclusion ..... 237
References ..... 240

**Blueprint for a Computer Immune System** ..... 242
*Jeffrey O. Kephart, Gregory B. Sorkin, Morton Swimmer, Steve R. White*
1 Introduction ..... 242
2 Requirements for a Computer Immune System ..... 244
3 Implementing an Immune System for Cyberspace ..... 246
4 Evaluation and Final Remarks ..... 256
References ..... 259

**An Anomaly Detection Algorithm Inspired by the Immune System** ..... 262
*Dipankar Dasgupta, Stephanie Forrest*
1 Introduction ..... 262
2 A Negative Selection Algorithm ..... 263
3 Anomaly Detection ..... 264
4 Experiments ..... 267
5 Conclusions ..... 273
References ..... 275

**Immunity-Based Management System for a Semiconductor Production Line** ..... 278
*Toyoo Fukuda, Kazuyuki Mori, and Makoto Tsukiyama*
1 Introduction ..... 278
2 Problem of Semiconductor Production System ..... 279
3 Immunity-Based System and Multi-Agent Nets ..... 281
4 Conclusion ..... 287
References ..... 288

**Indexed Bibliography** ..... 291

**Author Index** ..... 303

**Subject Index** ..... 304

# List of Contributors

**David H. Ackley**
Department of Computer Science
The University of New Mexico
Albuquerque, NM 87131, USA
*ackley@cs.unm.edu*

**Ruth Lev Bar-Or**
Department of Mathematics
and Computer Science
Weizmann Institute
Rehovot, Israel

**Hugues Bersini**
IRIDIA, CP 194/6
Université Libre de Bruxelles
50, av. Franklin Roosevelt
1050 Bruxelles, Belgium
*bersini@ulb.ac.be*

**Jorge Carneiro**
Theoretical Biology & Bioinformatics
Padualaan 8
3584 CH Utrecht
The Netherlands
*jorge@binf.biol.ruu.nl*

**Debashish Chowdhury**
Department of Physics
Indian Institute of Technology
Kanpur 208016, India
*debch@iitk.ernet.in*

**Denise Cooke**
Department of Computer Science
University of Wales, Aberystwyth
Penglais, Aberystwyth
Ceredigion, SY23 3DB, UK
*dzc@aber.ac.uk*

**Dipankar Dasgupta**
Department of Mathematical Sciences
The University of Memphis
Memphis, TN 38152-6429, USA
*dasgupta@msci.memphis.edu*

**Stephanie Forrest**
Department of Computer Science
The University of New Mexico
Albuquerque, NM 87131, USA
*forrest@cs.unm.edu*

**Toyoo Fukuda**
School of Policy Studies
Kwansei Gakuin University
2-1 Gakuen Sanda
Hyogo 669-13, Japan
*fukudat@mars.dti.ne.jp*

**John Hunt**
Department of Computer Science
University of Wales
Aberystwyth
Penglais, Aberystwyth
Dyfed, SY23 3DB, UK
*jjh@aber.ac.uk*

**Akio Ishiguro**
Department of Computational
Science and Engineering
Graduate School of Engineering
Nagoya University
Furo-cho, Chikusa-ku
Nagoya 464-01, Japan
*ishiguro@bioele.nuee.nagoya-u.ac.jp*

**Jeffrey O. Kephart**
IBM Thomas J. Watson
Research Center
30 Saw Mill River Rd.
Hawthorne, NY 10532, USA
*kephart@watson.ibm.com*

**Clive King**
Department of Computer Science
University of Wales, Aberystwyth
Penglais, Aberystwyth
Ceredigion, SY23 3DB, UK
*cmk@aber.ac.uk*

**Kalmanje KrishnaKumar**
Department of Aerospace
Engineering and Mechanics
The University of Alabama
Tuscaloosa, AL 35487-0280, USA
*kkumar@coe.eng.ua.edu*

**Kazuyuki Mori**
Industrial Electronics and
Systems Laboratory
Mitsubishi Electric Corporation
Amagasaki, Hyogo 661, Japan
*mori@soc.sdl.melco.co.jp*

**Mark Neal**
Department of Computer Science
University of Wales, Aberystwyth
Penglais, Aberystwyth
Ceredigion, SY23 3DB, UK
*mjnl@aber.ac.uk*

**James Neidhoefer**
Department of Aerospace
Engineering and Mechanics
The University of Alabama
Tuscaloosa, AL 35487-0280, USA
*james@coe.eng.ua.edu*

**Alan S. Perelson**
Theoretical Division
Los Alamos National Laboratory
Los Alamos, NM 87545, USA
*asp@t10.lanl.gov*

**Lee A. Segel**
Department of Mathematics
and Computer Science
Weizmann Institute, Rehovot, Israel
*lee@wisdom.weizmann.ac.il*

**Derek Smith**
Department of Computer Science
University of New Mexico
Albuquerque, NM 87131, USA
*dsmith@cs.unm.edu*

**Gregory B. Sorkin**
IBM Thomas J. Watson
Research Center
P.O. Box 704,Yorktown Heights
NY 10598, USA
*sorkin@watson.ibm.com*

**John Stewart**
COSTECH, Departement Technologie
et Sciences de l'Homme
Université de Technologie de Compiégne
BP 60649, F-60206
F-60206 Compiegne cedex, France
*John.Stewart@utc.fr*

**Morton Swimmer**
IBM Thomas J. Watson
Research Center
P.O. Box 704,Yorktown Heights
NY 10598, USA
*swimmer@watson.ibm.com*

**Wai-Yuan Tan**
Department of Mathematical Sciences
The University of Memphis
Memphis, TN 38152-6429, USA
*TANWY@mathsci.msci.memphis.edu*

**Jonathan Timmis**
Department of Computer Science
University of Wales, Aberystwyth
Penglais, Aberystwyth
Ceredigion, SY23 3DB, UK
*jot@aber.ac.uk*

**Makoto Tsukiyama**
Industrial Electronics
& Systems Laboratory
Mitsubishi Electric Corporation
Amagasaki, Hyogo 661, Japan
*tsukiyama@soc.sdl.melco.co.jp*

**Yoshiki Uchikawa**
Department of Computational
Science and Engineering
Graduate School of Engineering
Nagoya University, Furo-cho
Chikusa-ku Nagoya 464-8603, Japan
*uchikawa@bioele.nuee.nagoya-u.ac.jp*

**Yuji Watanabe**
Department of Information Electronics
Graduate School of Engineering
Nagoya University, Furo-cho
Chikusa-ku Nagoya 464-8603, Japan
*yuji@bioele.nuee.nagoya-u.ac.jp*

**Steve R. White**
IBM Thomas J. Watson
Research Center
30 Saw Mill River Rd.
Hawthorne, NY 10532, USA
*srwhite@watson.ibm.com*

**Zhihua Xiang**
Department of Mathematical Sciences
The University of Memphis
Memphis, TN 38152-6429, USA
*xiang@mathsci.msci.memphis.edu*

# Part I
# **Introduction**

# An Overview of Artificial Immune Systems and Their Applications

Dipankar Dasgupta

Mathematical Sciences Department
The University of Memphis
Memphis, TN 38152, USA.

**Abstract.** The natural immune system is a subject of great research interest because of its powerful information processing capabilities. From an information-processing perspective, the immune system is a highly parallel system. It provides an excellent model of adaptive processes operating at the local level and of useful behavior emerging at the global level. Moreover, it uses learning, memory, and associative retrieval to solve recognition and classification tasks. This chapter illustrates different immunological mechanisms and their relation to information processing, and provides an overview of the rapidly emerging field called Artificial Immune Systems. These techniques have been successfully used in pattern recognition, fault detection and diagnosis, computer security, and a variety of other applications.

## 1 Introduction

The natural immune system is a very complex system with several functional components. It employs a multilevel defense against invaders through non-specific (innate) and specific (acquired) immune mechanisms. The main role of the immune system is to recognize all cells (or molecules) within the body and categorize those cells as self or non-self. The non-self cells are further categorized in order to stimulate an appropriate type of defensive mechanism. The immune system learns through evolution to distinguish between foreign antigens (e.g., bacteria, viruses, etc.) and the body's own cells or molecules.

According to the Immunologists [30,32,37], our body maintains a large number of immune cells which circulate throughout the body. The lymphocyte is the main type of immune cell participating in the immune response that possesses the attributes of specificity, diversity, memory, and adaptivity. Other cells called phagocytic cells – neutrophils, eosinophils, basophils, monocytes – are accessory immune cells whose primary function is to provide facilities to eliminate antigens. There are mainly two types of lymphocytes, namely T cells and B cells. The primary lymphoid organs provide sites where lymphocytes mature and become antigenically committed. In particular, T lymphocytes develop in bone marrow and travel to the thymus to mature, whereas B lymphocytes develop and mature within the bone marrow. The secondary lymphoid organs function to capture antigen and to provide sites where lymphocytes interact with that the antigen to stimulate an immune response [34]. However, these two types of lymphocytes play different roles in the immune response, though they may act together and control or affect one another's function. For example, T cells can either enhance or suppress the B cells' response to a stimulus.

When an antigen invades the body, only a few of these immune cells can recognize the invader's peptides.[1] This recognition stimulates proliferation and differentiation of the cells that produce matching clones (or antibody).[2] This process, called clonal expansion, generates a large population of antibody-producing cells that are specific to the antigen. The clonal expansion of immune cells result in destroying or neutralizing the antigen. It also retains some of these cells in immunological memory, so that any subsequent exposure to a similar antigen leads to rapid immune response (secondary response).

Different populations of lymphocytes recirculate at primary and secondary lymphoid organs and are carefully controlled to ensure that appropriate populations of B and T cells (naive, effector, and memory) are recruited into different locations. This differential migration of lymphocyte subpopulations at different locations (organs) of the body is called *trafficking* or *homing*. These organs provide specialized environments to support the clonal expansion and differentiation of antigen-activated lymphocytes into effector and memory cells. Interestingly, memory cells exhibit selective homing to the type of tissue in which they first encountered an antigen. Presumably this ensures that a particular memory cell will return to the location where it is most likely to re-encounter a subsequent antigenic challenge.

The regulation of immune responses can broadly be divided into two branches – the humoral immunity which is mediated by B cells and their products, and the cellular immunity mediated by T cells. Both branches follow a similar sequence of steps for defense – proliferation, activation, induction, differentiation and secretion, attack, suppression, and memory; however, they do it in different ways. Specifically, regulation of both humoral and cellular immunity is conducted by a population of T cells referred to as either helper or suppressor cells, which either augment or suppress immune responses.

The purpose of this chapter is to provide an overview of the rapidly emerging field called Artificial Immune Systems (also called *Immunological Computation*). It also explores different immunological mechanisms and their relation to information processing and problem solving. So far, Artificial Immune Systems have received very little attention as compared to other techniques based on biological metaphors, such as neural networks and evolutionary algorithms . In the next section, the computational aspects of the natural

[1] Antigen presenting cells or macrophages present pieces of the antigen (called peptides) on its surface, to bring the attention of B and T cells for recognition.

[2] Affinity maturation occurs when the mutation rate of a cell clone increases in response to a match between the clone's antibody and an antigen. Those mutant cells that bind more tightly are stimulated to divide more rapidly.

immune system is highlighted. Section 3 addresses the differences and similarities between the nervous system and the immune system. Section 4 discusses different models based on various mechanisms of the immune system. Section 5 provides the applications of these models in the fields of science and engineering. The last section summarizes with some remarks.

## 2 Computational Aspects of the Immune System

The natural immune system is a subject of great research interest because of its powerful information processing capabilities. In particular, it performs many complex computations in a highly parallel and distributed fashion [17]. So the overall behavior of the immune system is an emergent property of many local interactions.

According to Rowe [40], the immune system functions as a kind of "second brain" because it can store memories of past experiences in strengths of the interactions of its constituent cells, and it can generate responses to new and novel patterns (antigens). Furthermore, the immune response develops in time and the description of its time evolution is an interesting problem in dynamical systems [39]. The key features of the immune system which provide several important aspects to the field of information processing may be summarized under the following terms of computation:

- *Recognition*: The immune system can recognize and classify different patterns and generate selective responses. Recognition is achieved by intercellular binding – the extent of this binding is determined by molecular shape and electrostatic charge. Self-nonself discrimination is one of the main tasks the immune system solves during the process of recognition.
- *Feature Extraction*: Antigen Presenting Cells (APCs) interpret the antigenic context and extract the features, by processing and presenting antigenic peptides on its surface. Each APC servers as a filter and a lens: a filter that destroys molecular noise, and a lens that focuses the attention of the lymphocyte - receptors [5].
- *Diversity*: It uses combinatorics (partly by a genetic process) for generating a diverse set of lymphocyte receptors to ensure that at least some lymphocytes can bind to any given (known or unknown) antigen.
- *Learning*: It learns, by experience, the structure of a specific antigen. Making changes in lymphocyte concentration is the mechanism for learning and takes place during the primary response (first encounter of the antigen). So the learning ability of the immune system lies primarily in the recruitment mechanism (IRM [2]) which generates new immune cells on the basis of the current state of the system (also called *clonal expansion*).

- *Memory*: When lymphocytes are activated, a few of each kind become special memory cells which are content-addressable. The inherent longevity of immune memory cells is dynamic and requires continued stimulation by residual antigens. The immune system keeps an ideal balance between economy and performance in conserving a minimal but sufficient memory of the past (using short-term and long-term memory mechanisms).
- *Distributed Detection*: The immune system is inherently distributed. The immune cells, in particular lymphocytes, undergo constant levels of recirculation through the blood, lymph, lymphoid organs, and tissue spaces. As lymphocytes recirculate, if they encounter antigenic challenges , they stimulate specific immune responses.
- *Self-regulation*: The mechanisms of immune responses are self-regulatory in nature. There is no central organ that controls the functions of the immune system. The regulation of immune responses can be either local or systemic, depending on the route and property of the antigenic challenge.
- *Threshold mechanism*: Immune response and the proliferation of the immune cells takes place above a certain matching threshold (strength of the chemical binding).
- *Co-stimulation*: Activation of B cells are closely regulated through co-stimulation. The second signal (from helper T cells) helps to ensure tolerance and judge between dangerous and harmless invaders or false alarm.
- *Dynamic protection*: Clonal expansion and somatic hyper-mutation allow generation of high-affinity immune cells (called affinity maturation). This process dynamically balances exploration versus exploitation in adaptive immunity . Dynamic protection increases the coverage provided by the immune system over time.
- *Probabilistic Detection*: The cross reaction in immune response is a stochastic process. Also the detection is approximate; hence, a lymphocyte can bind with several different kinds of (structurally related) antigens.

Other related features like adaptability, specificity, self-tolerance, differentiation etc. also perform important functions in immune response. All these remarkable information-processing properties of the immune system provide several important aspects in the field of computation.

## 3 The Nervous System and the Immune System

One principal difference between the nervous system and the immune system is in their interaction with the external environment. Although the I/O behavior of lymphocytes *in vivo* is not known with certainty, it is most likely some simple, nonlinear function [38]. Lymphocytes can be connected to external antigens (I/O lymphocytes), or to each other via antiidiotypic interactions [43]. According to Vertosick and Kelly [43], the clonal expansion and affinity maturation that accompany an immune response are reminiscent of Hebbian learning. In the immune system, learning occurs through the modification of the number and affinities of the receptors. However, connections within a nervous system are deterministic, whereas the cross reaction in immune response is a stochastic process.

The nervous system is commonly decomposed into sensory and motor parts. An analogous separation into recognition and effector functions can be made in the immune system where effector mechanisms lead to the elimination of the antigen. In neural system, assimilation of memories appear to be achieved by alteration of the strengths of connections between neurons, rather than change within the neurons themselves. Further, the brain allows memories to be addressable by content, the frequent death of individual neurons does not drastically affect performance of the brain as a whole. Similarly, cross-reactive memory, variable cell division and programmed cell death rates allow the immune system to allocate resources (cells) dynamically as needed in a distributed environment.

Though the models of neural networks and their applications have received wide attention, immune system models are of limited use. Also as compared to neurophysiology, where the Hodgkin-Huxley equations have provided a basis for modeling, there are no agreed upon generic equations describing the behavior of single immune cells [39]. However, both neural system and immune system share many common features as basic cognitive mechanisms. Table 1 summarizes the similarities and the differences between these two systems (as illustrated in [4,12,44]).

Many biologists believe that the immune system is in principle more complex than the brain-nervous system. Different theories have been suggested based on experimental evidences. Some of these theories are contradictory regarding the way cellular interactions occur in the immunological response. Because of the lack of understanding, there is still no unified model or view that accounts for all known immunological phenomena. Also there remains open questions whether the immune system operates at steady state, oscillates or chaotic.

## 4 Immune System Based Models

There exist several theories [31,36] and mathematical models [38,42] to explain immunological phenomena. There is also a growing number of computer models [43,45] to simulate various components of the immune system and the overall behavior from a biological point of view. These approaches include differential-equation models [38], stochastic-equation models [4], cellular-automata models [3,41], shape-space models [46], etc. However, the natural immune system is also a source of inspiration for developing intelligent methodologies toward problem solving, but there is not much research in this direction. In particular, more research is needed to extract information processing mechanisms which are of direct practical use.

| Features | Neural System | Immune System |
| --- | --- | --- |
| Similarities: | | |
| Basic Unit | Neurons are basic processing units in the brain. Each neuron has three parts: *soma* - the cell body, *dendrites* for carrying in information, and *axon* for carrying out information from the neuron. | Lymphocytes (B cell, T cell etc.) are an important class of immune cells. Each lymphocyte has about 100,000 receptors on its cellular membrane that enable it to recognize one specific antigen. |
| No. of Units | There are approximately $10^{10}$ neurons in the brain. | Humans have lymphocytes of the order of $10^{12}$. |
| Interaction | The synaptic junctions between neurons can be excitatory (stimulating) or inhibitory (depressing) which give rise to many different activity patterns. | The inter-lymphocyte interactions via cell-cell contact, or via chemical mediators have varying strengths which can be helping or suppressing. |
| Recognition | Recognize visual, auditory and other signal patterns. | Recognition occurs at the molecular level and is based on the complementarity in shape between the receptor and patterns stored in the epitope of the antigen. |
| Task perform | Distinguish between the stored patterns and conscious imagination. | Distinguish between foreign antigens and the cells or tissues of the host. |
| Learning | A combination of global/local learning rule occurs, where the global mechanism performs certain tasks and then uses the local mechanism for training/ learning (to tune the strength of synaptic links). | Changes in lymphocyte concentration are the mechanism for learning and takes place during the primary response according to the mutual recognition and inter-cellular binding. |
| Memory | Patterns of synaptic strengths constitute a memory which is auto-associative and non hereditary. | When lymphocytes are activated, a few of each kind become special memory cells which are content-addressable, but not hereditary. |

| Features | Neural System | Immune System |
|---|---|---|
| Similarities Continued... | | |
| Threshold | There is a threshold of connection strength for firing of neurons. The average strength is proportional to the weight of each connection. | Immune response and the proliferation of the immune cells takes place above a certain matching threshold. The matching depends on the strength of the chemical reaction. |
| Robustness | Very flexible and damage-tolerant. | Scalable and self-tolerant, but not well understood. |
| Differences: | | |
| Location | Position of the neurons are fixed. | Lymphocytes are positioned throughout the body. |
| Unit Type | Neurons are assumed to be homogeneous. | Immune cells are heterogeneous agents. |
| Communications | Takes place through the linkage hardware e.g. axons, dendrites as electrical signals. | Transient cell-cell contacts and/or via secretion of soluble molecules. |
| State | Activation level of the neural system. | Free antibody/antigen concentration. |
| Control | Brain controls the functioning of the nervous system. | No such central organ controls the functions of the immune system. |

**Table 1.** The table shows the similarities and differences of the *Neural System* and the *Immune System*.

The few computational models developed that have been based on immune system principles, seem to have chosen a different set of principles to emulate. Among these, the following models are often used by researchers [7].

### 4.1 Immune Network Model

Jerne [30,31] hypothesized that the immune system is a regulated network of molecules and cells that recognize one another even in the absence of antigen. Such networks are often called *idiotypic networks* which present a mathematical framework to illustrate the behavior of the immune system. His theory is modeled with a differential equation which simulates the dynamics of lymphocytes - the increase or decrease of the concentration of a set of lymphocyte clones and the corresponding immunoglobins. The idiotypic network hypothesis is based on the concept that lymphocytes are not isolated, but communicate with each other among different species of lymphocytes through interaction among antibodies. Accordingly, the identification of antigens is not done by a single recognizing set but rather a system-level recognition of the sets connected by antigen-antibody reaction as a network.

Jerne suggested that during an immune response antigen would directly elicit the production of a first set of antibodies, $Ab_1$. These antibodies would then act as antigens and elicit the production of a second set of "anti-idiotypic" (anti-id) antibodies $Ab_2$ which recognize idiotopes on $Ab_1$ antibodies. Similarly, a third set of antibodies, $Ab_3$ could be elicited that recognized $Ab_2$ antibodies, and so forth.

The key postulate of his theoretical framework is that one cell makes only one type of antibody, and this leads to several predictions which include (i) allelic exclusion, (ii) all antibody-like receptors displayed by a lymphocyte should be identical or at least have identical light chains and identical heavy variable regions, and (iii) all antibodies produced by a single cell and its progeny should have the identical idiotype. In formulating the framework, Jerne discusses formal and functional networks. The formal network discusses repertoire, dualism, and suppression. In the discussion of functional networks, a quantitative picture of the theory is presented.

Based on Jerne's work, Perelson [38], presented a probabilistic approach to idiotypic networks. Perelson's approach is very mathematical, discussing more about phase transition in idiotype networks. Perelson divided phase transition in idiotopic networks to pre-critical region, transition region and post-critical region.

Jerne's proposed immune network theory [31] received a lot of attention among the researchers [38,42,43] over the last two decades and many computational aspects of this model are derived for practical use [23,25,29].

## 4.2 Negative Selection Algorithm

Forrest et al. [16] developed a negative-selection algorithm for change detection based on the principles of self-nonself discrimination [37] in the immune system. This discrimination is achieved in part by T-cells, which have receptors on their surface that can detect foreign proteins (antigens). During the generation of T cells, receptors are made by a pseudo-random genetic rearrangement process. Then they undergo a censoring process, called negative selection, in the *thymus* where T cells that react against self-proteins are destroyed, so only those that do not bind to self-proteins are allowed to leave the thymus. These matured T cells then circulate throughout the body to perform immunological functions to protect against foreign antigens. The negative-selection algorithm works on similar principles, generating detectors randomly, and eliminating the ones that detect self, so that the remaining T-cells can detect any nonself. This algorithmic approach can be summarized as follows:

- Define *self* as a collection $S$ of strings of length $l$ over a finite alphabet, a collection that needs to be protected or monitor. For example, $S$ may be a program, data file (any software), or normal pattern of activity, which is segmented into equal-sized substrings.[3]
- Generate a set $R$ of *detectors*, each of which fails to match any string in $S$. Instead of exact or perfect matching,[4] the method uses a partial matching rule, in which two strings match if and only if they are identical at at least $r$ contiguous positions, where $r$ is a suitably chosen parameter (as described in [16]).
- Monitor $S$ for changes by continually matching the detectors in $R$ against $S$. If any detector ever matches, then a change is known to have occurred, because the detectors are designed to not match any of the original strings in $S$.

In the original description of the algorithm [16], candidate detectors are generated *randomly* and then tested (censored) to see if they match any self string. If a match is found, the candidate is rejected. This process is repeated until a desired number of detectors are generated. A probabilistic analysis is used to estimate the number of detectors that are required to provide a certain level of reliability. The major limitation of the random generation approach appears to be computational difficulty of generating valid detectors, which grows exponentially with the size of self. Subsequently,

[3] This is analogous to the way, proteins are broken up by the immune system into smaller subunits, called peptides, to recognize by T-cell receptors.

[4] For strings of any significant length a perfect match is highly improbable, so a partial matching rule is used which rewards more specific matches (i.e., matches on more bits) over less specific ones. This partial matching rule reflects the fact that the immune system's recognition capabilities need to be fairly specific in order to avoid confusing self molecules with foreign molecules.

a more efficient detector generation algorithm is proposed by Helman and Forrest [20] which runs in linear time with the size of self. Other methods for generating nonself detectors have also been suggested [11] which have varying degrees of computational complexities.

This algorithm relies on three important principles: (1) each copy of the detection algorithm is unique, (2) detection is probabilistic, and (3) a robust system should detect (probabilistically) any foreign activity rather than looking for specific known patterns of changes. Further studies show [11,10] many insights of the algorithm. The algorithm seems to have many potential applications in change-detection, some of these are discussed in the next section.

### 4.3 Other Models

There exist other computation models [13,15] which emulate different immunological aspects, for example, its ability to detect common patterns in a noisy environment [15], its ability to discover and maintain coverage of diverse pattern classes, and its ability to learn effectively, even when not all antibodies are expressed and not all antigens are presented [21]. In some studies, genetic algorithms have been used to model somatic mutation – the process by which antibodies are evolved to recognize a specific antigen. Hoffman [22] has compared the immune system and the nervous system. He has shown many similarities in the two systems, at the level of system behavior (though differ at the respective building-block level). He postulated a symmetrical neural network model that can produce desired stimulus-response behavior similar to immune response. Farmer et al. [13], and Bersini and Varela [2,1] have compared the immune system with learning classifier systems.

## 5 Some Applications of Artificial Immune Systems

The models based on immune system principles are finding increasing applications in the fields of science and engineering.

### 5.1 Computer Security

Stephanie Forrest and her group at the University of New Mexico are working on a research project with a long-term goal to build an artificial immune system for computers. This immunity-based system has much more sophisticated notions of identity and protection than those afforded by current operating systems, and it would provide a general-purpose protection system to augment current computer security systems. The security of computer systems depends on such activities as detecting unauthorized use of computer facilities, maintaining the integrity of data files, and preventing the spread of computer viruses.

The problem of protecting computer systems from harmful viruses is viewed as an instance of the more general problem of distinguishing *self* (legitimate users, uncorrupted data, etc.) from dangerous *other* (unauthorized users, viruses, and other malicious agents). This method is intended to be complementary to the more traditional cryptographic and deterministic approaches to computer security. As an initial step, the negative-selection algorithm (discussed in the previous section) has been used as a file-authentication method on the problem of computer virus detection.

**Virus Detection.** In this application, Forrest et al. [16] used the negative-selection algorithm to detect changes in the protected data and program files. A number of experiments are performed in a DOS environment with different viruses, including file-infector and boot sector virus samples. Reported results showed that the method could easily detect the modification that occurred in the data files due to virus infection. Compared to other virus detection methods, this algorithm has several advantages over the existing change detection methods: it is probabilistic and tunable (the probability of detection can be traded off against CPU time), it can be distributed (providing high system-wide reliability at low individual cost), and it can detect novel viruses that have not previously been identified.

However, since the stored information in a computer system in volatile in nature, the definition of self in computer systems should be more dynamic than in the case of natural immune systems. For example, computer users routinely load in updated software systems, edit files, or run new programs. So this implementation seems to have limited use - only to protect static data files or software.

**UNIX Process Monitoring.** As an on-going research on computer security, Forrest et al. [14] studied the proposed negative selection algorithm to monitor UNIX processes. The purpose is to detect harmful intrusions in a computer system. This implementation aimed at identifying a *sense of self* for UNIX processes, they redefined self to accommodate the legitimate activities in dynamic computer environment so that the definition is sensitive to malicious attacks.

This work is based on the assumption that the system calls of root processes are inherently more dangerous to cause damage than user processes. Also root processes have a limited range of behavior, and their behavior is relatively stable over time. The *normal or self* is defined by short-range correlations in a process' system calls. This definition of self seems to be stable during normal behavior for several standard UNIX programs. Further, it is able to detect several common intrusions involving *sendmail*. Their reason of monitoring *sendmail* is that its behavior is sufficiently varied and complex that it provides a good preliminary test, and there are several documented attacks against sendmail that can be used for testing. The experiments generated traces of three types of behavior that differ from that of normal sendmail: traces of successful sendmail attacks, traces of sendmail intrusion attempts that failed, and traces of error conditions. They have been able to execute and trace two attacks.

These experiments [14] suggest that short sequences of system calls provide a stable signature that can detect some common sources of anomalous behavior in *sendmail.* Because the current measure is easy to compute and is relatively modest in storage requirements, it would be plausible to implement it as an on-line system, in which the kernel checks each system call made by processes running as root. Under this scheme, each site would generate its own normal database, based on the local software/hardware configuration and usage patterns. One advantage of using local usage patterns is that every site would then have its own unique identity, slightly different from everyone else. This would mean that a successful intrusion at one site would not necessarily be successful at all sites running the same software, and it would increase the chance of at least one site noticing an attack. This work appears to be very promising and opens new venue in computer security research.

**An alternative approach to Virus Detection.** Kephart proposed [33] a different immunologically inspired approach (based on instruction hypothesis) for virus detection. In this approach, known viruses are detected by their computer-code sequences (signatures) and unknown viruses by their unusual behavior within the computer system. This virus detection system continually scans a computer's software for typical signs of viral infection. These signs trigger the release of *decoy programs* whose sole purpose is to become infected by the virus.

Specifically, a diverse suit of *decoy programs* are kept at different strategic areas in memory (e.g. home directory) to capture samples of viruses. Decoys are designed to be as attractive as possible to trap those types of viruses that spread most successfully. Each of the decoy programs is examined from time to time, to see if it has been modified. If one or more have been modified, it is almost certain that an unknown virus is loose in the system, and each of the modified decoys contains a sample of that virus. In particular, the infected decoys are processed by - *the signature extractor* - so as to develop a recognizer for the virus. It also extract information from the infected decoys about how the virus attaches to it's host program (attachment pattern of the virus), so that infected hosts can be repaired. The signature extractor must select a virus signature (from among the byte sequence produced by the attachment derivation step) such that it can avoid both false negatives and false positives while in use. In other words, the signature must be found in each instance of the virus, and it must be very unlikely to be found in uninfected programs. Once the best possible signature is selected from candidate signatures of the virus, it run against a half-gigabytes corpus of legitimate programs to make sure that they do not cause false positive. The repair information is checked out by testing on samples of the virus, and further by the human expert.

Finally, the signature and the repair program is stored in archive of the anti-virus database, and the updated (new) version is needed to be distributed to the customers. According to Kephart, this approach will also be used to stop the spreading of viruses in networked computers, where infected machines send out "kill signals" to warn other computers of the rampant virus. The signals tell how to kill the new virus as well as similar one.

### 5.2 Anomaly Detection in Time Series Data

Dasgupta and Forrest [9,6] experimented with several time series data sets (both real and simulated) to investigate the performance of the negative selection algorithm [16] for detecting anomaly in the data series. The objective of this work is to develop an efficient detection algorithm that can be used for noticing any changes in steady-state characteristics of a system or a process. In these experiments, the notion of self is considered as the normal behavior patterns of the monitored system.[5] So, any deviation that exceeds an allowable variation in the observed data, is considered as an anomaly in the behavior pattern. This approach relies on sufficient enough sample of normal data (that can capture the semantics of the data patterns) to generate a diverse set of detectors that probabilistically detect changes without requiring prior knowledge of anomaly (or faulty) patterns.

They applied the algorithm for "The Tool Breakage Detection" in a milling operation [8]. The tool breakage detection problem is formulated as the problem of detecting temporal changes in the cutting force pattern that results from a broken cutter. That is, the new data patterns are monitored to check for whether or not the current pattern is different from the established normal pattern, where a difference (i.e. a match in the complement space) implies a shift in the cutting force dynamics.

This detection algorithm was successful in detecting the existence of broken teeth from simulated cutting force signals in a milling process. The results suggest that the approach can be used as a tool for automated monitoring of safety-critical operations.

### 5.3 Fault Diagnosis

Ishida [26,27] studied the mutual recognition feature of the immune network model [31] for fault diagnosis. In his implementation, fault tolerance was attained by mutual recognition of interconnected units in the studied plant. That is, system level recognition was achieved by unit level recognition.

[5] It is assumed that the normal behavior of a system or a process can often be characterized by a series of observations over time. Also the normal system behavior generally exhibit stable patterns when observed over a time period.

The model has the following properties: (a) it has the ability to do parallel processing, (b) can handle incomplete information and data, (c) it is self-organizing, and (d) no feedback loop is necessary in the failure propagation. Ishida and Mizessyn [25] presented an application of this mutual recognition model to the process instrumentation system of a chemical plant. Using the relationship among sensors, sensor network are constructed by bi-directional arcs, in order to apply the model for fault diagnosis. The results are very promising and worth further investigation.

Ishiguro [29] applied the immune network model [31] to on-line fault diagnosis of plant systems. To apply the immune network to plant fault diagnosis, the following assumptions were made: (a) Sensors are not equipped with all components of the plant systems, and they inform the state of the equipped component as binary states, i.e fault-free (normal) or faulty (abnormal), (b) the number of failure origins is assumed to be one (namely, simultaneous and complex failure are not taken into account), (c) failure states propagate through branches without exceptions, and (d) no feedback loop exists in the failure propagation. This work attempts to develop an integrated fault diagnosis method which can be used in industrial plants.

### 5.4 AIS for Pattern Recognition

Hunt and Cooke [23,24] investigated an Artificial Immune System (AIS) based on the theory of immune network [31] within the context of machine learning. The AIS offers noise tolerant, unsupervised learning within a system which is self-organizing, does not require negative examples and explicitly represents what it has learnt. Such a system combines the advantages of learning classifier systems with some of the advantages of neural networks, machine induction and case-based retrieval.

The operation of the AIS comprises a root object, a network of cells, a teaching data set and a test data set. Each cell in the network possess a pattern matching element which is generated by mimicking the genetic mechanisms by which antibodies are formed in the natural immune system. This enables complex vocabularies and promotes diversity of the pattern matching elements. The system exhibits two types of response: primary and secondary. The primary response is the learning phase when the AIS learns about patterns in the input teaching data. The secondary response represents a pattern recognition process during which the AIS attempts to classify new data relative to the data it has seen before.

To apply the AIS to a particular problem, it is first taught with a sample teaching set in a one shot or an incremental manner (depending on the problem). The information learnt can then be exploited in a number of ways. They have shown the potential of AIS on a pattern recognition problem. The AIS was applied to the recognition of promoters in DNA sequences, i.e.

to determine whether new sequences were promoter containing or promoter negative. Their immune system algorithm has the following steps:

```
Randomly initialize initial B cell population
Load antigen population
Until termination condition is met do
  Randomly select an antigen from the antigen population
  Randomly select a point in the B cell network
                to insert the antigen
  Select a percentage of the B cells local
                to the insertion point
  For each B cell selected
    Present the antigen to each B cell and
               request immune response
    Order these B cells by stimulation
    Remove worths 5% of the B cell population
    Generate n new B cells (where n equals
               25% of the population)
    Select m B cells to join the immune network
          (where m equals 5% of the population)
```

Hunts and Cooke's work [24] demonstrated that how the AIS can represent a powerful example of learning within an adaptive non-linear network that contains an explicit content addressable memory. Their research objective is to develop a immunity-based toolkit for machine learning applications.

### 5.5 Other applications

Bersini and Varela [2] used the recruitment mechanism of the immune system to accelerate the parallel and local hill-climbing. Ishida investigated immunity-based methods as majority network, agent systems, and self-identification process [28]. Gilbert and Routen [18] experimented with immune network model to create a content-addressable auto-associative memory, specifically for image recognition. In this application, inputs to the system are black and white pictures of 64 by 64 pixels that are analogous to antigens. This approach seems very interesting, but their implementation failed to obtain a stable solution for the problem. McCoy and Devarajan applied the negative selection algorithm in Aerial Image Segmentation [35]. Hajela [19] recently used immune network based genetic search in structural optimization problems.

## 6 Summary

The natural immune system is a subject of great research interest because of its powerful information processing capabilities. In particular, it performs many complex computations in a completely parallel and distributed fashion. Like the nervous system, the immune system can learn new information, recall previously learned information and performs pattern recognition tasks in a decentralized fashion. Also its learning takes place by evolutionary processes similar to biological evolution. The paper reviews the models that have been developed based on various computational aspects of the immune system. Because of the page restrictions, we are unable to provide a detailed account of each of the models and their applications. However, the existing immunity-based methods emulate one or the other mechanisms of the natural immune system. Further study should integrate all the potentially useful properties in a single framework in order to develop a robust immunity-based system.

There are many potential application areas in which immunity-based models appear to be very useful. They include fault detection and diagnosis, machine monitoring, signature verification, noise detection, computer and data security, image and pattern recognition, and so forth. It is to be noted that the mechanisms of the immune system are remarkably complex and poorly understood, even by immunologists. Understanding the immune system is important, both because of determining its role in handling complex diseases and because of potential applications to computational problems. Moreover, if we can understand the functionalities and the inherent mechanisms of various components of the immune system from the computational viewpoint, we may gain better insights about how to engineer massively parallel adaptive computations.

## Acknowledgments

This work was partially supported by the Faculty Research Grant of the University of Memphis. A short version of this chapter appeared in the proceedings of the IEEE International Conference on Systems, Man, and Cybernetics, October 1997.

## References

1. H. Bersini and F. J. Varela. Hints for adaptive problem solving gleaned from immune networks. In *Proceedings of the first workshop on Parallel Problem Solving from Nature*, pages 343–354, 1990.
2. H. Bersini and F. J. Varela. The immune recruitment mechanism: A selective evolutionary strategy. In *Proceedings of the fourth International Conference on Genetic Algorithms*, pages 520–526, San Diego, July 13-16 1991.
3. Franco Celada and Philip E. Seiden. A computer model of cellular interactions in the immune system. *Immunology Today*, 13(2):56–62, 1992.
4. Debashish Chowdhury and Dietrich Stauffer. Statistical physics of immune networks. *Physica A*, 186:61–81, 1992.
5. Irun R. Cohen. The cognitive paradigm and the immunological homunculus. *Immunology Today*, 13(12):490–494, 1992.

6. Dipankar Dasgupta. Using Immunological Principles in Anomaly Detection. In *Proceedings of the Artificial Neural Networks in Engineering (ANNIE'96)*, St. Louis, USA, November 10-13 1996.
7. Dipankar Dasgupta and Nii Attoh-Okine. Immunity-based systems: A survey. In *Proceedings of the IEEE International Conference on Systems, Man, and Cybernetics*, pages 363–374, Orlando, Florida, October 12-15 1997.
8. Dipankar Dasgupta and Stephanie Forrest. Tool Breakage Detection in Milling Operations using a Negative-Selection Algorithm. Technical Report CS95-5, Department of Computer Science, University of New Mexico, 1995.
9. Dipankar Dasgupta and Stephanie Forrest. Novelty Detection in Time Series Data using Ideas from Immunology. In *ISCA 5th International Conference on Intelligent Systems*, Reno, Nevada, June 19-21 1996.
10. P. D'haeseleer. An immunological approach to change detection: theoretical results. In *Proceedings of IEEE Symposium on Research in Security and Privacy*, Oakland, CA, May 1996.
11. P. D'haeseleer, S. Forrest, and P. Helman. An immunological approach to change detection: algorithms, analysis, and implications. In *Proceedings of IEEE Symposium on Research in Security and Privacy*, Oakland, CA, May 1996.
12. J. D. Farmer. A rosetta stone for connectionism. *Physica D*, 42:153–187, 1990.
13. J. D. Farmer, N. H. Packard, and A. S. Perelson. The immune system, adaptation, and machine learning. *Physica D*, 22:187–204, 1986.
14. S. Forrest, S. A. Hofmeyr, A. Somayaji, and T. A. Longstaff. A sense of self for unix processes. In *Proceedings of IEEE Symposium on Research in Security and Privacy*, Oakland, CA, 1996.
15. S. Forrest, B. Javornik, R. Smith, and A. S. Perelson. Using genetic algorithms to explore pattern recognition in the immune system. *Evolutionary Computation*, 1(3):191–211, 1993.
16. S. Forrest, A. S. Perelson, L. Allen, and R. Cherukuri. Self-Nonself Discrimination in a Computer. In *Proceedings of IEEE Symposium on Research in Security and Privacy*, pages 202–212, Oakland, CA, 16-18 May 1994.
17. Steven A. Frank. *The Design of Natural and Artificial Adaptive Systems*. Academic Press, New York, M. R. Rose and G. V. Lauder edition, 1996.
18. C. J. Gibert and T. W. Routen. Associative memory in an immune-based system. In *Proceedings of the 12th National Conference on Artificial Intelligence (AAAI-94)*, pages 852–857, Seattle, July 31-August 4 1994.
19. P. Hajela, J. Yoo and J. Lee. GA Based Simulation of Immune Networks - Applications in Structural Optimization. *Journal of Engineering Optimization*, 1997.
20. Paul Helman and Stephanie Forrest. An Efficient Algorithm for Generating Random Antibody Strings. Technical Report Technical Report No. CS94-7, Department of Computer Science, University of New Mexico, 1994.
21. R. Hightower, S. Forrest, and A.S. Perelson. The evolution of emergent organization in immune system gene libraries. In *Proceedings of the Sixth International Conference on Genetic Algorithms*, Pittsburg, 1995. Morgan Kaufmann, San Francisco, CA.
22. Geoffrey W. Hoffmann. A neural network model based on the analogy with the immune system. *Journal of Theoretical Biology*, 122:33–67, 1986.

23. John E. Hunt and Denise E. Cooke. An adaptive, distributed learning system, based on the immune system. In *Proceedings of the IEEE International Conference on Systems, Man and Cybernatics*, pages 2494–2499, 1995.
24. John E. Hunt and Denise E. Cooke. Learning using an artificial immune system. *Journal of Network and Computer Applications*, 19:189–212, 1996.
25. Y. Ishida and F. Mizessyn. Learning Algorithms on an Immune Network Model: Application to Sensor Diagnosis. In *Proceedings of International Joint Conference on Neural Networks*, volume I, pages 33–38, China, November 3-6 1992.
26. Yoshiteru Ishida. Fully distributed diagnosis by PDP learning algorithm: Towards immune network PDP model. I:777–782, June 17-21 1990.
27. Yoshiteru Ishida. An Immune Network Model and its Applications to Process Diagnosis. *Systems and Computers in Japan*, 24(6):38–45, 1993.
28. Yoshiteru Ishida. The Immune System as a Self-Identification Proces: A survey and a proposal. Presented at IMBS workshop on Immunity-Based System, December 1996.
29. A. Ishiguru, Y. Watanabe, and Y. Uchikawa. Fault Diagnosis of Plant Systems Using Immune Networks. In *Proceedings of the 1994 IEEE International Conference on Multisensor Fusion and Integration for Intelligent Systems (MFI' 94)*, pages 34–42, Las Vegas, October 2-5 1994.
30. N. K. Jerne. The immune system. *Scientific American*, 229(1):52–60, 1973.
31. N. K. Jerne. Towards a network theory of the immune system. *Ann. Immunol. (Inst. Pasteur)*, 125C:373–389, 1974.
32. N. K. Jerne. The generative grammar of the immune system. *The EMBO Journal*, 4(4):847–852, 1985.
33. Jeffrey O. Kephart. A biologically inspired immune system for computer. In *Proceedings of Artificial Life*, Cambridge, M.A., July 6-8 1994.
34. Janis Kuby. *Immunology.* W. H. Freeman and Co., second edition, 1994.
35. David McCoy and Venkat Devarajan. Artificial immune systems for aerial image segmentation. In *Proceedings of the IEEE International Conference on Systems, Man, and Cybernetics*, pages 867–872, Orlando, Florida, October 12-15 1997.
36. Ronald R. Mohler, Carlo Bruni, and Alberto Gandolfi. A System Approach to Immunology. *Proceedings of the IEEE*, 68(8):964–990, 1980.
37. J. K Percus, O. Percus, and A. S. Person. Predicting the size of the antibody combining region from consideration of efficient self/non-self discrimination. *Proceedings of the National Academy of Science*, 60:1691–1695, 1993.
38. Alan S. Perelson. Immune network theory. *Immunological Reviews*, (10):5–36, 1989.
39. Alan S. Perelson and Gerard Weisbuch. Immunology for physicists. *Preprint for Review of Modern Physics*, June 1995.
40. Glenn W. Rowe. *The Theoretical Models in Biology.* Oxford University Press, first edition, 1994.
41. Rira M. Z. Santos and Américo T. Bernardes. The stable-chaotic transition on cellular automata used to model the immune repertoire. *Physica A*, 219:1–12, 1995.
42. Franciso J. Varela and John Stewart. Dynamics of a class of immune networks I. Global Stability of idiotype interactions. *Journal of Theoretical Biology*, 144(1):93–101, 1990.
43. Frank T. Vertosick and Robert H. Kelly. Immune network theory: a role for parallel distributed processing? *Immunology*, 66:1–7, 1989.

44. Frank T. Vertosick and Robert H. Kelly. The immune system as a neural network: A multi-epitope approach. *Journal of Theoretical Biology*, 150:225–237, 1991.
45. Richard G. Weinand. Somatic mutation, affinity maturation and antibody repertoire: A computer model. *Journal of Theoretical Biology*, 143(3):343–382, 1990.
46. Gerard Weisbuch. A shape space approach to the dynamics of the immune system. *Journal of Theoretical Biology*, 143(4):507–522, 1990.

**Dr. Dipankar Dasgupta** is an Assistant Professor of Computer Science in Mathematical Sciences department at the University of Memphis, Tennessee, USA. His research interests are broadly in the area of scientific computing, tracking real-world problems through interdisciplinary cooperation. His areas of special interests include Artificial Intelligence, Genetic Algorithms, Neural Networks, Computational models of Immune System, and Their Applications. He published more than 40 research papers in book chapters, journals, international conferences, and technical reports. He is also the co-editor of the book "Evolutionary Algorithms in Engineering Applications" published by Springer-Verlag, 1997.

Dr. Dasgupta obtained his Bachelors degree (1981) in Electrical Engineering and the Masters degree (1987) in Computer Engineering, from India. He received Ph.D (1994) in Computer Science from the University of Strathclyde, Glasgow. After finishing his Ph.D, he joined the University of New Mexico as a Post Doctorate researcher and worked there on various projects until August, 1995. He was a visiting faculty at the University of Missouri – St. Louis before coming to the University of Memphis in January 1997. He is a member of IEEE/IEEE Computer Society, ACM and other professional Societies. Dr. Dasgupta is also a member of the editorial board of an international journal and serve as a program committee member in many international conferences. He organized a special track (with 2 sessions) on Artificial Immune Systems and Their Applications at the IEEE International Conference on Systems, Man, and Cybernetics (SMC'97) held in Orlando, October 12-15, 1997. He is also organizing such a track at SMC'98, San Diego, October 11-14, 1998 and offer a tutorial on this topics.

# The Endogenous Double Plasticity of the Immune Network and the Inspiration to be Drawn for Engineering Artifacts

Hugues Bersini

IRIDIA - CP 194/6
Université Libre de Bruxelles
50, av. Franklin Roosevelt
1050 Bruxelles - Belgium

**Abstract.** Although for reasons that are discussed, immunology have had a weak influence so far on the design of artifacts, one key aspects of immune networks, namely their endogenous double plasticity could be of interest for future engineering applications facing complex, hard to model and time-varying environments. In immune networks, this double plasticity allows the system to conduct its self-assertion role while being in constant shifting according to the organic's ontogenic changes and in response to the environmental coupling. We argue that the development of complex systems, adaptive both at a structural and parametric levels, should comply with the following basic operational principles: - the structural adjustments intermittently occur following a longer time scale than the parametric adjustment - the structural plasticity amounts to the addition of new elements in the system and the suppression of redundant elements from it - the structural adjustments are dependent on the temporal evolution of the internal parameters being subject to some learning i.e. when and how to perform a structural change should depend on data related to the dynamics of the parametric change so that the network endogenous behaviour and no exogenous criteria will guide these structural changes - these structural alterations have to be done in a "collective" spirit namely by applying heurisitics like "help the weakest elements (or compensate for them)", "maintain diversity", "fill the blank spaces", "suppress redundant elements". Three applications are briefly discussed: neural network classification, autonomous agent learning by reinforcement learnig and the control of chaos, where these principles are in full play and seem to have positive effect.

## 1 Introduction

### 1.1 Immunology and its weak influence so far on the design of artifacts

Biological studies have always constitute a large pool of inspirations for the design of engineering systems. These last years, two biological systems have provided a formidable source of inspirations for the development of new types of algorithms for engineering applications as classical as non-linear modeling and optimization: they are neural networks and evolutionary algorithms .

Through neural networks new ideas, like multilayer hierarchical decomposition, parallel processing, use of saturated activation functions, which all originate in basic knowledge of the brain structure and functions, have complemented old ways of coping with non-linear modeling and pattern recognition. Evolutionary algorithms have led to two capital insights: first the combined use of parallel type of search with selective mechanism and random proposal of new candidates around existing promising ones but, above all, the use of recombination as a very clever way to generate new candidates from promising ones for problems of combinatorial optimization. In both cases, I would be inclined to characterize this influence as strong since the road to this new algorithms had to go through the biological knowledge. These new non-linear modeling and optimization methods would never have existed in the absence of some sufficient understanding of their biological sources of inspiration.

Has our biological knowledge of the immune system influenced in the same strong and direct way the design of new algorithms or artifacts. Not yet, at least to my knowledge. A lot of algorithms, methods or artifacts whose authors claim to be directly inspired by their understanding of how the immune system works could have been proposed by others (and have been proposed in various cases) without the least idea of what all this immunological stuff is about. This is certainly not to be taken as a criticism addressed to researchers whose works, however deep and original they appear to be, are influenced by their knowledge of immunology (and indeed I am one of them) but rather as a will to separate strong biological influence from weak one. In the same way, this helps to explain why the engineering developments inspired by the immune system have not gained the same popularity as neural networks and genetic algorithms. It could be just because there seem to be other roads to conduct to these same developments, roads for which knowing immunology is of no real necessity.

One other key reason for this weak influence is that our basic and common knowledge of the immune system is to some extent already expressed in quite an engineering not to say a military way: the immune system recognizes intruders (classical pattern recognition), eliminates it and memorizes this encounter (classical memorization mechanism). This is what a national army or police is supposed to do and people have for long invented way to provide their house with such safety and defensive measures before knowing that our immune system had the same type of worry. Even the way the immune system is doing it is, as traditionally described in the literature, not so original once you have resolved the fundamental problem of why an intruder is indeed classified as being an intruder : the self/non-self discrimination famous problem (problem which simply disappears in a lot of applications). So any defensive application of whatever system, computers or others i.e. the main type of artifacts that appear to result from inspirations drawn from immunology [9] [18] [23], seem to have benefit very little from knowing anything more than the immune system also is known in part as defending an organism. In other words, we could say that both the immune system and the protection of whatever artifacts are similarly inspired by some abstract conception of what a defensive system could be, without perceiving today how they do or they could mutually strongly influence each other.

Accordingly, in the work presented in this chapter, I would certainly not claim that the immunological influence was so strong as to make the development of algorithms to be shown in the following sections impossible without good knowledge of immunology. Here again the influence is, I recognize, pretty weak. However, if any the originality lies in the fact that the perception of the immune system from which the design of engineering artifacts is weakly derived is not the classically admitted one of a defensive system but rather a self- assertional system [25] [35] [37]. This self-assertion, in response to continuous interactions with the environment, is underlied by an continuous endogenous re-organization of the system both at a structural and parametric level.

## 1.2 The endogenous double plasticity of immune networks

In nature biological systems capable of adaptation based upon parametric and structural adjustments are legion. "Parametric plasticity" is the name given to the adaptive mechanism allowing the system to adjust its parameters while executing a certain task so as to improve its performance. A new classical parametric plasticity is the learning of the synaptic weights which has became inseparable of any effective use of neural networks. "Structural plasticity" allows one level more of adaptability. In systems structured as networks of interacting elements, the structural plasticity amounts to the integration and the disappearance of some of these elements from the network. Keeping with neural networks, this additional plasticity is provided by the possibility for neurons to disappearing or appearing in time [20], then for the whole neural net not only to adjust its synaptic weights but also to alter, while performing, its whole architecture. It is a different type of change since, if describing the system as a set of differential equation, the parametric changes will not modify this set whereas the structural changes will cause the suppression or addition of some of these equations.

Immune networks are members of this family of biological systems (see Farmer [16] for a convincing attempt to underline the similarities among the systems and to create a common language to describe this family). They are structured as networks of interacting units and present this double level of plasticity: the units already present in the network can vary their concentration, but also simply appear or disappear (see [6] [12] [10] for biologically-oriented simulations). Ecosystems as well are subject to this double plasticity: the parametric plasticity is due to the species density which varies according to the interactions with other species of the network, and also as consequence of environmental impacts. The introduction of new species is caused by crossover and mutations of genetic material already present in the network.

In both systems, a crucial issue is the fact that the network as such, and not the external interactions, exerts the selective pressure on the new elements to be integrated and the old ones to be suppressed. This double plasticity take place in an endogenous way i.e. in response to internal aspects and needs, instead of in an exogenous way i.e. as a direct response to external interactions. The environmental impact on this selection is diffused and transmitted by the network. The network re-organises itself to handle this interaction but indirectly, through the effect of this interaction on itself. Never this re-organization is a one-to-one function of the interaction. In engineering and quite naturally, the re-organization needs are often imputed restrictively to the external world interaction while in biology it has to be imputed to the network as a whole. This exogenous vision is also well diffused in immunology since the acceptance of the system as basically defensive emphasizes, in a capital way, the interaction with the external intruders. On the other hand, perceiving with Varela, Stewart and Coutinho [3] [7] [12] [25] [35] [37], the immune system as self-assertional with main finality to preserve some form of communication and homeostasis in the somatic identity of the organism, turn the scale in favour of an endogenous vision.

Besides this fundamental resemblance between evolutionary and immune systems, we do think that a key distinction has to be pointed out. While immune networks have a collective function and the way they perform can be considered at a global level, ecosystems have no collective responsibility. Instead each individual of the network tries to improve the way it behaves in a somehow "selfish" way (to borrow the famous "selfish gene" expression of Dawkins) taking into account both the network interactions and the environmental influence. The other members of the network are just there to hamper or to help each individual to better survive, but the survival of the network as a whole is of no consideration by each of the member. In an immune network, functions whatever they really are, appear as collective, while they must be appreciated at an individualistic level in ecosystems. The next section will present the immune double plasticity in a very simple way and show how the endogenous re-organization, while integrating response to external interactions, can result in an emergent form of memory.

These last years John Holland's classifiers systems (CFS [8] [13] [19] [21]) have received an increasing attention. They are among the first and the most interesting attempts to develop a methodology for integrating the two levels of plasticity in a distributed system which interacts with a complex, dynamic and unpredictable environment. Roughly, classifiers are sensory-motor units which can self-modify while acting (the bucket-brigade algorithm, a form of temporal difference reinforcement learning [8] [13] [33], is responsible for this progressive adaptation) their probability of being selected when the environment matches their sensory part. This is the parametric plasticity, and it evolves in time as a function of the punishments and rewards returned by the environment subsequently to the units execution. The most efficient unit will receive more and more positive reinforcement with final result to be always selected when matching the current situation. In addition, new units can be created by mutating and recombining the best units acting so far in the population.

This structural plasticity is in the hands of the famous Genetic Algorithms (GA, [8] [19]). While the innovative and pioneering Holland's developments will remain as an important inspiration for future works dedicated to the conception of adaptive mechanisms in autonomous complex systems, we believe that to some extent the biological inspiration i.e. ecosystems have led CFS to address the structural plasticity in an unsatisfactory way. Artificial GA like natural evolution indeed aim at generating new individuals by focusing mainly on the best individuals to be found so far in the current system. This is a very "individualistic" strategy, well appropriate when each individual selfishly tries to improve its chance of survival in an environment constituted by the other individuals. This also explains the popularity of GA today, when isolated from CFS, as an interesting optimization strategy. To combine the building blocks possibly responsible for the good performance of current actors is an intuitively appealing approach on the road to generate still better actors (perhaps the best). However, why should it be so when the behaviour of interest is not attached to any actor in particular but rather to their collective actions.

As an alternative, we hypothesize that, when interested in the collective performance of a system which indeed exhibits emergent functionalities, its structural adjustments should be achieved in a "collective spirit", more precisely: by compensating for the weakest actors of the system, by maintaining diversity and by filling the empty regions not occupied yet by the current actors, and finally by suppressing the redundant ones. The fact of focusing on the weakest member of the population so as to generate new compensatory ones is diametrically opposed to the part played by GA in CFS. GA focus on the best members and generate new ones very similar to them. We suggest in contrast to focus on the worst members and to generate new ones quite distinct from them. The operational philosophy which lies beyond is that the behaviour of a collective system is much more dependent on its weak part than its strong part, like the final sound of a complete stereo which is fully conditionned by its weakest part. If you have to replace one element of your stereo, rationally you'll begin with the worst one rather than with the best one.

A lot of engineering systems become operational provided both their structure and their parameters have been tuned in a satisfactory way. This is the case for polynomials, neural networks, fuzzy systems etc. In the majority of cases, even if the structural tuning always remains a problem, the structure is chosen randomly or richly enough for entrusting the parametric plasticity with all the adaptive needs. It is enough to observe the usual practice with neural networks, where the selection of the architecture looks very much like cooking recipes. Several problems can be raised by this lack of attention for the structural choice. Whatever parametric adjustment, the selected structure can turn out not to be a correct one, it can be not rich enough, or on the contrary, the selected structure can be satisfactory but too heavy (not a minimal one) and leads the parametric plasticity to consume too much computations and memory, or to be responsible for biasing effects such as the well known overfitting for neural networks. As a rule, a minimal structure has to be favoured and if the discovery of this structure can be automated while doing the task, so much the better.

Withdrawing some inspiration from our knowledge of the immune network, the construction of engineering complex adaptive systems which, while in the operational phase, self-modify their structure and adjust their parameters, could comply with the following basic principles:

1. the structural adjustments intermittently occur following a longer time scale than the parametric adjustment
2. the structural plasticity amounts to the addition of new elements in the system and the suppression of redundant elements from it
3. the structural adjustments are dependent on the temporal evolution of the internal parameters being subject to some learning or of other internal aspects of the system. When and how to perform a structural change should depend on data related to the dynamics of the parametric change. So the network endogenous behaviour and no exogenous criteria will guide these structural changes.
4. these structural alterations have to be done in a "collective" spirit namely by applying simple heuristics like "help the weakest elements (or compensate for them)", "maintain diversity", "fill the blank spaces", "suppress redundant elements".

To help making the point, this chapter will rely on three practical illustrations of systems capable of evolving in time their structure and parameters while executing their task: neural net classifiers, autonomous agents which adapt by reinforcement learning, and controllers of chaotic systems. Since each applications and its practical results has already been separately the object of complete papers, here we will shorten their presentation in a way which reflects sufficiently their relying on the biologically-inspired principles introduced above. Nevertheless, besides this sketchy presentation, a detailed understanding of any of these applications will require a dedicated complementary reading. Although each particular problem requires associate particular mechanisms, several principles they comply with have turned out to be similar enough to convince us that these principles might be at the basis of a very large set of potential applications.

### 1.3 A brief overview of these three applications

In the third section, a new algorithm for self-structuring neural net classifiers is presented. It is called EMANN for Evolving Modular Architecture for Neural Networks [32]. This algorithm allows to maintain a minimal size architecture thus a small number of parameters (the synaptic weights) to be trained together with, for this architecture, a satisfactory set of parameters. It extensively uses network internal local variables and the way the parametric learning modifies them to guide the construction of the structure.

Section four will be dedicated to reinforcement learning type of algorithm namely Watkins' Q-learning [1] [2] [5] [34] [38] [39] for the maze type of problems [33]. We will in part rely on a very nice work of Munos et al. [28] and show how the double level plasticity leads to an acceleration of the reinforcement learning discovery of good policies in large problem spaces. This acceleration is obtained by a simultaneous search of a satisfying minimal structural representation and, within this minimal representation, of the discovery at a computationally reduced cost of the optimal solution. In addition, like originally stated by Holland [21], the structural plasticity makes the system to exhibit a larger degree of adaptivity thus escaping from the brittleness of classical artificial intelligence methods. Since Q-learning added with structural adaptation results in a complete methodology endowed with the same double plasticity as CFS (Bucket Brigade + GA, see [8] for a discussion about this equivalence), how the structural plasticity differs in the two cases will easily come to light.

In recent years, methods have been proposed for controlling chaotic systems around unstable orbits embedded in chaotic attractors. These methods require linear feedback control in a small region around the desired trajectory. With my colleagues of IRIDIA, Antoine Duchateau and Nick Bradshaw [14], we have developed a non-linear local model-based approach to the control of chaos which gradually adds new local linear controller. The two main benefits with respect to the original OGY[1] method [29] is to first effectively enlarge the region of control and thus to reduce the time needed to stabilize the chaos. In section five, the control of the chaotic Henon map by gradual increase of local linear controller will be briefly illustrated.

## 2 An Elementary Immune Network and the Basic Principles to be Obeyed by a Double Plastic Adaptive System

In 1974, Jerne imagined an appealing possible explanation of how the immune system might do for maintaining the memory of an encounter with an antigen, and thus for being able of an improved reaction if encountering this

[1] OGY stands for the initials of the conceptors of the method – Ott, Gerbogi, Yorke.

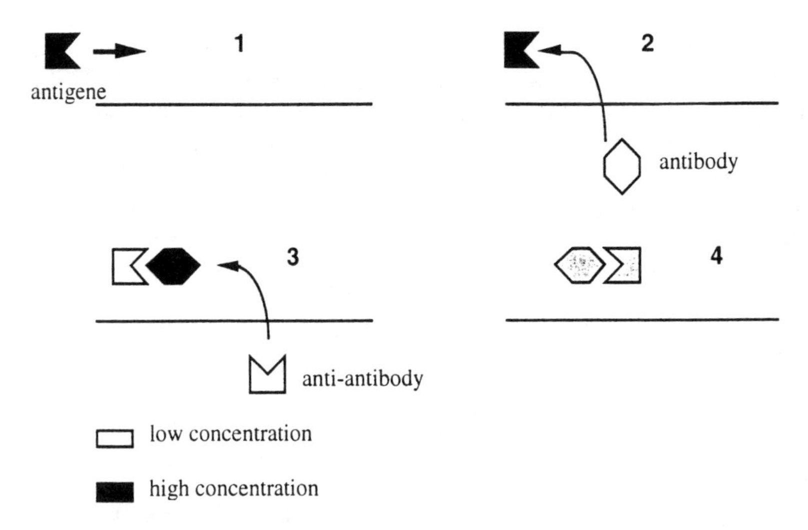


**Fig. 1.** The elementary network for the immune memory

same antigen a second time [22]. This explanation is illustrated in fig.1. The memory might result from the existence of an elementary network comprising two elements: the antibody which binds the antigen and the anti-antibody which binds the antibody. The explanation is the following. The antigen gets inside the body, if in sufficient concentration it generates a domain of affinity for the antibody with a complementary shape thus able to bind the antigen. Then one antibody is recruited and, being stimulated by the antigen, it grows in concentration. Their mutual binding causes the decreasing of the antigen together with the decreasing of the antibody. Now the presence of this second antibody, provided it reaches a sufficient concentration, also generates a domain of affinity which causes the recruitment of a second antibody binding to the first one namely an anti-antibody which, if the binding requires complementarity, turns out to be the replica of the antigen (often called the internal image of the antigen). What is interesting in the first place is that the presence of these two antibodies and their mutual sustain, due to a delicate balance between their mutual stimulation, is sufficient to explain memory. In fact the first antibody, necessary to suppress the antigen as soon as it intrudes on the body, will be maintained at an average concentration through this elementary network interactive effect. In brief, memory emerges from the endogenous equilibration of the network by mutual sustain.

Since this original vision, Varela, Stewart, Coutinho [35] [36] [37], Perelson [30] [31], De Boer [10], Weisbuch [40] and others, while preserving and propagating this view of the immune system as being in part structured as a network of antibodies, have made important contributions on the way to an improved modelling of the network and a deeper understanding of its functionalities. It would be too long and out of the scope of this paper to give an overview of their contributions. We just need to say that they all share with Jerne this view that the immune network could indeed be responsible for collective and emergent functionalities. In the small explanation given in the previous paragraph, memory is the result of the network taken as a whole (although being restricted to its minimal form: two elements). Several investigators of the immune network have the strong feeling that the whole network function might amount to the maintenance of a certain coherence or viability, a form of homeostasis preventing the network neither to collapse nor to explode despite external and internal interactions (external and self antigen). In contrast, all these interactions could imprint the network in such a way as to allow it to keep traces of all these imprints in an harmonious and not destabilizing way. Whatever kind of self-maintenance ability this network has, even the elementary example given as introduction of the section is already representative of the basic principles an adaptive distributed system endowed with a double plasticity is likely to obey:

- the structural changes (i.e. the recruitment of a new antibody in the system) occur following a longer time scale than the parametric changes (the varying concentration of the antibodies).
- the structural changes depend on the temporal evolution of the system parameters. Only when the concentration of the first antibody reaches a sufficient level can the second antibody be recruited.
- the nature of these structural changes depends on the whole network and not just on the external interactions. In the simple network above, it is the first antibody which is responsible for the recruitment of the second one, and not the antigen directly (although it is at the origin of the chain). In case of a bigger network, with more than two nodes, the next antibody to be recruited will have to show a good sensitivity with the whole network (see [6] [10] [12] for computer simulations of this type of network-based selection).
- the new added actors show complementarity rather than resemblance with the actors already present in the network. This is an important difference between immune recruitment and GA type of recruitment.

We expect this simple example, whatever biological likelihood, to be illustrative enough of the principles a double plastic adaptive system has to respect when, in contrast with ecosystems, the collective behaviour of the network is responsible for a benefic function, thanks or despite the environmental interactions.

## 3 The Endogenous Double Plasticity in Neural Net Classifiers

We have developed a new algorithm called EMANN for self-structuring neural net classifiers and have presented it in [32]. A very similar approach has been presented in [11]. In this section, we will briefly present the key mechanisms in sufficient depth for reflecting the principles introduced in the previous section (for deeper details and complete experimental results see the original paper). Here the classification problem must be regarded as a problem of on line adaptation since the algorithm to be described simultaneously builds and trains the network while the patterns to classify are continuously presented. The basic idea is to extensively use the evolution in time of the local internal parameters subject to learning instead of external global variables to evolve the structure. We do believe that such an alternative can be profitable in improving the accuracy of the resulting classifier while maintaining the neural architecture to a minimal size. It must be better to look inside (the synaptic weights) and not outside (the error function, like done for instance in [20] and [11]) the network in order to realize how it is performing i.e. whether it is on the right track and where it seems to run into difficulties.

In our approach, like in [11] and [20], a network is built by suppressing and/or adding neurons without modifying the remaining part of the network structure (i.e. no modification of the synaptic weights). In so doing, the information captured in the synaptic weights isn't lost at every structural change (and thus needs no complete re-learning). As a result, this preservation may speed up the whole process. In contrast, when using genetic algorithms for structural optimization as described in [27], the whole network is reinitialized and total learning is needed for each new structure. In the incremental approach, the one adopted by EMANN, the initial structure is too poor and the addition of further neurons is required. We do suspect that this incremental approach allows to better preserve the essential generalization capacities of the network. Besides, it seems to avoid better local minima: by adding new neurons, the algorithm continuously increases the dimension of the weight space allowing the system to easily find new path to escape from local minima. The main part of our methodology amounts to an incremental approach, fresh neurons being continuously added onto an initially small network. However some intermittent pruning also occurs, as described later, for suppressing unsettled neurons.

Inspired from Fahlman's cascade correlation method [15], there is a further incremental operation since the neural architecture to be evolved is a hierarchy of modules (see fig.2). However and departing from Fahlman's method, each module is a classical one hidden layer network (with a number of neurons depending on the previous incremental operation). The inputs of the problem are connected to the inputs of all superior modules, that is all the modules share the same task inputs. This avoids any module to be fed in only with the outputs of modules which may not have processed the network inputs correctly. Secondly, the outputs of each module are connected to the inputs of all the upper modules and thus the final coding of the task solution turns out to be the top module outputs. This second heuristic relates to the incrementally of our approach. When a fresh module is superimposed to the old ones, it must act in a complementary way and has to extract very informative data from the inferior ones. We believe this information to be appropriately captured by the output units. The new module can then efficiently use the results obtained by the lower structure after being trained.

To train the synaptic weights i.e. the parametric plasticity, EMANN uses an heuristically modified version of the standard backpropagation algorithm called "extended delta-bar-delta" and described by Fombellida in [17]. This learning algorithm tunes the step and momentum parameters during the training period. Each connection has its own learning parameters. We no longer have to tune them manually before training and the resulting method gains in autonomy since, in spite of the intermittent structural changes, these parameters can better fit a new problem due to a new structure.

The key local variable used to evolve the structure is the Connection Strength ($CS$) of a neuron defined as the average absolute value of the weights connected to N. Let $n$ be the number of weights connected to a neuron, let $W_i$ be the value of the $i$th weight connection to this neuron, then the $CS$ is given by:

$$CS = \frac{\sum_{i=1}^{n} |W_i|}{n}$$

The fact that a neuron which contributes efficiently to the classification present weights with great value is only due to the use, as activation function, of the sigmoid which saturates at 1 for great values of its input. We define a settled neuron as a neuron presenting a $CS$ above a certain settling threshold fixed initially. A settled neuron sharply truncates its input space. According to experimental results, such neurons are the most useful to the classification task and their associated hyperplane seem stable.

When all neurons of a module are settled, all the associated hyperplanes become almost motionless. Such a stabilized module can't improve its performances anymore. EMANN manages to always keep a pool of non-settled neurons in the evolving module so as to maintain sufficient potential for improvement. A neuron with a low $CS$ gives a same output ($\pm$ 0.5) for a wide range of points in the synaptic weight space, the exact position of the associated hyperplane does not matter much and keeps on changing. We define a useless neuron as a neuron with a $CS$ below the uselessness threshold parameter, here again initially fixed. Therefore two thresholds summarize the influence of $CS$: a low one - the uselessness threshold - and a high one - the settling threshold. A large amount of experimental tests for one hidden layer module convinced us that the useless neurons can be pruned without deteriorating in a significant way the module behavior. Consequently this pruning occurs in the module prior to the addition of a new upper module.

When adding a new neuron in the hidden layer of a module, we found fruitful not to initialize its synaptic weights randomly but, here again, keeping in line with the principles stated in the previous sections, to select the new neuron as being complementary to the ones in the current module. In order to help the neurons which seem to be in trouble i.e. presenting low $CS$, the

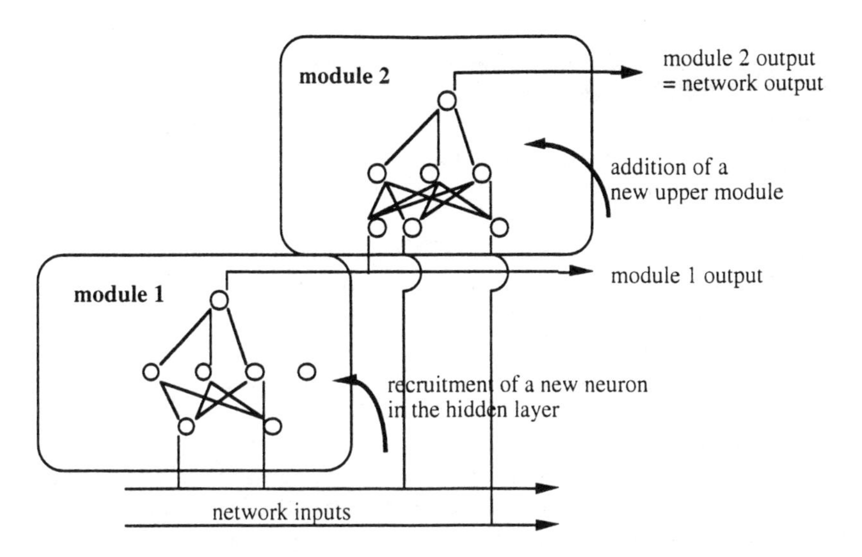


**Fig. 2.** The general type of architecture EMANN evolves (here with just two modules)

new neuron is initialized in such a way that its outputs are as different as possible from those of the troubled neuron. This is achieved by providing the new neuron with a weight combination showing a maximum number of sign inversions with respect to the neuron having the lowest $CS$. However when this sign configuration already exists elsewhere in the module, another configuration has to be chosen, still close to the opposite of the worst neuron but not yet present in the module.

EMANN starts with the smallest structure: one module with only one neuron in the hidden layer. The number of neurons both in the input layer and in the output layer is determined by the task. The evolution of one module follows four phases: ascension, improvement, pruning and recovery. First, the ascension phase consists in adding a neuron at each ascension threshold (this is another parameter to be tuned initially) epochs. It ends as soon as a first neuron is settled but only by having one connection from the network inputs to the current module above the settling threshold. This condition guarantees that at least one of the new neurons is really engaged in treating the problem and not just copying the results found by an inferior module (this problem is discussed below).

Secondly, in the improvement phase, a fresh neuron is added every time a neuron settles. When neurons start settling, the module is trying to reach a solution. As the number of settled neurons increase, this solution is getting better. The improvement phase stops when no further neuron has succeeded to settle during a number of epochs called the patience parameter (this is still a further parameter of the method). Thirdly, the following pruning phase suppresses all the neurons with $CS$ below the uselessness threshold. Finally, the recovery phase releases the learning algorithm in the remaining module for a small number of epochs, just to recover the previous accuracy on the training set slightly deteriorated by the pruning phase.

After these four phases, the treated module is frozen and EMANN starts building a new module constituting an upper layer, but only if the just treated one improved sufficiently on the network solution reached until its integration. Observation of the improvement phase indicates that the size of the non-settled neurons pool is kept constant. It is proportional to the number of ascension threshold epochs needed by the module to settle a first neuron, and appears as a very nice indication of the difficulty of the task. A large pool means a high diversity of neurons needed to perform the task. A kind of regulation occurs for free: the pool size increases with the complexity of the task helping the learning algorithm to reach a solution.

One major difficulty EMANN has to face is the copy problem. When a new module is added, it tends first to replicate the outputs of the module below. It then has strong connections with the outputs of the lower module. This leads to the settlement of neurons performing a purely copying work. In order to solve this problem EMANN, during the ascension phase, waits for one connection of the neuron with the task inputs to be strong enough first to start the improvement phase. This further requirement insures that the ascension phase ends when a new way of solving the task is being explored by the new module. Finally, the ascension threshold differs whether EMANN is running on the first module or not. It is higher for upper modules than for the first one. EMANN stops building the whole network (then add no new module) when the last module leads to no major gain of accuracy on the training set.

We tested EMANN on a classification benchmarks with results interesting enough to encourage us in believing that algorithms for self-structuring neural networks should give more attention to local internal variables at the expense of global external ones. Such algorithms should be capable of "introspective" regards on how the network behaves and, if necessary to improve it, on how and where to help it by enriching its current structure.

## 4 The Endogenous Double Plasticity in Autonomous Agents Learning by Reinforcement

Reinforcement learning concerns a family of problems in which an agent acting in a given environment aims at maximizing the cumulative outcome of its actions just on the basis of poorly informative responses coming from the environment. No complementary guidance is provided for helping the exploration/exploitation of the problem space, and therefore the learning agent can rely only on a trial-and-error strategy. Q-learning [1] [2] [4] [7] [13] [24] [34] [38] [39] and classifier systems (CFS, [8] [13] [19] [21]) have been separately proposed as two general frameworks for treating reinforcement learning problems. Some works have been done to show the large resemblance existing between these two frameworks [13]. Q-learning learns to select, for each environmental state, which action to execute, so that, at the end of the actions sequence, the selected action policy maximizes a utility function computed over the full sequence. Inherent to the recursive mechanism which characterizes this algorithm, the evaluation of an action for a particular state will only depend on information obtained in the immediate future, namely the immediate environmental response composed with the same evaluation but computed in the next state. Since Q-learning boils down to a weak search method, it is very slow and exponentially dependent on the size of the problem space. Various ways of accelerating it by means of structural generalization [26], hierarchical task decomposition and incremental increase of the size of the problem space, have been proposed and tested with different degrees of success. Speeding up the algorithm convergence for large problem space remains one of the most substantial improvements which a lot of current research has set as its goal. Provided the space of the problem has been initially partitioned in a certain number of cells N, within each cell an action has to be selected among a certain number of them K (fig.3). The classical Q-learning algorithm can be described as follows. Let's call the quality or Q-value of action $j$ when taken in cell $x$. The selection of the action in cell $Q_x^j$ is generally based on a Boltzmann distribution of these Q-values, then favoring probabilistically the highest Q-values. Initially set to 0, the Q-value of an action $j$ which drives the agent from cell $x$ to cell $x+1$ changes according to the formula:

$$\triangle Q_x^j = \alpha \left( r_t + \gamma . MAX_i Q_{x+1}^i - Q_x^j \right)$$

where $r_t$ is the immediate feedback given by the environment in response to the action $j$, $\alpha$ $(0 < \alpha < 1)$ is the learning rate, $\gamma$ $(0 < \gamma < 1)$ is the discount factor used in general to exponentially discount future rewards in the final cost function $E = \sum_{k=0}^{m} \gamma^k . r_{t+k}$, in order to minimize the number of successive steps for positive rewards and to maximize this number for negative ones, or just to bound the cost. Since its original presentation by Watkins, this algorithm has largely been exploited and analyzed both practically and theoretically [1] [2] [34] [38] [39]. The Q-learning algorithm amounts to the parametric plasticity of the whole framework. After convergence, the best action (i.e. the one whose local effect is to maximize the cost function E) will always be selected in each cell.

The computational cost of this weak search method is exponentially dependent on the number of cells N and the number of actions K. Then any attempt to keep small either the number of cells or the number of actions can induce important computational economies. As a matter of fact, the two mechanisms of structural plasticity to be presented now will aim at respectively keep the number of partitions N and the number of actions K small. To be a viable tool for real world applications, reinforcement learning techniques need effective methods to partition the state-action space. This point has been the subject of research by both the CFS and the Q-learning communities. In CFS generalization has been addressed by the use of the don't care (#) operator. A classifier attribute occupied by a don't care is considered to be irrelevant, and it is therefore by means of don't cares that generalization over classes of equivalent state-action pairs is achieved. However, it is still an open problem how to develop set of rules which can effectively exploit this generalization possibility. Moreover, CFS are inherently discrete systems which makes it difficult to achieve the kind of generalization in which a similar input should cause a similar output. This is more easily achieved in Q-learning systems enriched by neural nets, like in Lin's system [24].

Overviewing reinforcement learning algorithms able to adapt the partition of their problem space, we are in presence of the two traditional and opposite ways: bottom-up and top-down. In the bottom-up approach, the problem space is initially very fine grained, and the partitions are created by clustering together input regions showing similar properties [26]. In the top-down approach, the initial problem space is uniformly coded and is progressively subdivided in finer parts. Since top-down methods amount to an incremental structural alteration of system, they better comply with the principles associated with the structural plasticity.

Holland's biological inspiration, that is ecosystems and genetic mechanisms, led him to address this structural plasticity by GA. In CFS, the GA is responsible for two types of structural changes, depending on whether it applies to the condition or to the consequent part of the classifiers: a change in the coding of the state space and a change in the set of actions. These two types of changes have also been investigated in the Q-learning community, but within the more appropriate "collective and compensatory" perspective discussed above. Aware of the exponential dependency of the search duration with respect to the size of the state-action space, a very interesting method by Munos, Patinel and Goyeau [28] has been proposed in order to progressively partition the space such that Q-learning discovers a final satisfactory solution in the smallest possible space.

The algorithm they have developed is roughly the following (for a more detailed description see the presentation of the authors themselves in [28]). The problem starts with a very coarse partition of the space i.e. a small number of cells. Then in an intermittent way, a cell is split if the reinforcement received by the action acting in that particular cell presents variations of great amplitude indicating that a same action is not adequate for covering the whole cell (see fig.3b). Consequently a splitting turns out to be necessary together with the setting of distinct actions in the resulting smaller cells. In brief, when the update of the Q-values in a cell presents an important pseudo-standard deviation, this indicates that the cell is not homogeneous enough, and that a finer division is necessary so as to create two homogeneous regions out of this heterogeneous one.

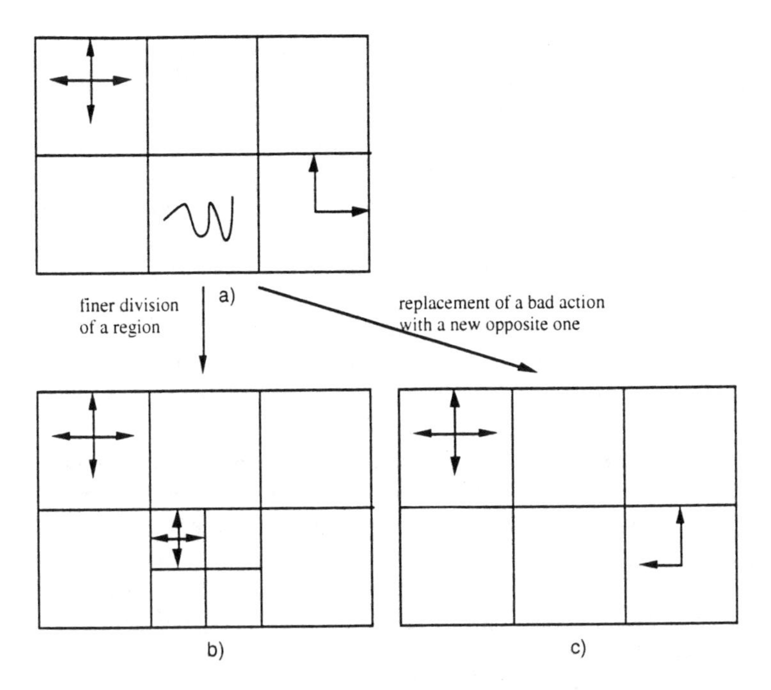


**Fig. 3.** The two types of structural plasticity for Q-learning - b) finer division of a cell and c) replacement of a bad action with a new opposite one

For the same kind of application and despite a shared interest for reinforcement learning in distributed complex adaptive system (Q-learning is very close to the parametric plasticity of CFS i.e. the bucket brigade algorithm), this form of structural plasticity appears very distinct from the part played by GA in CFS. It focuses on the current unsatisfactory part of the system to expect some improvements by structural additions. Besides, the authors propose a method for eliminating splitting that would turn out to be unnecessary. Since the partitioning should be maintained at a minimum level, a mechanism to regroup resembling regions and to eliminate useless subdivisions has been added: a finer region is kept as far as no general region lodging action with higher Q-value can be found. This algorithm was implemented on a maze type of problem with very satisfactory results. We find herewith again the basic principles introduced above:

- the structural changes are executed at a lower frequency, and in function of the time evolution of the Q-learning
- just the "weakest" cells i.e. the one presenting oscillating Q-values will be subject to structural modification by means of their splitting
- redundant splitting is suppressed

Regarding the action part, another strategy aiming at accelerate the discovery of a solution has been developed (fig. 3c) in which again the adaptation relies on the parametric and structural types of change occurring at different time scales [3] [4] [5] [7]. Now the partition is determined from the beginning and will not change. The new scope is to find the best action in each cell out of a set of actions whose cardinality has to be kept low. First, the Q-learning tries to find in each cell the best action among a preliminary small set of actions (the same in each state) and this during a certain number of Q-learning iterations. Then and expecting the convergence of Q-learning, new actions are recruited in the cells in which the current actions show bad Q-values as compared with other actions acting in the same cell or actions acting in neighboring cells. These new actions are selected so as to be the opposite of the bad ones they replace (for instance move left instead of move right or a negative value instead of a positive one) and they are given the Q-value of the best action already acting in the cell (so that new actions are immediately tested). Q-learning is then released again on the basis of the new set of the unchanged number of actions. This alternation between Q-learning and substitution of actions is carried on up to reach a satisfactory solution. In [4] and [5], it is shown how the control of the cart-pole is correctly realized after several generations of new actions. Here again the same principles apply: slower structural changes depending on the parametric adjustments, attention paid for the weakest elements, the suppression of bad elements and their replacement with new ones opposite to them.

## 5 The Endogenous Double Plasticity for the Control of Chaos

In [29] Ott, Grebogi and Yorke (OGY) proposed a method for controlling chaotic systems about fixed points (or, in principle, higher-period orbits) which are embedded in the attractor but are unstable. This method relies on a local linear model of the system, which can be obtained either theoretically or empirically, and employs standard linear optimal control techniques to control the system in the neighbourhood of the fixed point. The novelty of the approach was that a control action of limited magnitude (only small perturbations are exerted) can be used to good effect if it is applied in the region of a pre-existing, unstable fixed point. The region of control is dependent on both the allowed range of the control parameter and on the accuracy of the model used. Because the control law is only valid in a small neighbourhood of the point to be stabilized, the approach relies on the uncontrolled system passing near to the fixed point of its own accord. This can normally be guaranteed as the unstable fixed point is densely surrounded by other points of the attractor.

In order to minimize the expected time the system will wander around the attractor before coming under control it is desirable that the region of effective control can be extended over a wider area. An aim of the work currently under progress, with my colleagues Antoine Duchateau and Nick

Bradshaw [14], is to increase the size of the area of the attractor in which our controller is valid. We call these areas ZECs (zones of effective control) and by gradually adding these ZECs, we allow the controllable area to encompass as much of the state space of the chaotic system as possible. To achieve this goal, we must build a controller that has two main characteristics: First, it must be globally non-linear because the system we try to control is highly non-linear and a linear approximation around the fixed point will not hold elsewhere in the state. Second, as the size of the control action is strictly limited by assumption, the search for the control law has to be done in such a way that the resulting controller is able to lead the system to convergence using only small a perturbation at each time-step.

The ZECs are placed gradually along an uncontrolled convergent trajectory (this is the structural plasticity) and the linear controller inside each ZEC has to learn to force the chaotic process to follow this trajectory (this is the parametric plasticity). We fix the next controller in the trajectory as the target for the current one, so a small deviation from the uncontrolled trajectory could be canceled by a control action that would not exceed the maximum value. The first ZEC is centered on the fixed point (which for this work we assume is given). It can be seen as the fundamental zone of control since without it no control is possible. A control policy (very similar to OGY one) is learned for this rule so that each time the state of the process falls into, it is captured and the system converges. In our work, we basically extend this principle by gradually adding other controllers to the system. These structural additions remain endogenous since the new controllers are added on the natural trajectories of the chaotic system.

When the system has spent a previously stated number of consecutive steps (for the experiments here we used 200) in this ZEC it is said to have converged satisfactorily, and is considered to have been satisfactorily learnt. We then start to add new ZECs. To do this we must wait for another trajectory to converge, by chance, at which moment we define a sequence of ZECSs with centers at those points of the trajectory which lie outside the first ZEC. These new ZECs are numbered upwards so that a system whose state is at the center of one ZEC will pass in the next time-step to the next ZEC. In fig.4, you can see a succession of ZECs which together have for responsibility to stabilize the Henon chaotic map around its fixed point.

Following the structural additions of these new ZECs, the parametric learning take place in each of them and each hosted controller has to learn to direct the system towards the center of the next ZEC. After a certain amount of parametric learning steps, new ZECs can again be installed on experimented trajectories so as to gradually cover as much as possible of the state space. What is gradually evolved is a network of ZECs embedded in the chaotic trajectory. Their interconnection is due to the fact that each ZEC has for responsibility to transfer the system into the neighbouring one. The

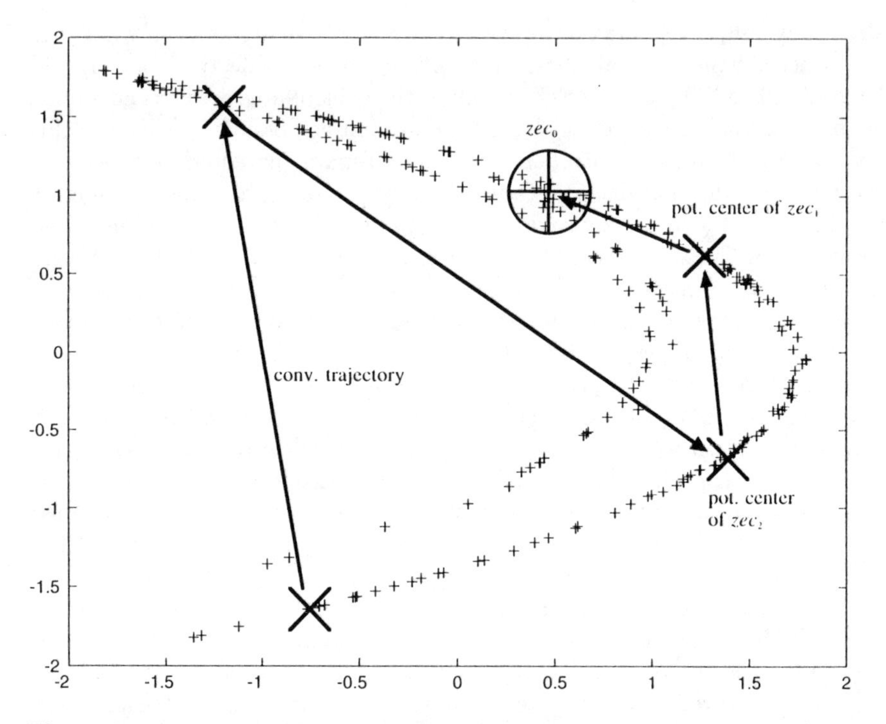


**Fig. 4.** A network of 5 ZECs aiming at stabilizing the Henon chaotic map at its fixed point (in the center of ZEC0). When a trajectory is found which converges to the fixed point, the centers of the new ZECs are located at the states of the trajectory which lie outside ZEC0

final scheme is very reminiscent of the network of antibodies embedded in an universe of somatic interaction and antigen encounters.

## 6 Conclusions

We have just described three practical applications in which the endogenous double level of adaptability, weakly inspired by our knowledge of this same double plasticity in immune networks, allows to learn rapidly a satisfactory solution, by parametric and structural adaptation, and to keep small the structure of this solution. In all three cases, the way the double plasticity was implemented respected principles originating from biological systems: while the system is in its operational phase, the structural changes occur at a lower frequency and as a function of the parametric changes, these changes aim at compensating for the weakest parts of the system, at maintaining the diversity and filling the empty spaces, and at preserving a low size structure. The contrast of such principles with the well known association of genetic mechanisms with classifiers systems was largely commented. We have illustrated how these same principles were respected in the three applications in which the structural changes respectively were: the addition and suppression of new neurons in a neural network classifier, the refinement or recoarsening of the partition of the problem space of an autonomous agent learning by reinforcement and the addition of adaptive linear controllers aiming at controlling chaos in the whole state space. We do expect that a huge amount of engineering system whose performance is highly sensitive to the structure and the values of tunable parameters could similarly benefit from their relying on such principles.

In a closed future, the conception of complex systems showing important autonomy and intended for interacting with realistic environments impossible to model and to predict with precision, will naturally require a substitution of optimization criteria by "satisfying" ones, of precise targets by viable ones, of teaching by weakly supervised guidance. This in fact will demand highly flexible systems, both at a parametric and structural level, capable of important internal and undirected re-organisation. Like the environment they will be designed to interact with, these systems will keep a large degree of autonomy, an important emancipation with respect to the designer, a potentiality slowly revealed through their interaction with the world to control, an identity not pre-determined but constantly in the making. In more practical words, and related to our three applications, the more complex, hard to model, time varying the classification problem, the autonomous agent environment or the dynamic system will be, the more naturally will the engineering solutions adopt the biologically-inspired algorithmic principles discussed in this chapter.

## References


1. Barto, A. (1990), Connectionist Learning for Control. In Neural Networks for Control (Thomas Miller III, Richard Sutton and Paul Werbos eds.) MIT Press, pp 5-58.
2. Barto, A. and Singh, S.P. (1990), Reinforcement Learning and dynamic programming. In Proceedings of the Sixth Yale Workshop on Adaptive and Learning Systems, New Haven, CT., K.S. Narendra (Ed).
3. Bersini, H. and F. Varela (1990), Hints for adaptive problem solving gleaned from immune networks. In Proceedings of the first conference on Parallel Problem Solving from Nature - Schwefel and Männer (Eds) - Springer Verlag. pp 343-354.
4. Bersini H., (1993), Immune Network and Adaptive Control. Toward a Practice of Autonomous Systems, In Proceedings of the First ECAL, Varela and Bourgine (Eds.), 217-225, MIT Press.
5. Bersini, H. (1992a), Reinforcement and Recruitment Learning for Adaptive Process Control - In Proceedings of the 1992 IFAC/IFIP/IMACS on Artificial Intelligence in Real Time Control pp.331-337.
6. Bersini, H. (1992b) The Interplay between the Dynamics and the Metadynamics of the Immune Network, Presented in the Third Conference on Artificial Life - Santa Fe 15-19 June.

7. Bersini H. and Varela F., (1994), The Immune Learning Mechanisms: Recruitment Reinforcement and their applications, In Computing with Biological Metaphors, R. Patton (Ed.), Chapman and Hall.
8. Booker, L.B, Goldberg, D.E. and J.H. Holland (1989) Classifier systems and genetic algorithms, Artificial Intelligence 40, Elsevier Science Publishers B.V. (North Holland) pp 235-282.
9. Dasgupta, D. and N. Attoh-Okine. (1996) Immunity-Based Systems: A Survey, Presented at the ICMAS workshop on Immunity-Based Systems, Japan (Dec'96).
10. De Boer, R.J. and A. Perelson. (1991), Size and Connectivity as Emergent Properties of a Developing Immune Network, In J. Theoretical Biology, Vol. 149, pp. 381-424.
11. Deffuant, G. (1992), Reseaux Connectionistes Auto-Construits - These D'Etat.
12. Detours, V., Bersini, H., Stewart, J. and F. Varela (1994), Development of an Idiotypic Network in Shape Space - in Journal of Theoretical Biology, Vol. 170, pp. 401-414.
13. Dorigo, M. and Bersini, H. (1994), A Comparative Analysis of Q-learning and Classifier Systems, In proceedings of SAB 94, MIT Press., pp. 248-255.
14. Duchateau, A., Bradshaw, N. and H. Bersini, H. (1997), A Multi-Model Solution for the Control of Chaos, Submitted to International Journal of Control.
15. Fahlman S. and C. Lebiere (1990), The Cascade-Correlation Learning Architecture, Advances in Neural Information Processing System, Vol 2, P.P. Morgan Kaufman Publishers, pp 524 - 532.
16. Farmer, D. (1991) A Rosetta Stone to Connectionism. In Emergent Computation, Forrest S. (Ed). MIT Press.
17. Fombellida M. (1992), Méthodes heuristiques et méthodes d'optimalisation non contraintes pour l'apprentissage des perceptrons multicouches, Proceedings of the fifth Int'l Conf. on Neural Networks & their application : Neuro-Nimes, pp 349-366.
18. Forrest, S., Hofmeyr, S.A., Somayaji, A. and T.A. Longstaff. (1996). A sense of self for unix processes. In Proceedings of IEEE Symposium on Research in Security and Privacy, Oakland, CA.
19. Goldberg, D.E. (1989), Genetic Algorithms in search, optimization and machine learning. Addison-Wesley Publishing Company, Inc.
20. Hirose Y., Yamashita K.and Hijiya S. (1991), Back-propagation Algorithm Which Varies the Number of Units, Neural Networks, Vol 4, pp 61-66.
21. Holland, J.H., Holyoak, K.J., Nisbett, R.E. & Thagard, P.R. (1986) Induction: Processes of inference, learning and discovery. Cambridge: MIT Press.
22. Jerne, N. (1974), Ann. Inst. Pasteur Immunol. 125C, pp. 435-441.
23. Kephart, J.O. (1994), A biologically inspired immune system for computer. In Proceedings of Artificial Life - MIT Press.
24. Lin L-J., (1992), Self-improving reactive agents based on reinforcement learning, planning and teaching. Machine Learning, 8, 3-4, 293-322.
25. Lundkvist, I., Coutinho, A. , Varela, F. and D. Holmberg (1989) Evidence for a functional idiotypic network among natural antibodies in normal mice, In Proc. Natl. Acad. Sci. USA, Vol. 86, pp. 5074-5078.
26. Mahadevan, S. and J. Connel (1992), Automatic programming of behavior-based robots using reinforcement learning, In Artificial Intelligence 55, Elsevier Science Publishers B.V. (North Holland) pp. 311-365.

27. Miller G., Todd P. and Hedge S. (1989), Designing Neural Networks using Genetic Algorithms, In Proceedings of the third Int'l Conf on Genetic Algorithms, pp 379-384.
28. Munos R., Patinel J. and Goyeau P., 1994. Partitioned Q-learning. CEMAGREF Technical Report, Paris, France - In proceedings of SAB 94 Conference, MIT Press, pp. 354-363.
29. Ott, E., Gerbogi, C. and J.A. Yorke. (1990), Controlling Chaos, Phys. Review Lett. 64(1196):292-295.
30. Perelson, A.S. (1988) Towards a Realistic Model of the Immune System, In Theoretical Immunology, Part Two, edited by A.S. Perelson. SFI Studies in the Sciences of Complexity, vol. 3, Reading, MA: Addison-Wesley, pp 377-401.
31. Perelson, A.S. (1990), Theoretical Immunology, In Lectures in Complex Systems - SFI Studies in the Sciences of Complexity, Lect. Vol. II, Edited by Erica Jen, Addison-Wesley, pp 465 - 500.
32. Salomé, T. and H. Bersini. 1994. An Algorithm for Self-Structuring Neural Net Classifiers - In proceedings of the Second IEEE Conf. On Neural Network - ICNN'94 - pp. 1307-1312.
33. Sutton, R.S. (1990) Reinforcement Learning Architectures for Animats. In Proceedings of the First SAB Conference - Meyer and Wilson (Eds.) - MIT Press - pp.288-296.
34. Tsitsiklis J.N, (1993), Asynchronous Stochastic Approximation and Q-learning. Internal Report from Laboratory for Information and Decision Systems and the Operations Research Center, MIT.
35. Varela, F., A. Coutinho, B. Dupire and N. Vaz. (1988) Cognitive networks: Immune, neural and otherwise, in A. Perelson (Ed.), Theoretical Immunology, Vol.2 SFI Series on the Science of Complexity, Addisson Wesley, New Jersey pp 359-375.
36. Varela, F., V. Sanchez and A. Coutinho (1989), Adaptive strategies gleaned from immune networks, in B. Goodwin and P. Saunders (Eds.), Evolutionary and epigenetic order from complex systems: A Waddington Memorial Volume. Edinburgh U. Press.
37. Varela, F.J. and A. Coutinho. (1991), Second Generation Immune Network - in Immunology Today, Vol. 12 No 5.- pp. 159-166.
38. Watkins C. J. C. H., (1989), Learning with delayed rewards. Ph. D. dissertation, Psychology Department, University of Cambridge, England.
39. Watkins C. J. C. H. and Dayan P., (1992), Technical Note: Q-learning. Machine Learning, 8, 3-4, 279-292.
40. Weisbuch, G. , De Boer, R.J. and A.S. Perselson. (1990), Localized memories in idiotypic networks, J. Theor. Biol. 146 - pp. 483-499.

**Dr. Hugues Bersini** has an MS degree (1983) and a Ph.D in engineering (1989) both from Université Libre de Bruxelles (ULB). He is member of the IRIDIA laboratory (the AI laboratory of ULB) and assistant professor teaching computer science and AI. He is partner of various industrial projects and EEC esprit projects involving the use of adaptive fuzzy and neuro controllers. Over the last 10 years, he has published about 80 papers on his research work which covers the domains of cognitive sciences, AI for process control, connectionism, fuzzy control, lazy learning for modeling and control, reinforcement learning, biological networks, the use of neural nets for medical applications, frustration in complex systems, chaos and epistemology. He is quite often asked for giving tutorials covering the use of neural networks and fuzzy systems and the behavior of complex systems. He co-organized at ULB the second conference on Parallel Problem Solving from Nature (PPSN) and the second European Conference on Artificial Life (ECAL). He co-organized the three European Workshops on Reinforcement Learning (EWRL 95 and 96 and 97). He co-organized the first International Competition on Evolutionary Optimization algorithms (ICEO' 96). He is the coordinator of the FAMIMO LTR European Project on fuzzy control for multi-input multi-output processes.

# Part II

# Artificial Immune Systems: Modeling & Simulation

# The Central and the Peripheral Immune Systems: What is the Relationship?

John Stewart[1] and Jorge Carneiro[2]

[1] Université de Technologie de Compiégne, France.
[2] Institute Gulbenkian of Science, Oeiras, Portugal.

**Abstract.** This chapter discusses the concept according to which the immune system is composed of two distinct compartments, a Central Immune System (CIS) and a Peripheral Immune System (PIS). The PIS is composed of disconnected lymphocyte clones which remain in a resting state unless they are specifically activated by an antigen giving rise to a classical immune response. The CIS is composed of a network of clones which display autonomous activity and integrates antigens into its ongoing regulatory dynamics. Functionally, the PIS is appropriate for reactions to immunizing antigens, whereas the CIS is appropriate for body antigens. Second generation immune network (SGIN) models are systematically reviewed; we conclude that they are unable to account satisfactorily for the CIS/PIS distinction. A third generation immune network model, incorporating B-T cell co-operation, is able to accommodate both the structural and the functional properties of CIS and PIS in a coherent account, and moreover to explain how the CIS/PIS distinction can be generated by the self-organizing properties of the network. Finally, we emphasize that the difficulty in establishing a productive relationship between theory and experiment is a hallmark of the whole network approach to the immune system, and is perhaps the reason why, at the present time, the immunological community regards idiotypic networks with skepticism.

## 1 Introduction

The aim of this chapter is to discuss the concept, first put forward by Coutinho and colleagues (Huetz et al., 1988; Coutinho, 1989), according to which the immune system is composed of two distinct compartments, a Central Immune System (CIS) and a Peripheral Immune System (PIS). The PIS is composed of lymphocyte clones which do not interact with each other; they remain in a resting state unless they are specifically activated by an antigen. In this case, clonal selection of the reactive lymphocytes gives rise to a classical immune response which triggers destruction of the antigen. The CIS is composed of a network of clones which activate each other by idiotypic interactions. Thus, the CIS displays autonomous activity even in the absence of antigenic stimulation. The CIS does of course interact with antigens; typically, however, it does not produce massive immune responses, but rather integrates the antigens into its ongoing regulatory dynamics. Functionally, it is clear that the PIS is appropriate for reactions to immunizing antigens, whereas the CIS is appropriate for body antigens.

The issue we wish to discuss is how the frontier between the CIS and PIS can be defined, and by what mechanisms the two systems and the frontier between them are generated. We shall base this discussion on the assumption, which it is nevertheless useful to make explicit, that any given lymphocyte clone, at a particuliar point in time, belongs either to the CIS or to the PIS; i.e., in clonal terms, the two systems are mutually exclusive but together make up the totality of all lymphocytes present in the system the so called available repertoire. On this basis, we shall examine several specific models of the immune system, seeking in each case to characterize the relationship between the CIS and the PIS that they represent. Perhaps the most appealing aspect of the CIS/PIS hypothesis is that it draws a clear and explicit relationship between the *structure* of the immune system and its *function*:

```
CIS = Network = Tolerance
PIS = Independent Clones = Immunity
```

As we shall see, most models in the literature can accommodate either the structural or the functional features of the CIS and the PIS, but fail to account simultaneously for both. The bottom line is that a fully fledged CIS and PIS distinction, displaying appropriate structure-function correlates, requires invoking specific co-operation between B and T lymphocytes.

## 2 Second Generation Network Models

The first set of models we shall discuss is the class of "second generation idiotypic networks" (SGIN) (Varela & Coutinho, 1991). The term referes not only to a certain class of mathematical network models, but designates an entire research programme which aimed at modelling the natural, autonomous behaviour of the immune system. The first model which was designed with this concern was that of Varela et al. (1988). This model shares many common features with most of the contemporary and later network models, notably those proposed by De Boer et al. (De Boer & Hogeweg, 1989a, 1989b, 1989c; De Boer & Perelson, 1991; De Boer et al., 1993a), Weisbuch et al. (1990, 1993), Faro & Velasco (1993c), and Sulzer et al. (1993). In the present paper, the term SGIN will be restricted to this class of mathematical models, independently of the aim of their design.

The uniqueness of the SGIN models as compared with other idiotypic network models is the following set of qualitative postulates.

First, the immune network is made up of B lymphocyte clones that are connected through idiotypic interactions. The participation of T lymphocytes is typically neglected or ignored.

Second, the distinction between parotopic and idiotopic interactions in the original proposal of Jerne (1974) has been dropped, following the suggestion of Hoffman (1975, 1980). The affinities and consequences of the idiotypic interactions are assumed to be symmetric, and the "helper" or "suppressor" properties of lymphocytes are relational properties which depend on the extent of their interactions with the network.

Third, the degree of activation and the population dynamics of each lymphocyte clone is essentially controlled by the extent of receptor ligation by soluble Ig-molecules. The activation of the lymphocytes follows a characteristic log-normal function of the sensitivity or field, i.e. the sum of the concentrations of ligand weighted by the corresponding affinities for the receptor. This response curve is founded on the analogy with experimental LPS-responses (Coutinho, 1974), on the cross-linking of the membrane Ig receptors (Perelson & DeLisi, 1980; Perelson, 1984; Faro & Velasco, 1993a, 1993b), or on a competition between proliferation and maturation responses (Grossman & Cohen, 1980; Sulzer et al., 1993).

Fourth, and last, the soluble Ig-molecules are the main mediators of idiotypic interactions because they can rapidly diffuse through the body fluids, in numbers which are much higher than those present in the lymphocytes as membrane Ig-receptors.

The first SGIN model we shall discuss is that systematically employed by Weisbuch and Neumann, to which de Boer and Perelson have also contributed (De Boer, 1989; Neuman, 1992, Weisbuch et al., 1990). In its initial form, this model did not distinguish between free and cell membrane-bound immunoglobulins, but Anderson et al. (1993) have shown that making this distinction does not modify the essential conclusions. In the simple case of two complementary clones, this model possesses a characteristic fixed point attractor, in which one clone, present in high concentration, is in an "immune" state (further antigenic stimulation leads to expansion), and the other clone, present in low concentration, is present in a "suppressed" state (further antigenic stimulation leads to decrease; see (De Boer et al. 1993a, 1993b) for an extensive investigation of the conditions under which this dynamic pattern can be obtained). In order to study an extended network, Weisbuch et al use a Cayley-tree structure of connectivity, and privilege parameter settings which avoid percolation. Depending on the quantitative dynamics of antigen presentation and elimination, two basic patterns arise: "vaccination" (clones complementary to the eliciting antigen are in an immune state), and "tolerance" (clones complementary to the eliciting antigen are in a suppressed state). The network as a whole can demonstrate localized "memory" for a certain number of antigens (in either the vaccinated or tolerant mode), essentially independently of each other. What happens if we try and fit this model into the "CIS vs PIS" mould? In order to make functional sense, we have to identify "vaccination" with the PIS, and "tolerance" with the CIS. Neumann (1992) has made an interesting suggestion as to how the appropriate attribution of clones to the CIS and PIS might occur: "At prenatal and neonatal stages, when multi-specific clones and odd loops are present, localized tolerance attractors are established in response to early presented (self) antigens. As the immune system develops, the multispecific idiotypes are increasingly suppressed, odd loops vanish from the network, and exposure to antigen now generates immunity rather than tolerance. Those clones that remained virgin during early development are now able to respond to newly presented antigens and immunize the body against them. Nevertheless, the (self) antigens first presented to the network continue to be tolerated because the idiotypes that can react against them are still suppressed by their anti-idiotypes".

It is interesting to compare these results with those obtained by Detours et al. (1994). They have used the model proposed by Varela et al (1988) which distinguishes circulating and membrane immunoglobulins; however, with a sufficiently high source term the basic two-clone dynamics has the same asymmetric fixed-point attractor as the single-compartment model discussed above. In the extended network, the connectivity structure of the idiotypic interactions is derived from a "double sheet" version of a quasi-continuous 2-dimensional shape-space, in which each point corresponds to a pair of complementary clones. Under these conditions, percolation cannot be avoided. The presence of a constant antigen stimulates complementary clones, which in return stimulate idiotypes resembling the antigen; the result is a pattern of spreading "waves" of idiotypes and anti-idiotypes. When the two wavefronts meet, a quasi-stable "standing wave" of very high field is formed. This "wall" marks the frontier separating two uniform regions in shape-space, one of which is "tolerant" and the other "vaccinated". The introduction of a new antigen into a tolerant zone leads to a minimal alteration; by contrast, an antigen in the vaccinated zone provokes a strong immune response. Interestingly, if the ontogenesis of the system from a uniform virgin state occurs in the presence of a fixed antigen, this antigen is always incorporated into a tolerant zone. If we fit this model into the CIS/PIS schema, the tolerant zone clearly assumes the functions of the CIS, the vaccinated zone those of the PIS.

This model graphically illustrates a feature which is also characteristic of the Weisbuch model. In both cases, the idiotypic interactions underlying dynamic memory are such that CIS clones are sustained by complementary PIS clones, and vice versa. This implies not only that the CIS and PIS are interdependant with repertoires of essentially equal size, but that tolerance is equivalent to vaccination against molecular forms complementary to self-antigens, and conversely that vaccination is equivalent to tolerance with respect to molecular forms complementary to external antigens. To summarize, these models can readily account for the functions of the CIS and PIS, but the corresponding structures are entangled in a way quite contrary to immunological intuition and empirical observation.

A somewhat different picture emerges from the initial attempts to simulate the metadynamical recruitment of clones into an extended network of activated lymphocytes (Bersini, 1992; De Boer & Perelson, 1991; De Boer et al., 1992; Stewart & Varela, 1991). A distinguishing feature, compared to the models previously discussed, is that the relationship between mutually sustaining idiotypes is symmetric rather than asymmetric. Under these conditions, the principal result obtained by Stewart and Varela (1991), confirmed and extended in a more sophisticated version by de Boer et al. (1992), and also reproduced by Bersini (1992), is the following: after a rather chaotic initial period, one sees the emergence of characteristic quasi-stable configurations in shape-space comprising parallel chains of complementary clones (fig.1).

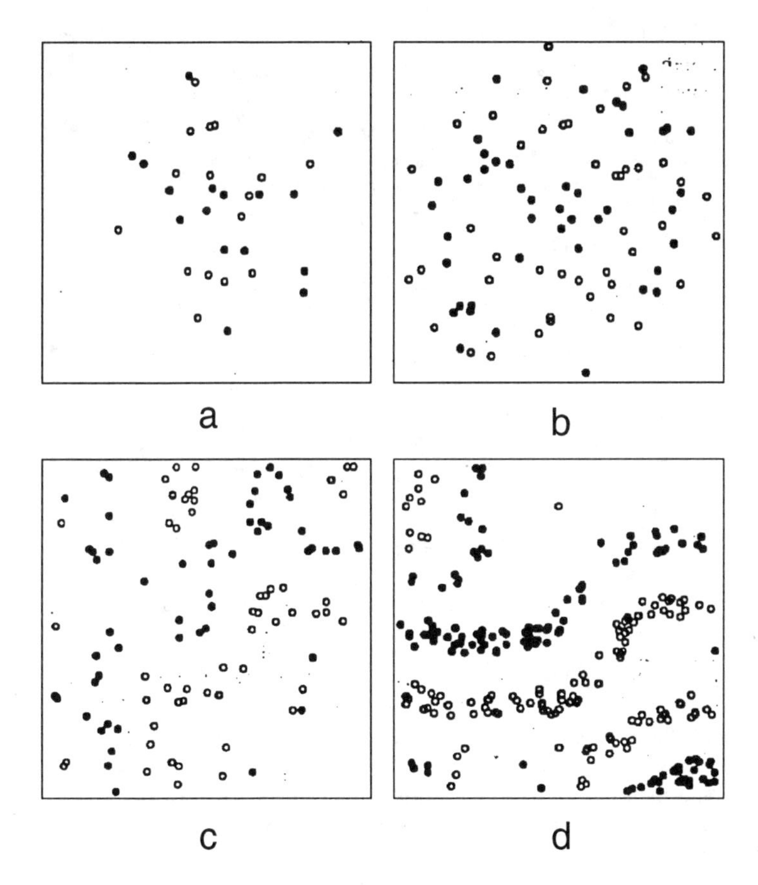


**Fig. 1.** Four successive stages in the self-organized constitution of an immune network, modelled by computer simulation in a 2-dimensional shape-space. After an initial chaotic period (1a and 1b), parallel chains of "black" and "white" clones appear (1c) and stabilize (1d). After Stewart & Varela (1991)

Fixed antigens are incorporated into chains of idiotypes that resemble them (fig.2). Since the field experienced by such antigens is moderate, this corresponds to tolerance. Consequently, in terms of CIS/PIS, the whole of the self-sustaining network corresponds to the CIS; the PIS is simply the residue of non-activated clones, freshly emerged from the bone-marrow, which are not recruited into the network because, being distant in shape-space, they fail to interact with it.

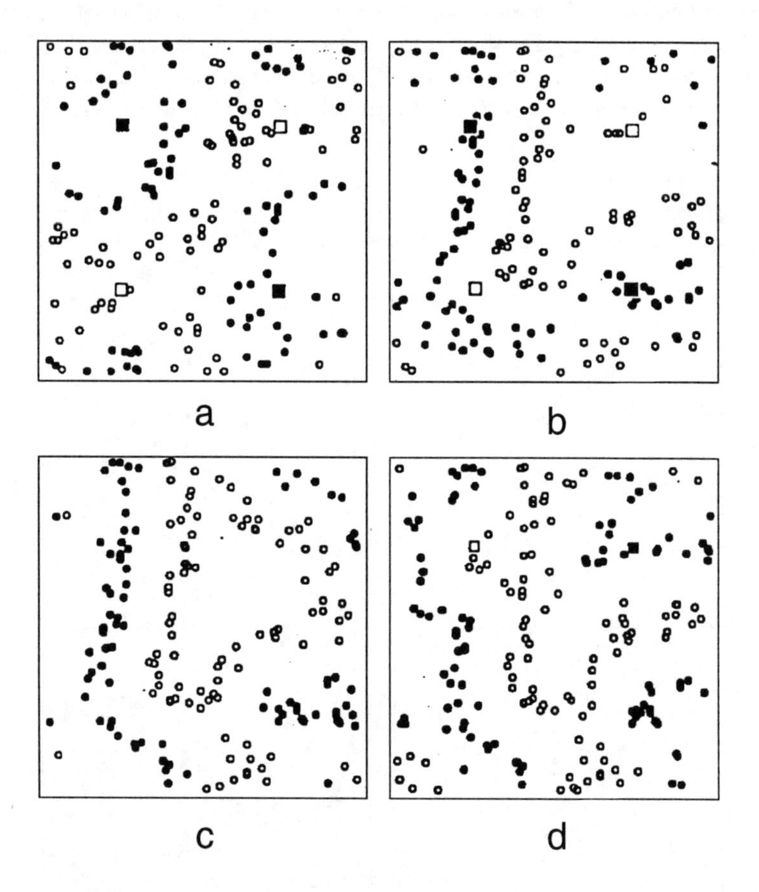


**Fig. 2.** The effect of coupling the immune network, simulated as in Figures 1 and 2, with fixed antigens (black and white squares). 2a and 2b: two examples which illustrate the incorporation of the antigens in chains of like-coloured clones. 3c: the configuration of 3b remains quasi-stable even after removal of the antigens, which corresponds to a form of "memory" in the system. 2d: The introduction of discordant antigens in the preceding situation (2c) leads to an adjustment of the chains. After Stewart & Varela (1991)

This picture is much more in accordance with the spirit of the CIS/PIS distinction as initially proposed by Coutinho (1989), particularly concerning the CIS as an instrument of self-assertion. However, there are substantial problems. In all the models simulated to date, the CIS network expands to fill the totality of available shape-space. The PIS, being "Totality - CIS", is thus reduced to a few percent.

This problem was first raised by de Boer and Perelson (1991), who suggested by extrapolation from results in 1- and 2-dimensional shape spaces that the fraction of disconnected naive clones could eventually be increased in shape spaces of higher dimension (1992). However, this suggestion has never been directly investigated, and all the results obtained so far seem to indicate that the tendency to reach "repertoire completeness" is a rather generic feature of the SGIN models[1].

First, in the studies in which the affinity coefficients are generated by bit-string matching — a procedure that is understood as a higher dimension "shape space" — the results were already unsatisfactory (De Boer & Perelson, 1991). Second, in our own simulations of the Varela et al. (1988) model using a procedure for the generation of continuous affinity coeficients with random topology (Detours et al., 1994; see Carneiro, 1996b for details), the network also develops into a "complete repertoire". Finally, by some kind of proof by negative induction, one should stress that the only extended SGIN models in which significant proportions of both "network" and "naive disconnected" clones have been shown to coexist, are based on a "Caylee tree" topology in which the affinity coeficients are binary (either null or a unique positive value) (Weisbuch et al., 1990; Anderson et al., 1993; Weisbuch & Oprea, 1994); whenever these topological constraints are relaxed the localised networks are lost (Neumann & Weisbuch, 1992a; de Monvel & Martin, 1995).

The tendency of the network to percolate and reach "repertoire completeness" is in apparent contradiction both with empirical estimates (in the spleen, at most 20% of lymphocytes are activated in uninfected animals, leaving 80% for the PIS), and with functional requirements: in order that pathological micro-organisms should not escape an immune response, the repertoire of the PIS should be practically "complete" (Perelson & Oster, 1979; De Boer & Perelson, 1993; Percus et al., 1993; Nemazee, 1996).

Morevoer, this is not the only problem in trying to fit the CIS into the network portion emerging from SGIN. The actual dynamical properties of

[1] Recently, De Boer et al. (1995) proposed a refinement of the activation function of lymphocyte clones based on receptor crosslinking, that confers an intrinsic advantage to higher affinity interactions. The implementation of this function in simulations in 2-dimensional shape space resulted in small localised networks in which the connections are of high affinity (De Boer et al., 1995). These small networks do not percolate because the lower affinity clones are not recruited, and because in the particular shape space formalism that has been used, each clonotype has one, and only one, high affinity complementary clone. If this strict constraint on the underlying topology of interactions is relaxed by allowing several high affinity connections per clone, then percolation and repertoire completeness seem to be again the main result (Takumi & De Boer, 1996).

the network, in particular its lack of robusteness to antigenic perturbations, pose additional difficulties. The main problem, closely associated with the symmetry of idiotypic interactions, was first raised by De Boer & Hogeweg (1989). A clone whose growth is sustained by a specific antigen can be easily uncoupled from the network, because it suppresses its complementary clone or clones. Carneiro (1997) redeployed the term "broken mirror", first put forward by Aubin, to refer to this situation so caracteristic of SGIN.

Many studies on SGIN models were focused on the regulation of immune responses and immunological memory (De Boer & Hogeweg, 1989a; Weisbuch et al., 1990; Neumann & Weisbuch, 1992a; Neumann & Weisbuch, 1992b; Sulzer et al., 1993; Weisbuch & Oprea, 1994; de Monvel & Martin, 1995). In most of these models, the clearance of the antigen is an explicit function of the responding clone. After the antigen is cleared, the responding clone will inevitably decay and go through the range of stimulatory clonal sizes and, in so doing will once again recruit its complementary clones. The sustained dynamics of this local nerwork in the absence of antigen is precisely what has been interpreted as immunologic memory (De Boer & Hogeweg, 1989a; Weisbuch et al., 1990; Neumann & Weisbuch, 1992a; Neumann & Weisbuch, 1992b; Sulzer et al., 1993; Weisbuch & Oprea, 1994; de Monvel & Martin, 1995). A "broken mirror" caused by antigen is not a problem in this particular context, however, it poses a serious problem for its functional interpretation as the CIS. Indeed, the decoupling from the network of the clones specific for body antigens must be interpreted as a break of natural tolerance and the onset of an autoimmune disease. It is important therefore to ask: how can antigen driven uncoupling of a clone from the network be avoided?

Uncoupling of clones driven by body antigens can be avoided if they always remain "suppressed" in an attractor which is qualitatively similar to the assymmetric fixed point in the model first described, i.e. in an attractor in which the two mirror clones do not switch their "immune" and "suppressed" status. Most situations in which a network was shown to develop and sustain some bounded dynamics in the presence of constant antigenic stimuli shared this general property, even if the underlying topologies were as different as a "Caylee tree" (Neumann & Weisbuch, 1992a; Anderson et al., 1993), a "shape space" (Detours et al., 1994), or some more complicated structures (such as the KS-network studied by Detours, 1996). As a corollary, any dynamic attractor in which antigen specific clones fluctuate between "suppressed" and "immune" states opens the door, at least transiently, to the uncoupling of antigen driven clones (De Boer & Perelson, 1991; Takumi & De Boer, 1996; Detours et al., 1994; Calenbuhr et al., 1994; Van Hammen, personal communication; Faro, personal communication; Neumann, personal communication; Carneiro, unpublished observations).

Alternatively, the specific clones can be maintained in the "suppressed" state because they are highly connected. The basic idea was first formalised by Stewart et al. (Stewart & Varela, 1989; Stewart et al., 1989), upon the analysis of the structure and dynamic implications of an experimental connectivity matrix (Kearney et al., 1987). More recently, Sulzer et al. (1994) have studied the behaviour of a model they proposed before (Sulzer et al., 1993). Using affinity matrices generated according to Stewart's ABCD topology, they concluded (Sulzer et al., 1994) that tolerance is only consistently observed if and only if the body antigens are coupled to the members of the highly connected A group; the structure in the remaining groups cannot reliably explain tolerance.

## 3 An Immune Network Incorporating B-T Cell Co-operation

Recently, we criticized the SGIN models along these lines, and questioned their basic assumption, according to which T-cell help is never a limiting factor for B-lymphocyte proliferation or Ig-production. In an amplified version of the model proposed by Varela et al. (1988), we made the activation of B-lymphocytes explicitly dependent on co-operation with activated T-lymphocytes.

In this model the main propositions in SGIN still hold, but some additional ones were introduced to describe the dynamics of T lymphocyte clones and their co-operation and interactions with B cell clones and the Igs they produce.

The process of B cell activation was divided in two steps. The first step is the induction which depends on the extent of receptor ligation by cross-linking agents such as the anti-idiotypic circulating Ig or native antigen. Since the induction process is analogous to the activation of lymphocytes in SGIN, it is described by the same characteristic log-normal function of the field. The second step is the co-operation between an induced B cell and an activated T cell which leads to full B cell activation. This process is described by a function that saturates on the total number of B or T cells weighted by their pairwise affinity; this function implements in this way the competition of B cells for T cell help. An induced B cell can co-operate with an activated T cell if it engages its TCR in either of two ways: by working as an antigen presenting cell or by being anti-idiotypic (fig.3).

The dynamics of T lymphocyte clones is very similar to the dynamics of the B cell clones, with the peculiarity that they are only driven by antigenic peptides presented by APCs. The presentation of specific peptides from the Igs expressed and produced by B lymphocytes are neglected because of their low individual concentration and frequency. Circulating Igs mediate idiotypic interactions amongst B cell clones, controlling their induction, much in the same way as they determined their activation in the SGIN models. Circulating Igs can only interfere with the dynamics of T cell clones if they have some affinity for they TCR, conditions in which they will inhibit their activation. In this model, circulating Igs are the only inhibitory influence on T cell acti-

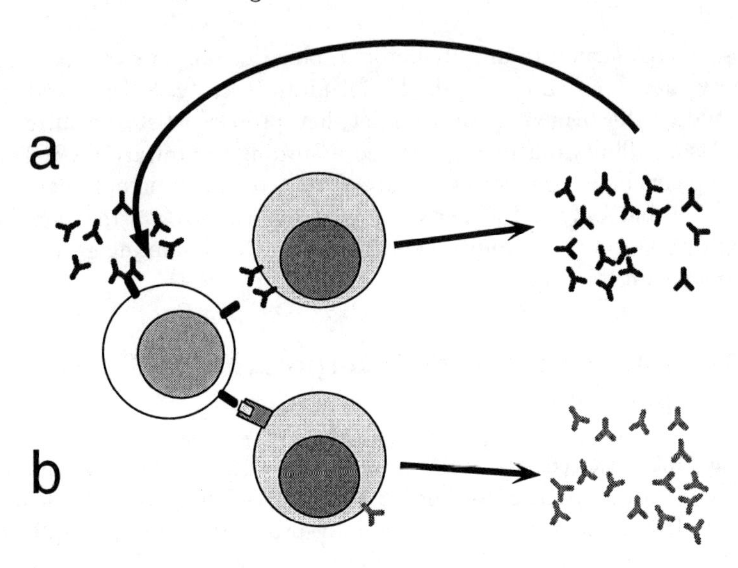


**Fig. 3.** The two modes by which a B lymphocyte can co-operate with an activated T lymphocyte: a) peptide presentation and b) idiotypic interaction

vation and growth. As a corollary, a bounded dynamics of the T cell clones can be achieved if and only if their TCRs are integrated into the idiotypic network.

The dynamics properties of this new model are critically dependent on the two modes of B-T cell co-operation depicted in fig.3. In the case where the members of a B-cell clone target the members of a given T-cell clone by presenting 'specific' peptides on their membrane MHCs, there is no particular relationship between the clonal receptors of the two types of lymphocytes. The Ig-molecules produced by the B-cell following activation do not interfere directly with the TCR of the T-cells, and so do not interfere with the state of activation of that clone. The consequence of this mode of B-T co-operation is immediate: both lymphocyte clones will grow exponentially as long as the other stimuli they need are maintained.

The second mode occurs when a B-cell clone co-operates with a T-cell clone through direct membrane Ig-TCR interactions. In this case, the Ig molecules produced by the activated B-lymphocytes specifically recognize the TCR of their T-cell counterparts. Since free anti-TCR Ig molecules are inhibitory for the T-cell, the B-T pair will be dynamically stabilized by a negative feed-back loop. Thus, even when the other stimuli they require are optimally stimulatory, the B-T pair will evolve towards a situation in which the anti-TCR Ig molecules (both free and membrane-bound) produced by the B-cells maintain a certain level of T-cell activity, which in turn is just sufficient to sustain the B-cells. This equilibrium is stable, because if the B-cell activity were to increase, the additional anti-TCR Igs would inhibit the

T-cells, and the reduced T-help would decrease the B-cell activity back to the equilibrium point.

It is clear that a model implementing these two modes of co-operation can exhibit two distinct modes of coupling with antigens: an "immune response" mode in which T- and B-cell clones grow exponentially; and a "tolerant" mode in which T-cell clones are controlled by inclusion of their TCRs in the repertoire of an idiotypic B-cell network. It is also clear that these two modes can be functionally mapped to the PIS and the CIS respectively. In summary, the co-operation between B and T cells breaks the symmetry in idiotype-antiidiotype interactions, and sets up a clear relation between the connectivity structure and the functions of tolerance and immunity.

It is now important to consider the results obtained by the simulations of an extended network in which there is a metadynamic interplay between these two modes of B-T co-operation (Carneiro et al., 1996b). Similarly to Detours et al. (1994) the simulation starts in a state where only antigens are present. The first event is necessarily the antigen-driven activation and expansion of T-lymphocyte clones, which is immediately followed by waves of antigen specific B-cell clones, and waves of anti-idiotypic B-cell clones, that both recognize some of the circulating idiotypes and the TCR of the antigen driven T cells. An idiotypic network forms, and, by recursive recruitment of new clones, diversifies its repertoire, until it becomes practically "complete" (fig.4). At this stage, the TCR of the antigen driven clones cannot escape being recognized by the idiotypic network, and therefore they are inhibited by the circulating anti-idiotypic Ig.

At this stage antigen-driven T-cells start to become a limiting factor for full B-cell activation, and the induced B-cells must now compete with each other for limited "T-cell co-operation sites" in order to obtain help. The simulations systematically reveal a stage of competitive exclusion, in which clones which bear higher affinity for the T cells compete out the less fit clones (fig.5). The result is a reduction of the number of species and connections in the idiotypic network, which "focuses" on the nodes anchored by antigen-activated T-clonotypes. The effective repertoire of the idiotypic network becomes restricted to just a fraction of the potential repertoire of the B-cells (fig.4). The result is a partition of the available B-cell repertoire into two compartments, represented respectively by the lymphocytes in the idiotypic network, versus all the other resting naive cells which are transiently available in the system (freshly produced by the bone-marrow, but not being activated, they are just waiting to die). These two compartments clearly correspond to the structural definition of the CIS and PIS as originally proposed by Coutinho.

Once again let us compare this result with the one obtained with the simulations of extended SGIN models. As long as T-cell help is not a limiting factor, the model by Carneiro et al. (1996a, 1996b) behaves like a SGIN[2].

[2] It is worth notice that the form of the activation function of B lymphocytes in Carneiro et al. (1996a, 1996b) reduces to the functional form in the classical

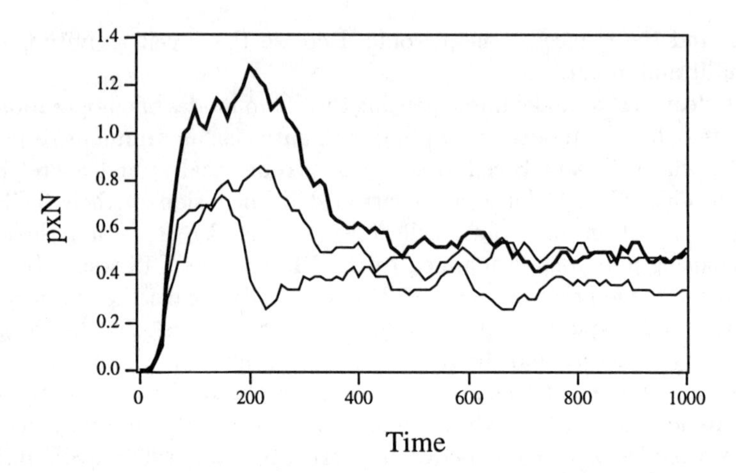


**Fig. 4.** The stable development of the immune network model always implies a shift from a phase in which the B-cell repertoire diversifies by recruitment of new clones to a phase in which the repertoire contracts and becomes restricted to a fraction of its potential. The time course of the product pxN during several simulation runs that develop stably are co-plotted, where p is the constant probability that an Ig recognizes another molecule and N is the number of B cell clones in the system. Their product is a measure of the "completeness" of the network repertoire. After Carneiro et al (1996b).

Hence, in both classes of models the idiotypic network reaches a state of repertoire "completeness". However, in standard SGIN this corresponds to the (metadynamic) steady state of the system, while in the model of Carneiro et al. this is a transient state, that is followed by a marked restriction of the network repertoire.

The metadynamic steady state — the state in which there is no net gain nor loss of network clones — is necessarily quite different in the two models. In SGIN, as the network repertoire diversifies a steady state is reached in which the average connectivity is minimal; the net recruitment of clones ceases because the new candidates, made available by the bone marrow, receive an average suppressive field. If the repertoire of the network is reduced by loss of clones, due to the internal activity of the network, than the new candidates can again "fit in" and compensate that loss (in fact in many simulations there is a continuous loss and recruitment of clones; in shape space this leads to a characteristic movement of chains).

In contrast, in the model of Carneiro et al., the steady state network is composed by those B cell clones that won the competition for cooperation with the available T cells; this steady state is stable because the network clones have maximal co-operation coefficients and therefore can compete out

Varela et al. (1988; Detours, 1994) in the limit when the number of activated T cells tends to infinity.

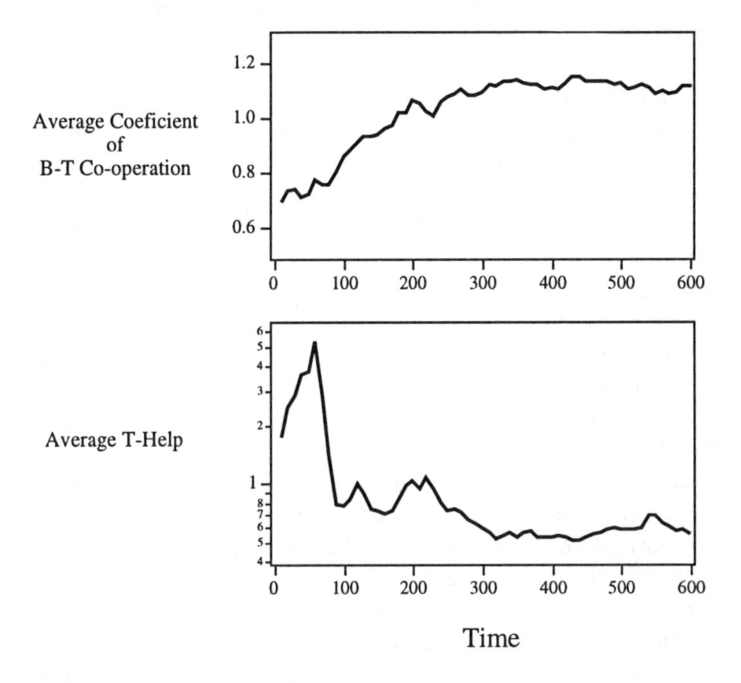


**Fig. 5.** Time courses of (top) the average coeficient of B-T cell interaction and (bottom) the average 'T-help' got per B-cell clone during a representative simulation run in which the model develops in a stable mode. Note the free availability of 'T-help' per B-cell clone in the early phase of development; a drop of the amount of 'help' available results in a progressive increase in the average interaction coeficient. After Carneiro et al (1996b).

any other candidates for T help. This steady state is not strongly affected by the characteristic of the clones produced by the bone marrow. Leon et al. (1998) make use of this metadynamic stability of the idiotypic network to explain how classical findings of induced tolerance could be achieved.

## 4 Concluding Remarks

In this article we have tried to analyse two classes of models of the immune network in terms of their capacity to substantiate the concept that the immune system is organized into a CIS and a PIS. We have pointed out that there are two distinct ways of interpreting the SGIN in terms of the CIS/PIS framework. The first way is based on what we call here a "structural definition"; on this view, the dynamically sustained network is interpreted as the CIS, while the clones that are disconnected are interpreted as the PIS. However, it is not easy to accommodate the functional properties of the CIS and the PIS in this account. There are several reasons for this: the proportions of the CIS and PIS are essentially inverted; and the operation of network fails to appropriately account for robust natural tolerance. The second interpretation is the one that results from mapping the functional definitions of the CIS and PIS into different sets of clones making a SGIN. The main difficulty in assuming this second view is that the corresponding structures are entangled in a way quite contrary to immunological intuition. Consequently, there is no clear, identifiable property that allows us to say whether a clone belongs to the CIS or the PIS, other than the response of that clone when stimulated by antigen.

We have discussed the possibility of overcoming these limitations of the SGIN by extending these models to include B-T cell co-operation (Carneiro et al., 1996a,b). We have argued that this extended version is able to accommodate both the structural and the functional properties of CIS and PIS in a coherent account, and moreover to explain how the CIS/PIS distinction can be generated by the self-organizing properties of the network. Since this new model represents a qualitative departure from all the previous SGIN models as a whole, we propose to call it a "third generation network model" (TGIN).

It is important to emphasise that although the TGIN model is able to account for the CIS and PIS distinction, whereas the SGIN models fail to do so, this does not allow us to make a rigorous judgement about their respective validities; they just represent two alternative hypotheses about the organization of immune system. In fact, Jerne's view of the idiotypic network was that of a complete network, that would perform multiple functions such as the selection of the pre-immune repertoire, tolerance and regulation of the immune responses, etc. (Jerne, 1974; Coutinho, personal comunication). Sophisticated SGIN models — illustrated by the work of Detours et al. (1994; 1996) — can be regarded as a mathematical implementation of Jerne's qualitative schema. In clear rupture with this more "classic" view, Coutinho's hypothesis represented an attempt to reconcile Jerne's network theory with the clonal selection theory, by postulating a dual organisation of the immune system into two compartments which are structurally and functionally distinct (for an extended discussion of the issue see: Carneiro, 1997). The TGIN model corresponds to a mathematically explicit formulation of this qualitative hypothesis.

We would like to conclude with a remark about the relationship between these models and empirical observations on natural antibodies. Perhaps the most striking difference between SGIN and TGIN models lies in their respective predictions about the size of the idiotypic network at the steady state. The SGIN models predict that the network should have a "complete repertoire", in the sense that practically every clone that is newly produced by the bone marrow should display measurable interactions with the circulating Igs. In contrast, the TGIN model predicts that the majority of the clones produced by the bone marrow or the thymus should exhibit no measurable interactions with the circulating Igs. It becomes an important question for empirical investigation as to whether the network (represented by the pool of circulating Igs) is "complete" or not. Empirical support for one or the other possibility is lacking in the literature, perhaps because the actual measurement of "completeness" of the antibody repertoire involves a whole set of conceptual and empirical pitfalls (Carneiro, 1997; Brissac et al., 1998). This difficulty in establishing a productive relationship between theory and experiment is a hallmark of the whole network approach to the immune system, and is perhaps the reason why, at the present time, the immunological community regards idiotypic networks with skepticism.

**Acknowledgements**

This paper would not have been possible without the stimulating discussions provided by Hugues Bersini, Chandrika Bhimarao, Caroline Brissac, Vera Calenbuhr, Antonio Coutinho, Vincent Detours, Kalet Leon, Olivier Martin, and Francisco Varela.

## References

1. Anderson, R.W., Neumann, A.U. and Perelson, A.S. (1993). A Cayley tree immune network model with antibody dynamics. Bull. Math. Biol. 55, 1091.
2. Bersini H. (1992). The Interplay between Dynamics and Metadynamics of the Immune Network. Artificial Life III Workshop, Santa Fe, 15-19 June 1992.
3. Calenbuhr, V. Bersini, H., Stewart, and J.Varela, F.J. (1994). Natural Tolerance in Simple Immune Network. J. Theor. Biol. 177, 199.
4. Carneiro, J., J.Faro, A.Coutinho, and J.Stewart. (1996a). A model of the immune network with B-T cell co-operation. I-Prototypical Structures and Dynamics. J. Theor. Biol. 182, 513.
5. Carneiro, J., A.Coutinho, and J.Stewart. (1996b). A model of the immune network with B-T cell co-operation. II-The simulation of ontogenesis. J. Theor. Biol. 182, 531.
6. Carneiro, J. (1997). Towards a comprehensive view of the immune system. PhD Thesis. University of Porto. Portugal.
7. Coutinho, A. (1974). Immune activation of B cells: an analysis of the triggering mechanisms. Stockholm: Akademisk Avhandling, Karolinska Institutet.
8. Coutinho, A. (1989). Beyond clonal selection and network. Immunol. Rev. 110, 63.
9. De Boer R.J. (1989). Clonal Selection versus Idiotypic Network Models of the Immune System: a Bioinformatic Approach. PhD thesis, University of Utrecht, The Netherlands.
10. De Boer R.J., Hogeweg P, and Perelson A.S. (1992). Growth and recruitment in the immune network. In Perelson A.S., Weisbuch G. & Coutinho A. (Eds), Theoretical and experimental insights into immunology. Springer, N.Y.
11. De Boer, R.J. and Hogeweg, P. (1989a). Memory but no suppression in low-dimensional symmetric idiotypic networks. Bull. Math. Biol. 51, 223.

12. De Boer, R.J. and Hogeweg, P. (1989b). Stability of symmetric idiotypic networks–a critique of Hoffmann's analysis. Bull. Math. Biol. 51, 217.
13. De Boer, R.J. and Hogeweg, P. (1989c). Unreasonable implications of reasonable idiotypic network assumptions. Bull. Math. Biol. 51, 381.
14. De Boer, R.J. and Perelson, A.S. (1991). Size and connectivity as emergent properties of a developing network. J.Theor. Biol. 149, 381.
15. De Boer, R.J., Segel, L.A. and Perelson, A.S. (1992). Pattern formation in one- and two-dimensional shape-space models of the immune system. J. Theor. Biol. 155, 295.
16. De Boer, R.J., Perelson, A.S. and Kevrekidis, I.G. (1993). Immune network behavior. I- From stationary states to limit cycle oscillations. Bull. Math. Biol. 55, 745.
17. De Boer, R.J., Perelson, A.S. and Kevrekidis, I.G. (1993b). Immune network behavior. II- From oscillations to chaos and stationary states. Bull. Math. Biol. 55, 781.
18. De Boer, R.J., and Perelson, A.S. (1993). How diverse should the immune system be? Proc.R.Soc.Lond.B. 252, 171.
19. De Monvel, J.H.B., and Martin, O.C. (1995). Memory capacity in large idiotypic networks. Bull. Math. Biol. 57, 109.
20. Detours, V. (1996). Modeles formels de la selection des cellules B et T. PhD Thesis, University Paris 6, France.
21. Detours, V., Bersini, H., Stewart, J. and Varela, F. (1994). Development of an idiotypic network in shape space. J. Theor. Biol. 170, 401.
22. Faro, J. and Velasco, S. (1993a). Crosslinking of membrane immunoglobulins and B-cell activation: a simple model based on percolation theory. Proc. R. Soc. Lond. B. 254, 139.
23. Faro, J. and Velasco, S. (1993b). Numerical analysis of a model of ligand-induced B-cell antigen-receptor clustering. Implications for simple models of B-cell activation in an immune network. J. Theor. Biol. 167, 45.
24. Faro, J. and Velasco, S. (1993c). Studies on a recent class of network models of the immune system. J. Theor. Biol. 164, 271.
25. Grossman, Z. and Cohen, I.R. (1980). A theoretical analysis of the phenotypic expression of immune response genes. Eur. J. Immunol. 10, 633.
26. Hoffman, G.W. (1975). A theory of regulation and self-nonself discrimination in an immune network. Eur. J. Immunol. 5, 638.
27. Hoffman, G.W. (1980). On network theory and H-2 restriction. Contemp. Top. Immunobiol. 11, 185.
28. Huetz, F., Jacquemart, F., Pena-Rossi, C., Varela, F. and Coutinho, A. (1988). Autoimmunity: The moving boundaries between physiology and pathology. J. Autoimmunity. 1, 507.
29. Jerne, N.K. (1974). Towards a network theory of the immune system. Ann. Immunol. (Inst. Pasteur). 125C, 373.
30. Kearney, J.F., Vakil, M. and Nicholson, N. (1987). Non-random VH gene expression and idiotype-anti-idiotype expression on early B cells. In: Evolution and Vertebrate Immunity: teh antigen receptor and MHC gene families. (Kelsoe & Schulze, eds.) pp. 174. Austin: Texas University Press.
31. Leon, K., Carneiro, J., Perez, R., Montero, E. and Lage, A. (1998). Natural and Induced Tolerance in an Immune Network Model. J.Theor.Biol. Submitted.
32. Nemazee, D. (1996). Antigen receptor capacity and the sensitivity of self-tolerance. Immunol. Today. 17, 25.

33. Neumann A.U. (1992). Dynamical Transitions and Percolation in Network Models of the Immune Response. PhD thesis, Bar-Ilan University, Israel.
34. Neumann, A.U., and Weisbuch, G. (1992a). Dynamics and topology of idiotypic networks. Bull. Math. Biol. 54, 699.
35. Neumann, A.U., and Weisbuch, G. (1992b). Window automata analysis of population dynamics in the immune system. Bull. Math. Biol. 54, 21.
36. Perelson, A.S. (1984). Some mathematical models of receptor clustering by multivalent ligands. In: Cell Surface Dynamics: Concepts and Models. (Perelson et al., eds.) pp. 377. New York: Marcel Dekker.
37. Percus, J.K., Percus, O.E., and Perelson, A.S. (1993). Predicting the size of the T-cell receptor and antibody combining region from consideration of efficient self-nonself discrimination. Proc. Natl. Acad. Sci. USA. 90, 1691.
38. Perelson, A.S. and DeLisi, C. (1980). Receptor clustering on a cell surface. I. Theory of receptor cross-linking by lignads bearing tow chemical dienticla functional groups. Math. Biosci. 64, 169.
39. Perelson, A.S., and Oster, G.F. (1979). Theoretical studies of clonal selection: minimal antibody repertoire and reliability of self-non-self discrimination. J.theor.Biol. 81, 645.
40. Stewart, J., and Varela, F.J. (1989). Exploring the meaning of connectivity in the immune network. Immunol. Rev. 110, 37.
41. Stewart, J., and Varela, F.J. (1991). Morphogenesis in shape-space. Elementary meta-dynamics in a model of the immune network. J. Theor.Biol. 153, 477.
42. Stewart, J., Varela, F.J., and Coutinho, A. (1989). The relationship between connectivity and tolerance as revealed by computer stimulation of the immune network: some lessons for an understanding of autoimmunity. Journal of Autoimmunity. 2, 15.
43. Sulzer, B., Van Hemmen, J.L., Neumann, A.U., and Behn, U. (1993). Memory in idiotypic networks due to competition between proliferation and differentiation. Bull. Math. Biol. 55, 1133.
44. Sulzer, B., Van Hemmen, J.L., and Behn, U. (1994). Central immune system, the self and autoimmunity. Bull. Math. Biol. 56, 1009.
45. Takumi, K., and De Boer, R.J. (1996). Self assertion modeled as a network repertoire of multi-determinant antibodies. J. Theor. Biol. In press
46. Varela, F.J., and Coutinho, A. (1991). Second generation immune networks. Immunol. Today. 12, 159.
47. Varela, F.J., Coutinho, A., Dupire, B., and Vaz, N. (1988). Cognitive networks: immune, neural and otherwise. In Theoretical Immunology. (Perelson, ed.) 3. pp. 359. Redwood City: Addison-Wesley.
48. Weisbuch, G., De Boer, R.J., and Perelson, A.S. (1990). Localized memories in idiotypic networks. J. Theor. Biol. 146, 483.
49. Weisbuch, G., Dos Santos, R.M., and Neumann, A.U. (1993). Tolerance to hormones and receptors in an idiotypic network model. J. Theor. Biol. 163, 237.
50. Weisbuch, G., and Oprea, M. (1994). Capacity of a model immune network. Bull. Math. Biol. 56, 899.

**Dr. John Stewart** did his PhD in Genetics from Cambridge University, 1966. His fields of research include physiological genetics, sociology of knowledge, epistemology of cognitive science, and theoretical immunology. He is currently working as a Research scientist at CNRS, France. He is the Director of a research team "Connaissance, Organisation, Systemes Techniques", Department of Technology and Human Science, Université de Technologie de Compiégne, France.

# Immunology Viewed as the Study of an Autonomous Decentralized System

Lee A. Segel and Ruth Lev Bar-Or

Department of Applied Mathematics and Computer Science
The Weizmann Institute of Science
Rehovot 76100, Israel

**Abstract.** Arguments are given for the tenet that although the immune system has no long term goals, it does have short term goals — which are often contradictory. Simple models illustrate how feedbacks can (i) harmonize conflicting goals, (ii) improve the performance of a given type of effector cell, (iii) cause the preferential amplification of more potent effectors. It is shown that spatial organization can allow non-specific chemical signals to select specific immune elements that contribute to system goals. Comparison is made with other autonomous decentralized systems.

## 1 Introduction

One of the most fruitful appositions in modern science is between natural and artificial life. Animal and computer vision, motor control and robotics — these are two examples of rapidly developing research spectra ranging from biology to applied mathematics and computer science. This article concerns aspects of a new example, natural and artificial immunology.

Some of the salient biology is reviewed, so that it can be seen how suitable the immune system is as a prototype of "bottom up" artificial intelligence. We stress that the immune system is entirely distributed (to first approximation). Its agents, the cells, are highly complex. Much is known about these cells and their interaction with each other and with pathogens, and the system is of high biological and medical interest.

Major questions to be addressed include the following. (i) What are the "goals" of the immune system, and how might feedback promote these goals? (ii) How can spatial organization allow non-specific chemical signals to select specific immune elements that contribute effectively to system goals? (iii) Can one make fruitful comparisons between the immune system and other autonomous decentralized systems?

## 2 A Nano-course in Immunology

To begin, we shall sketch a few aspects of adaptive immune systems (as found in vertebrates, but not lower creatures). A number of concepts and technical terms will be introduced, which is unavoidable if we are to know what we are talking about. There is no necessity to master the details however: for present purposes a general impression suffices. (Useful general references are texts such as that of Janeway and Travers [13], and a recent presentation of "Immunology for physicists" [24]).

Broadly speaking the principal function of the immune system is to limit damage to the host organism by *pathogens* (harmful bacteria, viruses, fungi, protozoa and worms). Such organisms, as well as large individual molecules, generate an immune response, and are thus called *antigens*. One type of response is the secretion of *antibody* molecules by so-called *B cells*. Secretion requires that the B cells become activated from their immature forms, undergo proliferation, and then finally *differentiate* (transform themselves) into antibody secreting *plasma cells*.

*Opsonization* (from the Greek for "buttering") is one way that antibodies lead to the destruction of bacteria. The antibodies *bind* (stick chemically) to the bacteria, providing that there is a complementary match between the shape of certain molecules on the bacteria and the shape of the "business end" (*variable region*) of a suitable type of antibody molecule. There are about 10 million antibody shapes (*specificities*). Initially only a few copies of each shape are present. The presence of an antigen encourages proliferation of those particular B cells that provide a good antibody-antigen match. The basic unit of an antibody molecule is Y-shaped, with identical variable regions at the top of the Y. At the bottom of the Y is the *constant region*. This comes in several forms, which are associated with different antibody *isotypes* (called IgG1, IgG2, IgM, IgA, etc). If many antibodies bind to a bacterium, then it looks like a porcupine with myriad tiny quills displaying their constant regions. IgG1 constant regions, are particularly "delicious" for *phagocytosing* "digesting cells" such as *macrophages*. These cells ingest bacteria that are opsonized by IgG1 antibody; many bacterial species can then be dismantled by various internal chemical means.

Some bacteria thrive in the interior of macrophages. An important way that such intracellular pathogens can be destroyed is via *cytotoxic* (cell killing) versions of another line of cells called *T cells*. (B and T refer to bone marrow and thymus, from which these cells emerge). Other kinds of T cells are called *helpers*. Suitable chemical signals from T helpers, typically diffusible hormone-like *cytokines* or *interleukins*, have profound effects on other cells of the immune system. For example cytokines influence the transition of B cells from dormant to proliferating to secreting, and they influence the isotype of the secreted antibody.

How do cytotoxic T cells know that they should kill a macrophage harboring an intracellular bacteria, or an epithelial cell (say) into which viruses have penetrated? This is done via complex intracellular machinery that displays on the surface of the cell under attack digested small pieces of bacterial or viral protein (*peptides*) embedded in special so-called *MHC molecules*.

T cells bear *receptor* molecules that "recognize" an MHC-protein combination that matches the special shape (*specificity*) of the receptor. Suitable recognition triggers an intracellular molecular cascade that leads to killing by the cytotoxic T cells (and under other circumstances to signalling by the T helpers). Note that in the process of combating pathogens the cytotoxic T cells damage the host. There are several other examples of pathogen killing that is accompanied by a degree of host damage. *Autoimmune disease* occurs when self-destruction by the immune system gets out of hand (whether or not the trigger is pathogen killing).

## 3 Overall Characterization of the Immune System

From our nano-survey and a few additional facts we can already draw important conclusions.

a) The cells of the immune system are highly complex living machines.
b) The immune system is completely distributed (Although there are connections with neuronal systems, these can be ignored to first approximation).
c) The elements of the immune system include various effector "combat troops" (such as macrophages, antibodies of various specificities and isotypes, and cytotoxic T cells) as well as a "signal corps" (exemplified by helper T cells and their cytokines).
d) Different tactical mixes are effective for different pathogens. Figure 9.33 of the Janeway-Travers text [13], for example, gives about 20 different mixes of four isotypes and two types of cell-mediated immunity that are used for combating 30 types of common pathogens.
e) To frustrate immune recognition, pathogens can alter their outermost "coat" — sometimes even during the course of a single attack. Pathogens can also employ various devices to sabotage immune signalling.
f) In the face of myriad possible "enemies", each with its own special "life style" and evasive tactics, the immune system must automatically choose which of the various fighting arms to deploy against a given pathogen, and must select the intensity of the response as a function of time.
g) Choosing the wrong mix of effectors wastes resources, may divert attention from more threatening attackers, and may blunt the weapon of choice (e.g. when too many antibodies block the relevant MHC-peptide combination and thereby diminish a necessary attack by cytotoxic T cells).

## 4 Postulating a Role for Feedback

Over millenia, evolution has forged an immune system that does a reasonably good job in combatting pathogens. The joint co-evolutionary development of the immune system and of the pathogens themselves inevitably mandates a certain lack of immune efficiency, since there is a compromise between the "desires" of the pathogens and those of the immune system. Evolution is constrained by cost and previous history. At least superficially, the size of the pharmaceutical industry is witness to imperfections in our immune responses.

Has evolutionary tinkering pieced together an immune system that tends toward optimal attainment of an overall goal? Experts on evolution would give a negative answer. They (and we) believe that the history of life on earth is equivalent to an enormous dynamical system that evolves according to physico-biochemical rules. There is no good reason to think that anything is optimized [16], [22].

Although there may not be an overall goal toward which the immune system "strives", still it may well be profitable for scientists to make the hypothesis that there is such a goal. Classic works on evolutionary theory demonstrate that it is productive to assume that under suitably restricted circumstances evolution assures that "fitness" is somehow maximized. (Fitness can be defined as long term reproductive success). Such an assumption is in fact a model of reality. As is characteristic of models the assumption of fitness maximization is incomplete and simplified, yet such an assumption can bring a measure of understanding to the complexities of evolution.

Assume then that the immune system has evolved to achieve the *evolutionary goal* of enhancing the long term reproductive success of the vertebrates in which it resides. *As such this evolutionary goal is too general and diffuse to be of any use in influencing the hour by hour operation of the immune system.* To achieve such an influence vertebrates must be constituted so that they interpret the evolutionary goal at a lower level. We hypothesize that such an interpretation can be approximated by the assumption that the immune system has the *physiological goal* of minimizing the net damage from pathogens together with the damage rendered by the immune system itself during the course of its attacks on pathogens. We shall describe here how this physiological goal might be expressed at the molecular and cellular level.

A key element of this expression is feedback. This feedback is not of the conventional type, wherein system control is based on the difference between a reference signal from a desired state and a feedback signal from the actual state. Rather there are known "good" and "bad" tendencies by means of which the immune system can learn during the course of a single disease how to make incremental improvements in its struggle with the pathogens that are causing the disease.

Analogous situations are ubiquitous in biochemistry where a variety of chemicals exert activating or inhibiting influences on a single enzyme. The precise purpose of these feedbacks is hard to discern, but one can say that the presence of a number of such multi-regulatable enzymes permit the organism to modulate "appropriately" the concentrations of a variety of important chemicals.

The immune system faces two challenges that feedback can help meet: (i) optimize individual effector performance; (ii) optimize effector choice. We will employ simple mathematical models to illustrate the problems involved in achieving these goals. Our purpose in this modeling is to illuminate strategic considerations. Such a broad focus is appropriate here because the present paper is just a first step in discussing the various issues, and because an overall view of natural immune systems, not a detailed one, is most likely to prove useful in constructing efficient artificial immune systems.

## 5 Optimizing Effector Performance

To illustrate some of the considerations involved in optimizing the performance of a given cell type, we will first consider efforts by a single clone of effector cells to control a single pathogen strain. The central aspect of our analysis will be an exploration of situations wherein the effector damages the host in the process of destroying pathogens. Pathogens also damage the host. The question thus arises, how should a balance be struck, given that strongly destructive effectors cause serious damage to the host, but weakly destructive effectors combat pathogens inefficiently and hence permit extensive host damage by pathogens.

To model damage, we assume that at rate $s$ the effector cells $E$ produce a noxious chemical $N$ (such as the cytotoxic chemical nitric oxide that is secreted by macrophages). If $N$ has a decay rate $g_N$ then

$$\frac{dN}{dt} = sE - g_N N \ . \tag{1a}$$

Pathogens $P$ are assumed to reproduce exponentially at rate $r$, and are killed by effectors $E$ at a rate that increases linearly with $EP$ (the probability of pathogen-effector encounter). What matters in pathogen killing is the local concentration of $N$ delivered by the effector to the pathogen. In our space-independent model, we will assume that the magnitude of this concentration is reflected in the average concentration of $N$. Thus the pathogen killing term is assumed to be jointly proportional to $E$, $P$ and $N$:

$$\frac{dP}{dt} = rP - aEPN \ . \tag{1b}$$

Effector proliferation is induced by pathogens, and effectors have a death rate $g_E$:

$$\frac{dE}{dt} = E(\mu_P P - g_E) \ . \tag{1c}$$

As a measure of performance in this context, we employ the average damage rate $\delta$:

$$\delta = \frac{1}{T}\int_0^T (h_P P + h_N N)dt \ . \tag{2}$$

According to this definition, the pathogens $P$ and the noxious chemical $N$ respectively cause damage at rates $h_P$ and $h_N$.

Equations (1a–c) and definition (2) comprise our first model, which we shall term Model A. For many sets of parameters we find that the solutions to Eqs. (1a–c) have the following behavior. The pathogen population grows for a while, and then decays when the pathogens have stimulated enough effectors. When the pathogen population reaches a low level, however, the consequent effector stimulation is far outweighed by effector death and thus the effector population drops. But this leads to a resurgence of pathogen growth and the whole process begins again. Thus solutions continually oscillate.

We neglect all bursts of pathogen growth except the first. Thus integration is terminated at time $T$, where $T$ is the period of the oscillation. [To be precise, $T$ was selected to be the time when $h_P P + h_N N$ was minimal. The same $T$ is used in (2)]. The reason is that in most instances the observed oscillations have no immunological significance. The resurgence of pathogen growth occurs from pathogen population levels that are so low that the differential equation model is no longer valid. At very low average pathogen levels $P$, most hosts contain no pathogens, and in those that do random events not considered in the basic model would usually wipe out the last vestige of infection. See Ref [9] for an earlier treatment of this epiphenomenon.

Figure 1A shows results obtained from a numerical solution to the differential Eqs. (1) of Model A. The damage rate $\delta$ is plotted as a function of the secretion rate $s$. As one would expect, there is an optimum secretion rate at which the appropriate balance between effector and pathogen destruction is achieved so as to minimize the damage measure $\delta$. The graphs in Figs. 1B and 1C demonstrate that the optimum depends on the initial pathogen population. At higher pathogen populations, more effector damage to the host should be accepted, in order to be able to enhance the killing of the more threatening pathogens.

Our simple calculation thus illustrates an obvious general point, once one thinks of it, that the way to obtain optimum performance is not absolute but varies with different conditions that the organism might be subject to. How can the immune system choose an appropriate balance between the levels of effector damage to the host and effector efficiency in pathogen killing, given that these levels vary with various factors such as the number and virulence of the pathogens? The answer is that the host must acquire and utilize devices that monitor the levels of decisive variables. In the present instance, therefore, we introduce a "kill indication" chemical $K$ that represents the level of pathogen destruction and a "damage" or "harm" chemical $H$ that expresses the level of harm to the host. Chemical $K$ is produced at a rate proportional to the rate of pathogen killing [compare Eq. (1a)] and has a decay rate $g_K$:

$$\frac{dK}{dt} = c_K(aEPN) - g_K K \; . \tag{3a}$$

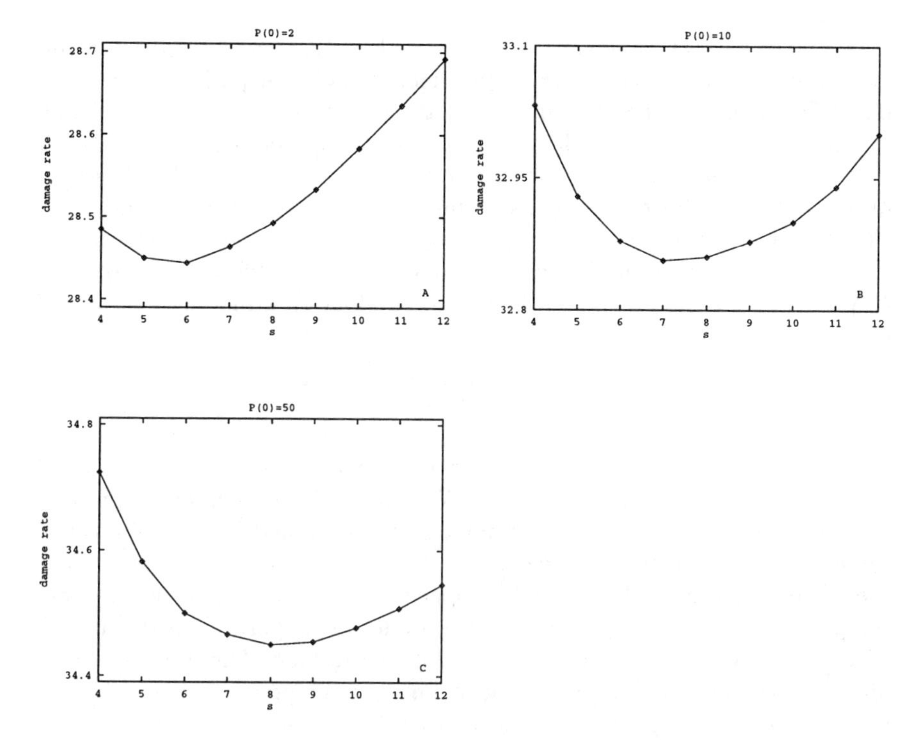


**Fig. 1.** Model A: Damage rate $\delta$ [see Eq. (2)] for three different initial pathogen levels, $P(0) = 2$ (A), $P(0) = 10$ (B), $P(0) = 50$ (C). Numerical solutions of (1). Parameters: $g_N = 30$, $r = 5$, $a = 0.02$, $\mu_P = 0.1$, $g_E = 3$, $h_P = 1$, $h_N = 1$, $E(0) = 1$, $N(0) = 0$.

Similarly, the harm chemical H is produced at a rate proportional to the rate at which damage to the host is done by both pathogens and effectors [compare (2)]. There is a decay rate $g_H$:

$$\frac{dH}{dt} = c_H(h_P P + h_N N) - g_H H \ . \tag{3b}$$

How can we estimate the amount $H_P$ of the damage that flows from pathogen action? A simple possibility is

$$H_P(H, N) = \frac{H}{1 + k_P N} \ . \tag{3c}$$

Definition (3c) has the favorable properties that $H_P$ tends to zero when $N$ is sufficiently large (so that all the damage is due to the effectors) while $H_P \approx H$ when $N$ is sufficiently small (all the damage must be due to the pathogens in the absence of effector-produced poison). Note that (3c) is easy to implement biochemically; it is the classical expression for the action of an inhibitor ($N$) on an agonist ($H$).

We now have at our disposal three variables that convey important information concerning the state of the struggle between pathogens and the immune system: the harm (damage) to the host from the pathogens ($H_P$), the harm to the host from the immune system (represented by $N$) and the rate of pathogen killing ($K$). We exemplify means that could be chosen to implement this information by assuming that the three chemicals alter the effector proliferation rate. (More precisely, $E$ represents effector efficacy, so that the chemicals are in fact hypothesized to alter proliferation and/or activation). Our hypothesis is enshrined in the following modified version of (1c):

$$\frac{dE}{dt} = E\left[\mu_P P\left(m_1 + \frac{q_{KH}KH_P}{1+m_2N+q_{KH}KH_P}\right) - g_E\right] . \tag{3d}$$

All other things being equal, effector damage, as represented by $N$, should down-regulate immune response. Thus $N$ inhibits effector activation/proliferation in (3d). By contrast, the immune response should be upregulated by evidence that damaging pathogens are being killed, i.e. by evidence that there is both pathogen killing and pathogen harm. The "and" translates into the product of $K$ and $H_P$ in (3d). This product is hypothesized to enhance effector activation/proliferation in a saturating fashion. The present model, Model B, is completed by adjoining to Eqs. (3) the previous Eqs. (1b) and (1a) for the pathogen $P$ and the noxious chemical $N$.

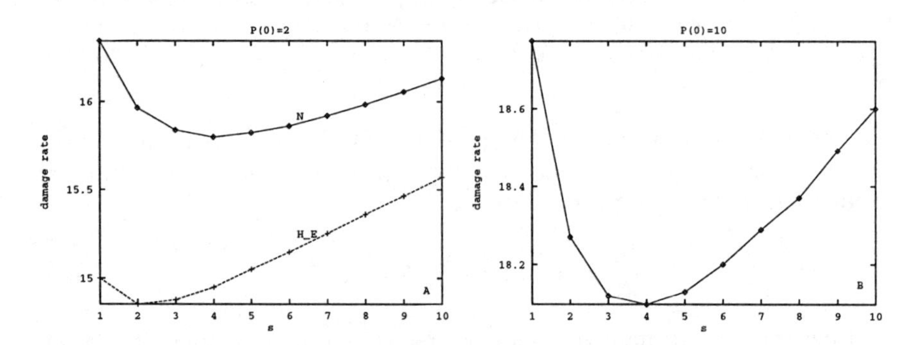


**Fig. 2.** Model B: Damage rate for two different initial pathogen levels, $P(0) = 2$ (A), $P(0) = 10$ (B). Numerical solutions of (1a–b) and (3). Parameters: $c_K = 5$, $g_K = 1$, $c_H = 1$, $g_H = 1$, $k_P = 1$, $\mu_P = 0.1$, $q_{KH} = 1$. Other parameters as in Fig. 1.

Figure 2 is the counterpart of Fig. 1 for Model B. We see that the optimal secretion rate is lowered significantly. Even for secretion rates that are not particularly close to optimal the damage rate $\delta$ has been cut almost in half. Figure 3 shows the reason. With the information that is provided in Model B the optimal system secretes $N$ more slowly than in the optimal "no information" system of Model A (Compare Fig. 1 and Fig. 2). Despite the lower secretion rate the total amount of $N$ is about the same in both cases (Fig. 3C) since the effector population is larger in Model B (Fig. 3B). Similar levels of $N$ mean similar host damage by the effector. But the significantly larger effector levels yield more rapid pathogen elimination (Fig. 3A) and hence markedly diminished pathogen damage to the host.

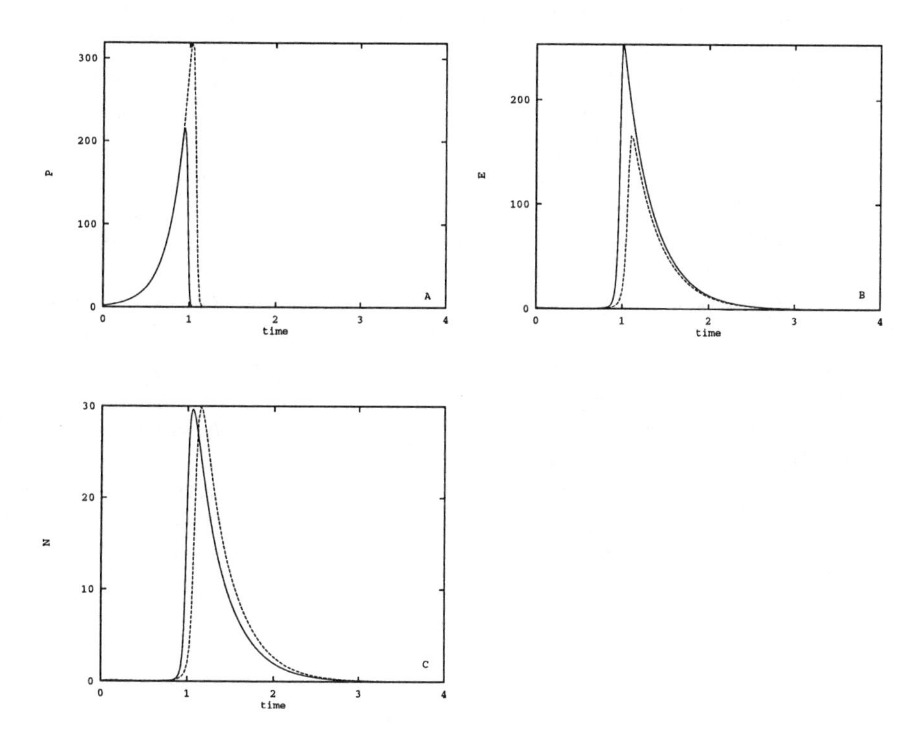


**Fig. 3.** Time course A – of pathogens ($P$); B – of effectors ($E$); and C – noxious chemical ($N$). Simulations of model A (solid line) and model B (dashed line). $P(0) = 2$. Other parameters in as Figs. 1 and 2.

In the preceding calculations we have used the chemical concentration $N$ as a measure of effector damage to the host. It would be more consistent, however, to estimate this damage by $H_E$, the complement of the pathogen damage estimate $H_P$:

$$H_E \equiv H - H_P = \frac{k_P N}{1 + k_P N} H \; . \tag{4}$$

Results obtained upon replacing $N$ by $H_E$ in Eq. (3d) are shown in Fig. 2A. We see that there is remarkably little change. This provides evidence that as far as selecting effective strategies is concerned there may be a variety of roughly equivalent ways that the immune system can translate concepts into the chemical discourse that is used for intracellular communication. (In this case, the concept in question is "all other things being equal, immune system damage to the host should decrease the immune response").

## 6 Optimizing Effector Choice

We now take for granted the "abilities" of each effector type, and turn to the question of how the immune system might select the more effective types.

Something starts the immune response, perhaps a rapidly increasing pathogen concentration [12] or perhaps "danger" [20]. The initial triggering mechanisms will not concern us here. We assume that a variety of different effectors is triggered and that the potency of the various effectors is somehow tested. Our purpose is to illustrate some of the issues involved in selecting the more potent effectors. For this purpose it will be sufficient to hypothesize that pathogen killing is an adequate measure of effector competence. We thus assume that the initially diffuse response becomes focussed because the number and activity of a given type of effector cell is increased to the degree that such a cell type is successful in killing pathogens. To see how this suggestion might be implemented by the immune system we will formulate a simple mathematical model of an interaction involving a pathogen $P$ and "competing" types of effector cells.

In the present discussion the variables $E$ and $F$ represent the efficacy of two different effector types. It will be seen that spatial effects are important. Thus, in the model there are two spatial compartments, represented by subscript $i$; $i = 1, 2$. Cells and chemicals diffuse between compartments. For each corresponding variable there is thus a diffusion coefficient $d$, with an appropriate subscript.

Pathogens $P$ reproduce exponentially at rate $r$, are killed by effectors $E$ and $F$ in their compartment with different efficiencies $a$ and $b$, and diffuse:

$$\frac{dP_i}{dt} = rP_i - (aE_i + bF_i)P_i + d_P(P_j - P_i) . \tag{5}$$

Here and below, there is one equation for each compartment $i$; $i = 1, 2$. The subscript $j = 1, 2$ is different from $i$; when $i = 1$, $j = 2$ and when $i = 2$, $j = 1$.

Generalizing Eq. (3a), we consider a "kill-indication" chemical $K$, which indicates how many pathogens have been killed. $K$ is produced at a rate proportional to the killing rate. In addition, $K$ decays, and diffuses. Thus

$$\frac{dK_i}{dt} = c_K(aE_i + bF_i)P_i - g_K K_i + d_K(K_j - K_i) . \tag{6}$$

For effectors $E$ and $F$, we write equations with terms for proliferation/activation, for death or another type of decay or removal (parameterized by $g$), and for intercompartmental diffusion. We adopt a saturating form to express our assumption that the proliferation/activation rate is an increasing function of the pathogen killing measure $K$. This gives

$$\frac{dE_i}{dt} = E_i \left[ \frac{qK_i}{n + K_i} - g_E \right] + d_E(E_j - E_i) , \tag{7a}$$

$$\frac{dF_i}{dt} = F_i \left[ \frac{qK_i}{n + K_i} - g_F \right] + d_F(F_j - F_i) , \tag{7b}$$

where $n$ is the half-saturation coefficient. Equations (5)–(7) constitute Model C.

The key activation/proliferation terms (proportional to $q$) are identical in (7a) and (7b). The reason is that these terms represent the action of signalling chemicals and helper cells concerning which there is no reason to assume preferential treatment of a particular effector type.

How can an effector-blind signal "reward" effectors that are superior pathogen killers? Here is where the geometry comes in. Suppose that initially effectors $E$ are concentrated near some point $P_1$ and abundant effectors $F$ occur only near $P_2$. (In our simple model, $E$ would be abundant in compartment 1 and $F$ in compartment 2). Suppose that $E$ cells but not $F$ cells are efficient pathogen killers. Then the "pathogen kill indicator" $K$ will be preferentially produced near $P_1$, and the effectors $E$ will proliferate faster than their rivals $F$. This behavior is illustrated in Fig. 4. Initially we place one unit of $E$ in compartment 1 and one unit of $F$ in compartment 2. These initial concentrations are very small compared to what $E$ and $F$ become later. Yet this initial small difference is responsible for the large later differences in $K_1$ and $K_2$, which in turn drive the sizably greater production of the more competent effector $E$ compared to the less competent effector $F$. ($E$ kills pathogens ten times faster than $F$). The preferential amplification of $E_1$ results from the positive feedback

$$\text{more killing of } P \text{ by } E \rightarrow \text{more } K \rightarrow \text{more } E .$$

In examining Model C we shall restrict ourselves to the matter of how to select the parameters connected to the informational chemical $K$ in order to obtain a better response. As a measure of response merit we shall first take the difference, $M$, in integrated output, from both compartments, between the more competent effector $E$ and the less competent effector $F$. Assuming that output is proportional to concentration we thus posit the following definition:

$$M = \int_0^T (E_1 + E_2 - F_1 - F_2) dt . \tag{8}$$

$T$ was chosen as the time at which $E(t)$ attains a preselected small value.

Here are the results concerning the behavior of M that we found from our simulations, together with explanations.

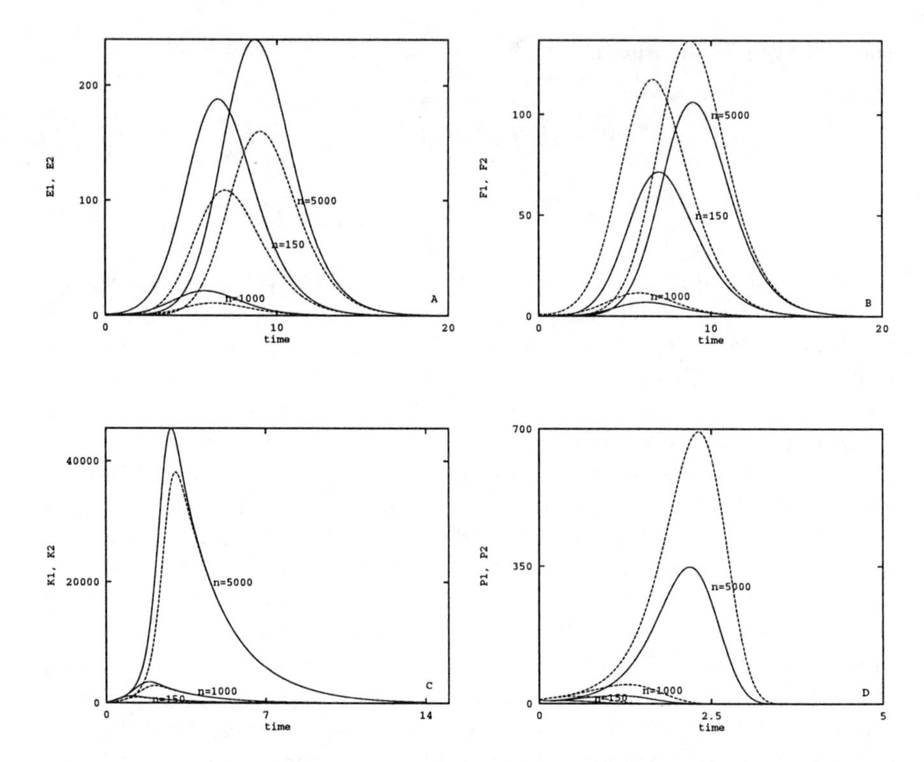


**Fig. 4.** Model C. A – effectors of greater potency ($E$); B – effectors of less potency ($F$); C – indicator chemical ($K$); D – pathogen level ($P$). Different values of the half saturation coefficient $n$ are examined. Solid line: Compartment 1. Dashed line: Compartment 2. Numerical solutions of Eqs. (5)–(7). Parameters: $r = 5$, $a = 8$, $b = 0.8$, $d_P = 5$, $c_K = 20$, $g_K = 0.5$, $d_K = 1$, $q = 2.5$, $g_E = g_F = 0.8$, $d_E = d_F = 0.1$. At $t = 0$: $P_1 = P_2 = 10$, $E_1 = F_2 = 1$, $E_2 = F_1 = K_1 = K_2 = 0$.

a) For the "kill indicator" diffusivity $d_K$ between 0.01 and 100, $M$ decreases as $d_K$ increases. (Stronger mixing between compartments blurs the difference between them).
b) For the $K$ half-life $1/g_K$ between 0.002 and 4, $M$ increases and then decreases as the half-life increases. (If $K$ has a very short half-life then its influence is negligible. But with too long a half life $K$ reflects the whole past history of effector action, and it has ample time to lose significance by diffusing to the other compartment).
c) As the $K$ production parameter $c_K$ increases from 0.1 to 20, there is a maximum in $M$ at about $c_K = 1$. (Too slow $K$ production means that $K$ will have no influence. Too fast $K$ production saturates the effector proliferation rate in both compartments, so that there is negligible difference in the proliferation rates of $E$ and $F$).

d) In contrast to the optimal value of $c_K$, the merit measure $M$ is minimized at an intermediate value of $n$. See Fig. 5. The explanation of this observation is somewhat lengthy, and thus is relegated to Appendix 1.

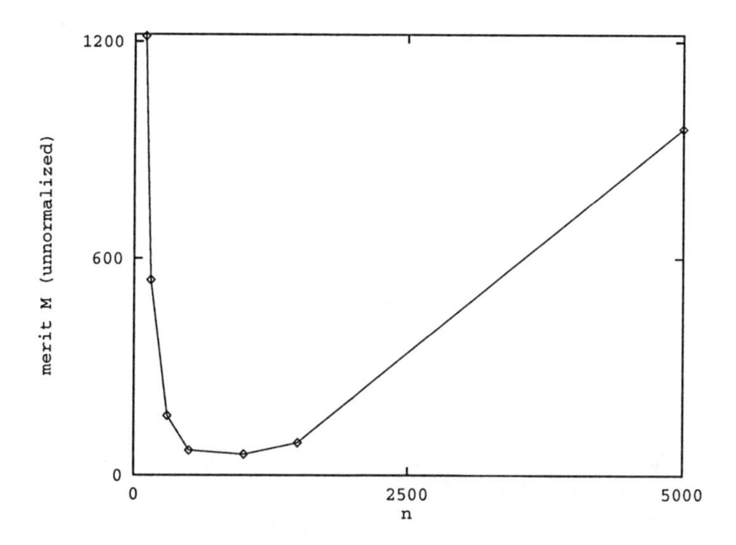


**Fig. 5.** Model C: The merit index $M$ of (8) as a function of the half-saturation constant $n$ in (7). Equations and parameters as in Fig. 4.

It is noteworthy that the dependence of the merit on $n$ is completely reversed if a somewhat different definition of merit is adopted, a normalized merit $\overline{M}$ wherein the difference in integrated effector levels is divided by their sum:

$$\overline{M} = \frac{\int_0^T (E_1 + E_2 - F_1 - F_2)dt}{\int_0^T (E_1 + E_2 + F_1 + F_2)dt} . \tag{9}$$

In contrast with the interior minimum found in Fig. 5, Fig. 6 shows that the normalized figure of merit $\overline{M}$ has an interior maximum. This behavior is a consequence of the low effector levels at intermediate values of $n$ (see Fig. 4). Which "figure of merit" better reflects the biological situation, $M$ or $\overline{M}$? $M$ monitors the absolute difference in outputs of more and less competent effectors, while the difference is normalized in $\overline{M}$. It is likely that the "competence per cell" measure $\overline{M}$ is more appropriate in situations where the cost of generating cells is important. By contrast one can envision life-threatening scenarios where a pathogen invasion must be suppressed regardless of expense; here $M$ might be the more appropriate measure.

The initial process of reinforcing the more potent $E$ cells becomes less efficient as time goes on, owing to the diffusive spreading of the informational

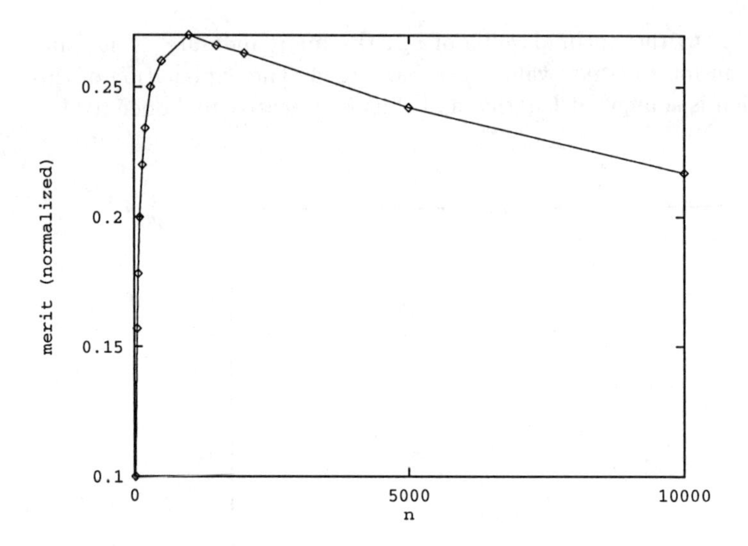


**Fig. 6.** Like Fig. 5, except that the index of merit $\overline{M}$ of (9) is employed.

chemicals and to the diffusive mixing of the $E$ and $F$ cells. The system would be more robust and reliable if the selection process were sharper. As is well known from the theory of pattern formation [21], a major path to sharp selection is via a combination of short range activation and long range inhibition.

Model C for optimizing effector choice contains activation, via the enhancement by $K$ of activation/proliferation in Eqs. (7). Here is one biologically reasonable way that the success of the $E$ cells can inhibit the $F$ cells. Suppose that the reinforcing signal to the $E$ cells is stimulated by $K$, as before, but that the signal is actually delivered by a cell type $A$. Suppose that $A$ cells are positively *chemotactic* toward $K$, i.e. that $A$ cells move preferentially toward relatively high concentrations of $K$. Then the initial build-up of $K$ will not only lead to the preferential reinforcement of $E_1$ cells in compartment 1 but also to the movement of $A$ cells from compartment 2 to compartment 1. The additional $A$ cells in compartment 1 will further reinforce the $E_1$ cells, bringing about further pathogen killing and hence production of more $K_1$. By contrast, the depletion of $A$ cells in compartment 2 will lead to decreased $K_2$. There will ensue yet more preferential movement of $A$ cells from compartment 2 to compartment 1. There are opposing components of random movement, but nonetheless the chemotaxis is expected to provide strong reinforcement to the more potent $E$ cells *and* strong inhibition of the less potent $F$ cells.

To model the scenario just sketched, we postulated an equation for the $A$ cells that contains a discrete version of standard terms for random motion and chemotaxis [14]. The overall number of $A$ cells was regarded as fixed. The necessity of $A$ cells for enhancing proliferation was modelled simply by introducing a factor $A_i$ after $c_K$ in (6). We found that the effects of chemotaxis indeed dramatically magnified the elevation of the $E$ cells and the suppression of the $F$ cells (not shown).

In unpublished work we have collected evidence that macrophages play the role assigned to $A$ cells, and indeed that a number of other conjectures made here have considerable biological plausibility. For example a chemical $K$ that can give evidence of bacterial killing might either be bacterial heat shock protein or certain palindromic immunostimulatory DNA sequences [26]. Another possibility is N-formyl methionine peptides that are characteristic of bacteria and are strong inducers of leukocyte chemotaxis [28].

## 7 The Importance of Geography

If functionally different antibody and T cell receptor shapes are taken into account, then the number of different kinds of effectors in the immune system is astronomical. It does not seem remotely feasible that there are a comparable number of different "signal corps" cytokines that could coordinate all these effectors. How then might one or several among myriad effectors be selected in suitable circumstances, given that there are only relatively few different possible chemical signals to monitor and guide effector actions?

It has been argued in Section 6 that selection can occur if there is spatial separation of groups of identical cells (e.g. $E$ initially predominates in compartment 1, $F$ in compartment 2). The positive feedback owing to overall success of a member of one of these groups, or negative feedback to failures, will be supplied preferentially to group members and at a much lower level to others.

At first sight, the required spatial organization might seem difficult to attain. One reason is that pathogens are often concentrated in tissues that are normally not heavily frequented by leukocytes. In addition, blood pathogens thrive in a turbulent medium where no precise cellular organization is possible. However much immune activity takes place in lymph nodes that are near the site of infection. "Samples" of the pathogens are physically brought to the lymph nodes by lymphatic fluids and/or by special *dendritic cells*. A controlled complex interwining of different types of lymphocytes develops in prescribed ways with the ongoing local immune response. It is thus reasonable to believe that in the lymph node a spatial arrangement exists that permits appropriate selection among the various responses. (The spleen plays a similar role, especially in the case of blood borne infections). Once appropriate responses have been selected in these "skirmishes" (or "simulations" in the well-chosen term suggested to us by R. de Boer) the chosen cells then can become the cadres of greater masses of effectors at the principal battlegrounds. Indeed, it is known that some B cells move from lymph nodes to the bone marrow where they proliferate and then migrate to the site of the infection.

Blood vessel surfaces near sites of infection are another possible locus of feedback modulated by spatial organization, since adhesion and penetration of cells is highly regulated [3].

## 8 Communication

Extracellular communication in the immune system is via scores of special molecules. Some of these are secreted, diffuse, and bind to receptors of the receiving cells, like hormones. Other messages require contact between messenger molecules that are displayed on cell surfaces. Intracellular communication is perhaps even more complex than extracellular. Cascades of coupled intracellular interactions follow the binding of a receptor. Eventually "action" results, typically via modulating the activity of selected genes. Another form of communication is indirect, via the "purposful" movement of cells to various destinations — whether for further maturation or for action against a concentration of antigen.

An important observation concerning all these messengers is that no type of messenger molecule seems responsible for just a single task, and that each task is regulated by a number of messengers. There is a network of influences. We believe that such *pleiotropy* is inevitable in the face of the many criteria that are used in assessing immune system performance. Evidence concerning this belief can perhaps be obtained by studying the "evolution" of model immune systems. Schemes such as genetic algorithms can be used to improve parameter settings so as to further predefined goals of the model systems. If the systems are complex, and/or if they are embedded in a complex environment, then we predict that pleiotropic signalling networks will emerge.

In immune signalling networks, both natural and artificial, it is probable that the emergent connection structure will be difficult to explain in detail. This has proved to be the case in the relatively simple problems of constructing neural networks to carry out defined tasks [7], [4]. Nonetheless we believe that considerations such as those suggested here can yield valuable overall understanding of a system whose detailed workings may forever be veiled in mystery.

## 9 A Brief Comparison to Some Other Approaches to Decentralized Systems

What can the immune system teach us concerning the general topic of how other collections of leaderless agents might be induced to perform "intelligent" actions? It must remain for the future to make a thorough comparison between the present ideas concerning the immune system and other ideas in the literature concerning intelligent distributed systems. Here a few remarks must suffice, to give the flavor of such a comparison.

The importance of spatial effects has been stressed by many, for example in Maes treatment [17] of "situated agents". (We have not seen any other presentation of the particular type of spatial reinforcement that was suggested here). Reminiscent of how the immune system seems to work is Maes discussion of how suitably spreading activation can help select among competing goals. Maes tries "to avoid having 'bureaucratic modules' whose only task is to influence the actions of other agents that effect concrete changes in their surroundings." The immune system on the other hand makes very important use of T helper "bureaucrats" in controlling effectors. (The role of T helpers is only implicit in our present simple models).

One of the central problems in organizing ensembles of agents to perform tasks is *credit assignment*, how to allocate rewards for successful attainment of a goal or subgoal (or a punishment for inappropriate action) among the agents. (A fine introduction is A.L. Samuel's classic paper on computer checkers [8]. Also see Refs. [2], [25] and [19]). Emphasized here as a major method for assigning credit for a given deed is reinforcing those agents who are in geographical proximity to the location where the deed was done. Another way that the credit assignment issue has arisen here is in connection with the allocation of somatic damage between pathogens and effectors. We have seen that the simple "associative" combination of variables (3c) can provide a sensible allocation. The fact that monitoring a multi-variable function can reveal subtleties of context is consonant with the numerous observations that in the immune system there is very considerable cross-influence among the cytokines.

Selecting among various pre-defined behaviors plays a central role in Matarić's investigation [18] of reinforcement learning among groups of robots. We have chosen this investigation as a case study to exemplify similarities and differences between the immune system and other decentralized systems.

The robots have a well-defined task, bringing scattered objects (pucks) to a predesignated "home" area. The task is done by means of mutually exclusive and learned

*behaviors*: safe-wandering, dispersion, homing.

(This simplified description omits certain features that are inessential for present purposes, and in particular neglects issues connected with recharging robot batteries). Behavior choices depend on

*states*: have-puck ($S_1$), near-neighbor ($S_2$).

Also, there is an automatic occurence of instantaneous

*actions*: grasp puck($A_1$),
drop puck at home ($A_2$),
drop puck away from home ($A_3$).

At any time $t$, with each behavior-condition pair is associated a *score*, which is a normalized weighted sum of (positive or negative) *reinforcements* received in the past by that pair. Reinforcements are updated after each

*event*: an action, or a behavioral switch.

Actions $A_1$ and $A_2$ give positive reinforcement, $A_3$ gives negative reinforcement. In states $S_1$ and $S_2$ there is positive reinforcement if the distance to home or the distance from a neighbor is increased; if the distances decrease, reinforcement is negative. Too small a reinforcement leads to cessation of the current behavior. For a given robot, behaviors are successively selected — an untried behavior if there is one, otherwise the behavior with the highest score.

Although "evaluating robot performance is notoriously difficult", such an evaluation was carried out [18], based on the closeness of learned matrices of behavior-state scores to a hand-derived "desired" matrix. In about 90% of the runs, the learning scheme fairly rapidly produced the desired matrix.

The following are points of comparison between the immune system and the puck-gathering robots of Ref. 15. Note: when (below) a property is attributed to the immune system, often the existence of this property has been suggested here but there has been no verification that natural immune systems possess the property in question.

a) The immune system does not have a well-defined overall goal.
b) Cells of the immune system do have behaviors, such as secreting, pathogen killing, dispersion (diffusion), and activation-proliferation.
c) The behaviors of the immune system occur concomitantly, not sequentially as in the puck-gathering robots.
d) Instead of using reinforcement to decide which behavior to select next (puck-gathering robots), the immune system uses a generalized proliferation function to influence the evolving intensity of each behavior.
e) Analogs of the puck-gathering robots progress-estimators are the concentrations of indicator chemicals such as $K$ and $H$. The robots have a clear goal. For the immune system "progress" is defined by reference to a fuzzily defined implicit goal, which might be approximated as "minimizing pathogen damage, both direct damage and damage caused by the immune system".
f) For the immune system events are continuous. (This seems not to be a major difference; for example, it would be easy to cast the above immune system models into discrete form).
g) For the immune system, interagent communication is via the "broadcast" of diffusible chemicals.

In the field of Artificial Intelligence, interactions of simple autonomous agents are not only of importance to applications such as coordinating the actions of a group of robots. An example of a high level system where such interactions play a major role is the Copycat analogy-making project of Hofstadter and Mitchell [23]. Here too, preliminary analysis indicates that analogies with the immune system are illuminating. Further study is planned.

Production of intentional systemic behavior is another high level topic wherein a study of the immune system can be helpful. In an important essay on intentional self organization, Atlan [1] writes that "a succcessful theory of self-organization should be able to explain the emergence of meaningful intentional behaviors from networks of non-intentional physical units defined by local laws only." He asks "is it possible to conceive of a machine where *the goal* to be reached, the task to be accomplished, would not be imposed from the outside but *produced by the machine itself*" (Atlan's italics)? We believe that our analysis provides elements of a theory of how evolution has crafted such a machine, the immune system. This system can be described as one wherein "meaningful functions" are "achieved on the basis of self-generated criteria for recognition" and thus is "strongly" self-organizing according to Atlan's definition. But the immune system is not "intentionally self organizing" since the interpretation of its behavior comes not from within but from scientists, who (intellectually, albeit not physically) are detached from the system under investigation.

## 10 Overview

There is enormous interest in the immune system, both as a biological entity of profound but accessible complexity and as a physiological complex of the highest medical importance. We contend that there is an additional major reason for interest in the immune system, its paradigmatic status as an example of a distributed intelligent system.

The immune system exemplifies the problem of guiding a huge distributed system to accomplish complex tasks. Moreover the immune system also offers us a solution to this problem, not a perfect solution but one that has been forged by evolution over eons. A very great deal is known, albeit a fraction of what is needed, concerning how details of agent (cellular) behavior in the immune system impact on accomplishing overall tasks. This is in contrast with neurobiology where there has been only relatively modest success in fathoming the connection between the cellular and behavioral levels — presumably because of the enormous complexity of the latter. All this means that careful study of the immune system can teach us a great deal about distributed intelligent systems.

One line of research uses methods of natural immunology to solve analogous "artificial" problems, such as combatting computer viruses [10]. Probably more important will be gleaning general insights from the workings of the immune system concerning the construction of distributed systems for carrying out complex tasks.

Interesting earlier attempts to understand cognitive aspects of immunology have been made [5], [6], [27]. Cohn and Langman have stressed that suitable effectors must somehow be chosen from an initial broad response, and they provided some ideas on how this might be done [15]. Grossman

[11] advocated the importance of "feedback signals, geared to the collective performance of the cells", noting that "the signal could be a local measure of 'stress' in the tissue, reinforcing an organization that becomes increasingly correlated to reduction in stress". Grossman [11], [12] emphasizes the tunable activation threshold and other possible intracellular devices for "learning" a better immune response, while the discussion here is centrally involved with selecting among a variety of pre-committed cells.

In the present work we would like to stress the matter of forging a more appropriate immune response without knowing what a good response is. The conventional approach to designing a system for carrying out a variety of tasks is to try to construct an overall measure of performance quality and then choose system structure and parameters to extremalize that measure. With respect to a complex entity such as the immune system, however, it is difficult (both for evolution and for the scientist) to construct a satisfactory scalar measure of quality in achieving an ensemble of goals.

The production of the damage-indicator chemical $H$ serves as one good scalar measure of immune system performance. But the inevitable processes of decay and diffusion mar the accuracy to which $H$ measures overall damage. With all its deficiencies, however, the level of $H$ provides invaluable information. Indeed, one message of our studies is that an imperfect performance measure can nonetheless help greatly toward achieving an ensemble of goals.

What are these goals? Minimizing the overall rate of damage is a step in the right direction. But should the average damage be minimized, or should its maximum be minimized (to avoid fatal attacks), or should it be some combination of the two? What of the fact that some organs are much more essential than others? Or that damage in some tissues rapidly heals? Over what ensemble of pathogen attacks should damage-minimization be based? Such queries encourage retreat to the evolutionary goal of maximizing long term reproduction rate.

There is thus profound difficulty in constructing a useful overall quality measure. Moreover, as has already been pointed out, even if such a measure could be constructed it is probably infeasible to use such a high level construction as a basis for modulating the behavior of low-level units. The alternative approach advocated here relies on *performance assessors* that (imperfectly) estimate low level spatially localized properties of system performance. These properties fall into two groups. *Good* properties (such as pathogen killing) are desirable attributes of system performance (all other things being equal) and *bad* properties are undesirable. If such a categorization is difficult then the properties being measured should in fact be ignored as not decisive in modulating the response. Some properties may be good or bad, depending on the circumstances. But we should attempt to discover a "basis set" of properties that are usually either good or bad.

In the simplest instantiation the good properties act as activators of local units that produce the behavior in question, and bad properties act as inhibitors. Although coefficients of activation and inhibition give an opportunity to weight the relative importance of the various properties nonetheless there is no decisive merit function, and in general even *post hoc* it is difficult to decide exactly how well the system is doing globally.

The good and bad properties often overlap and conflict. How does the immune system generate the required trade offs? We have suggested that this could be handled simply by arranging that the proliferation rate and/or the degree of activation of a given effector type is an increasing function of favorable factors and a decreasing function of unfavorable factors. For suitable parameter ranges (that have been mysteriously picked by "evolution"), feedback-guided intereffector dynamics can result in the selection of elements that forge an appropriate immune response.

We view the evolution of the immune system as combining with increasing sophistication elementary "good" and "bad" properties. An evolutionary twitch that yields such an elementary property should lead to something that remains in the species for many generations. This is because on balance a good property, or diminution of a bad property, somewhat enhances the survival of the organism. For example, "killing internal bacteria" on the whole seems desirable for vertebrates even though there are definite drawbacks to this policy (since many bacteria are benign or even helpful). Once the elementary properties are in place, evolution can hone interactions to obtain organisms that are increasngly more effective in that they tend to prevail as time goes on.

From our study there emerges a common-sense three-step path for guiding a complex distributed system toward better performance in spite of the absence of a clearly defined overall goal against which system "achievement" can be judged: (a) identify elementary subgoals, steps in the right direction; (b) monitor progress toward the subgoals; (c) effectively combine the evaluations of progress to regulate overall system performance. In biological systems, evolution somehow selects the effective combinations sought in step (c). If distributed systems for engineering applications are so complex that their overall goals cannot be explicitly formulated, then intelligent monitoring of extensive simulations under a variety of conditions may be a partial substitute for the "wisdom" of evolution in carrying out step (c).

## Acknowledgements

This chapter is an expanded and altered version of "The immune system as a prototype of autonomous decentralized systems", by Lee A. Segel which appeared in the proceedings of the IEEE International Conference on Systems, Man, and Cybernetics, October 1997, Orlando, FL. We have benefited from interactions with many colleagues, especially R. de Boer, I. Cohen, S. Forrest, G. Kelsoe, P. Matzinger and A. Perelson. T. Flash, S. Gielen and M. Matarić improved our understanding of decentralized systems. Thanks to

S. Fliegelmann for excellent word processing. Support is acknowledged from the US-Israel Binational Science Foundation, Grant 95-00526.

## References


1. H. Atlan, "Intentional self-organization. Emergence and reduction: towards a physical theory of intentionality", Thesis Eleven 1998, pp. 5–34.
2. A.G. Barto, "Reinforcement learning", in *Handbook of Brain Theory and Neural Networks* (M.A. Arbib, ed.), Cambridge: MIT Press, 1995.
3. E.C. Butcher and L.J. Picker, Lymphocyte homing and homeostatis, *Science*, Vol. 272, 1996, pp. 60–66.
4. G.A. Carpenter and A-H. Tan, "Rule extraction: From neural architecture to symbolic representation", *Connections Science*, Vol. 7, 1995, pp. 3–28.
5. I.R. Cohen, "The cognitive principle challenges clonal selection", *Immunol. Today*, Vol. 13, 1992, pp. 441-444.
6. I.R. Cohen, "A cognitive paradigm of the immune system", *Immunol. Today*, Vol. 13, 1992, pp. 490–494.
7. F. D'Alche-Buc, V. Andres and J-P. Nadal, "Rule extraction with fuzzy neural network", *Intern. J. Neural Systems*, Vol. 5, 1994, pp. 1-11.
8. E.A. Feigenbaum and J. Feldman, *Computers and Thought*, New York: McGraw-Hill, 1963.
9. M.A. Fishman and A.S. Perelson, "Modeling T cell-antigen presenting cell interactions", *J. thoer. Biol.*, Vol. 160, 1993, pp. 311–342.
10. S. Forrest, A.S. Perelson, L. Allen and R. Cherukuri, "Self-nonself discrimination in a computer", *Proc. 1994 IEEE Symp. on Research in Security and Privacy*, IEEE Computer Society Press, Los Alamitos, CA, 1994, pp. 202–212. Also see the paper of Kephart in this volume.
11. Z. Grossman, "Contextual discrimination of antigens by the immune system: towards a unifying hypothesis", in *Theoretical and Experimental Insights into Immunology* (A.S. Perelson and G. Weisbuch, eds.), NATO ASI Series, Vol. H66, Berlin, Heidelberg: Springer-Verlag, 1992, pp. 71–89.
12. Z. Grossman and W.E. Paul, "Adaptive cellular interactions in the immune system: The tunable activation threshold and the significance of subthreshold responses, *Proc. Natl. Acad. Sci. USA*, Vol. 89, 1992, pp. 10365-10369.
13. C.A. Janeway, Jr. and P. Travers, *Immunobiology*, Oxford: Blackwell Scientific Publications, 1994.
14. E.F. Keller and L.A. Segel, "The initiation of slime mold aggregation viewed as an instability, *J. Theor. Biol.*, Vol. 26, 1970, pp. 399–415.
15. R.E. Langman, *The Immune System*, San Diego: Academic Press, 1989.
16. S.A. Levin, "On the evolution of ecological parameters", in *Ecological Genetics: The Interface* (P.F. Brussard, ed.), *Proceedings in Life Sciences*, Springer, 1978, pp. 3–26.
17. P. Maes, "Situated agents can have goals", *Robotics and Autonomous Systems*, Vol. 6, 1990, pp. 49–70.
18. M.J. Matarić, "Reinforcement learning in the multi-robot domain", *Autonomous Robots*, Vol. 4, No. 1, Jan. 1997, pp. 73–83.
19. M.J. Matarić, "Using communication to reduce locality in distributed multi-agent learning", *Proc. AAAI-97*, Providence, Rhode Island, July 27–31, 1997.

20. P. Matzinger, "Tolerance, danger, and the extended family", *Ann. Rev. Immunol.*, Vol. 12, 1994, pp. 991–1045.
21. H. Meinhardt, *Models for Biological Pattern Formation*, London: Academic Press, 1982.
22. J.A.J. Metz, R.M. Nisbet and S.A.H. Geritz, "How should we define 'fitness' for general ecological scenarios?", *TREE* (*Trends in Ecology and Evolution*), Vol. 7, No. 6, June 1992, pp. 198–202.
23. M. Mitchell, *Analogy-Making as Perception*, Cambridge MA: MIT Press, 1993.
24. A.S. Perelson and G. Weisbuch, "Immunology for physicists", *Rev. Modern Phys.*, Oct. 1997.
25. D.E. Rumelhart and J.L. McClellend, *Parallel Distributed Processing*, Cambridge: MIT Press, 1986.
26. Y. Sato, M. Roman, H. Tighe, D. Lee, M. Corr, M-D. Nguyen, G.J. Silverman, M. Lotz, D.A. Carson and Y. Raz, "Immunostimulatory DNA sequences necessary for effective intradermal gene immunization", *Science* 273, 1996, pp. 352–354.
27. F. Varela, A. Coutinho, B. Dupire and N.N. Vaz, "Cognitive networks: immune, neural and otherwise", in *Theoretical Immunology* (A.S. Perelson, ed.), Part 2, Redwood City: Addison-Wesley, 1988, p. 359.
28. S.H. Zigmond and S.J. Sullivan, " Receptor modulation and its consequences for the response to chemotactic peptides", in *Biology of the Chemotactic Response* (J.M. Lackie and P.C. Wilkinson, eds.), Cambridge: Cambridge University Press, 1981, pp. 73–88.


## Appendix 1: Explaining Fig. 5

Figure 5 shows that the merit $M$ attains a minimum at an intermediate value of the half-saturation constant $n$ for the influence of $K$ on the proliferation rate. To understand this observation, we first examine, as indicators of their qualitative behavior, the maximum values that the various functions take during the course of time. The results of Fig. 4 show that as $n$ increases, $E_{\max}$ goes through a minimum. By contrast both $K_{\max}$ and $P_{\max}$ increase monotonically. Superficially there is a paradox. Compared to their values for small $n$, for intermediate values of $n$, the larger values of $P_{\max}$ and $K_{\max}$ are associated with smaller values of $E_{\max}$, but for still larger values of $n$ the further increases in $P_{\max}$ and $K_{\max}$ are associated with large values of $E_{\max}$.

To explain what is going on, we first note from Fig. 4 that at any given time $K$ is larger at larger values of $n$. The production of $K$ is driven by the product of $E$ and $P$. For fixed $K$ an increase of $n$ has opposite effects on $E$ and $P$; $E$ decreases, because its proliferation rate decreases, but a decrease in $E$ leads to an increase in $P$. The results of the simulation show that the latter effect predominates for the present model, which is responsible for the increase in $K$.

Given that an increase in $n$ increases $K$, there are competing effects on the growth of $E$. Let $p(K_1)$ denote the proliferation rate of $E_1$, where from (9a)

$$p(K_1) = qK_1/(n + K_1) \ . \tag{10}$$

The direct effect of increasing $n$ is to decrease $p$ but the relevant indirect effect of larger $n$, increasing $K_1$, tends to increase $p$. The plot of $p(K_1)$ in Fig. 7 shows that at intermediate values of $n$ it is the former effect that is more important ($p(K_1)$ decreases when $n$ is raised from $n = 150$ to $n = 1000$) but at higher values of $n$ it is the latter effect that dominates (overall, $p(K_1)$ is larger at $n = 5000$ than for $n = 150$ or $n = 1000$). In other words, although $K_{\max}$ increases as $n$ increases, a shift from $n = 150$ to $n = 1000$ does not produce a large enough increase in $K$ to outweigh the depressing effect on $p$ of elevating $n$.

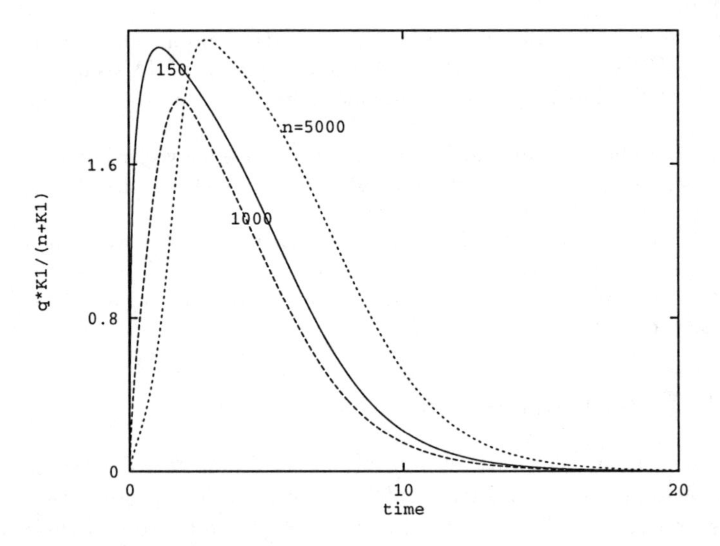


**Fig. 7.** Model C: The effector proliferation rate (10) for three values of $n$, calculated from simulations of Fig. 4.

**Dr. Lee Segel** was educated at Harvard College (A.B., 1953) and MIT (PhD, 1959), with an interim year as a Fullbright scholar at Cambridge University. After a post-doctoral period at the National Physical Laboratory (England) he became a member of the Applied Mathematics Department at Rensselaer Polytechnic Institute. In 1971-2 he was a Guggenheim Fellow at the Weizmann Institute in Israel; in 1973 he became a permanent member of their staff. His research interests originally were centered about nonlinear hydrodynamic stability theory. In 1969 he switched his main attention to problems of theoretical biology.

# Immune Network: An Example of Complex Adaptive Systems

Debashish Chowdhury

Physics Department
Indian Institute of Technology
Kanpur 208016, U.P.
India

**Abstract.** The phenomenon of immunological memory has been known for a long time. But, the underlying mechanism is poorly understood. According to the theory of clonal selection the response to a specific invading antigen (e.g., bacteria) is offered by a specific clone of the cells. Some of the lymphocytes activated during the primary response remain dormant and keep circulating in the immune system for a long time carrying the memory of the encounter and, therefore, these long-lived cells are called memory cells. Proponents of the alternative network theory maintain that the immune response is offered by a "network" of clones in a collective manner. In recent years several possible scenarios of the "structure" and function of the immune network have been considered. We have developed mathematical models for describing the population dynamics of the immunocompetent cells in a unified manner. We have incorporated intra-clonal as well as inter-clonal interactions in a discrete formulation and also studied a continuum version of this model.

## 1 Introduction

The latin word "immunitas" is related to the concept of exemption from a service or duty or from civil laws (e.g., "diplomatic immunity" of an ambassador of one country in another). It has been known for more than two thousand years [1] that individuals who recover from a disease become "immune" to it; this is the phenomenon of "acquired immunity". The scientific investigation of immunology, however, began much later when Jenner utilized this phenomenon of "acquired immunity" to develope a vaccine against small pox. The first breakthrough in understanding the mechanism of this remarkable phenomenon was made by Louis Pasteur in 1880. Over the last hundred years we have collected an enormous amount of information on the "hardware" of the immune system (e.g., the molecules and cells involved) [2–4] but we understand very little about the "software" that runs it, i.e., the principles governing various immunological processes.

Theoretical immunology [5,6] deals with the mathematical modelling of immunological processes at various levels, e.g., molecular level, cellular level and the level of cell populations. One of the major aims of theoretical immunology [7,8] is to predict "macroscopic" properties of the immune system from the properties and interactions among its elementary "microscopic" constituents; this problem is similar to those usually studied by physicists using the techniques of statistical mechanics. Theoretical immunologists develop mathematical models to understand how the immune system evolves over long time scales, how its size and inter-cellular interactions vary with time, how these interactions govern the dynamics of the populations of various types of cells during an immune response to a specific antigen and how it "learns" adaptively about new antigens (i.e., acquires new knowledge) and how it retains the newly acquired knowledge in its "memory" and, finally, how it retrieves information from its memory. Several mathematical models have been developed so far to capture the known immunological phenomena as well as to predict new ones. In this chapter we summarize some of the modern approaches to the mathematical modelling of the immune system and illustrate these with specific examples. We hope that some of the modelling strategy developed for the immune system may find applications in designing artificial immune systems.

## 2 A Brief Summary of Experimental Phenomena to be Modelled Theoretically

Millions of different varieties of lymphocytes are known to be produced by the immune system. However, according to the *clonal selection theory*, only a specific type can respond to a specific antigen. This is in sharp contrast to the non-antigen-specific response offered by the macrophages to the antigens. The body seemingly anticipates all the types of antigens it may encounter in the future and prepares accordingly by producing a large variety of lymphocytes. For an antigen-specific response the antigen must be, first of all, properly recognized by the specific lymphocytes. Different types of lymphocytes identify the antigens in different manners. Following the recognition of the antigen, a specific type of lymphocyte, which fit best with the antigen, proliferates rapidly through cell division into a clone (a population of genetically identical cells). The corresponding process is called clonal selection because the antigen selects which lymphocytes must develop into a clone [9].

There are several alternative and complimentary routes of immune response. In a humoral immune response a specific type of B-cell proliferates and the terminal differentiation of a fraction of this B-cell population leads to plasma cells. These produce antibodies, which react with the antigen and eventually lead to the elimination of the antigen from the host system. The remaining fraction of the proliferating B-cells become dormant and keep circulating in the bloodstream carrying a memory of the encounter with the antigen; the latter variety of the long-lived B-cells are called memory B-cells. In the cell-mediated immune response a specific type of T-cell becomes cytotoxic and kills the antigen directly. Memory of the encounter with the specific antigen is thereafter carried by the corresponding long-lived memory T-cells.

The helper T-cells play very crucial roles of regulating the immune response in both routes to immunity. The host carrying the memory cells is said to have acquired immunity against the specific antigen because the presence of the memory cells leads to a quicker and stronger secondary immune response when the host is stimulated again with the same antigen. In fact, this is the basic principle of vaccination. The humoral and cell-mediated routes to immunity are illustrated schematically in fig.1.

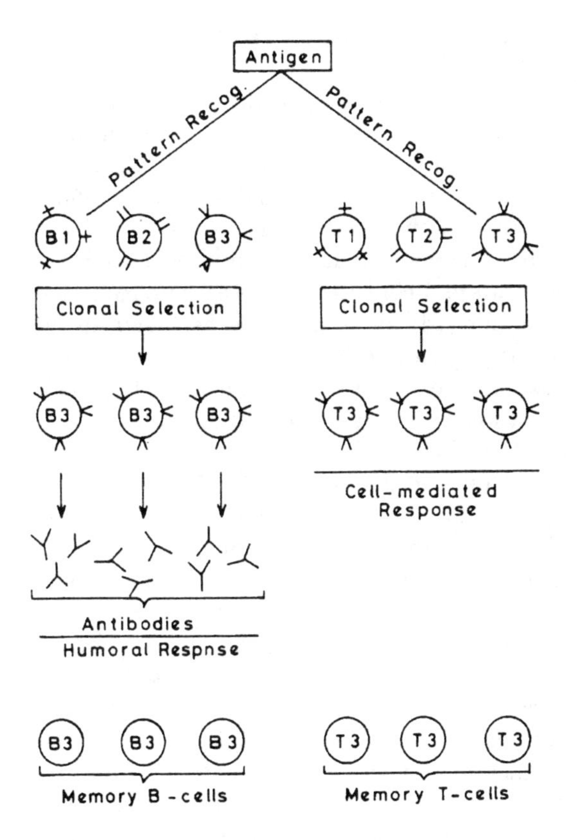


**Fig. 1.** A schematic description of the routes to immunity

Normally, the immune system can distinguish the cells and tissues of the host ("self") from the foreign invaders ("non-self"). A normal immune response (NIR) follows when the population of a foreign antigen in the body exceeds a tolerance level [10]. However, under special circumstances, the immune system mistakenly identifies a part of the host as a "foreign" substance because of some "error" [11]. Then, the immune response that follows against the host is called an auto-immune response (AIR) and such a response can lead to a auto-immune disease.

The human immunodeficiency virus (HIV) is an exceptional invader in the sense that, unlike other foreign antigens, it destroys the helper T-cells of the immune system which are known to be crucial for almost all types of immune response. Therefore, during the late stages of HIV infection the patient's immune system becomes disabled; this is the acquired immune deficiency syndrome (AIDS). Such a patient ultimately succumbs to a secondary infectious agent, raher than to the HIV itself [12].

## 3 Clonal Selection and Its Mathematical Modelling

The equations describing the population dynamics of the cells involved in immune response to a specific antigen can be formulated in two different ways. In the discrete approach, the population of each type of cells is modelled by a discrete variable which can take one of only two allowed values: 0 and 1 corresponding to low and high populations, respectively. In this approach, the dynamical equations are written as maps in discrete time. Moreover, the interactions between the various pairs of different cell types are also restricted to have only a few discrete set of allowed values. On the other hand, in the continuum approach, the populations of the cells, the interactions between the different cell types as well as time are assumed to be real variables, which can vary continuously; the population dynamics of the cells are now given by a set of differential equations.

The continuum approach was followed first by Bell [13,14], and subsequently by many other investigators, for developing mathematical models of clonal selection. But, since quite often the models are "underdetermined" by the available experimental data, i.e., more than one model can account for the known experimental facts, some authors have, in the recent years, advocated the use of a discrete language as a first step towards the formulation of the quantitative theories [15]. The advantage of a discrete language arises from the fact that the range of allowed values of the variables and the parameters is so narrow that one does not need to adjust too many free parameters to reproduce experimentally known facts. The discrete theories can satisfactorily account for the qualitative features of immune response. The discrete models are not intended to be a substitute for the more realistic continuum description; one can construct the continuum counterpart of the discrete model following well known mathematical prescriptions. The relative advantages and disadvantages of these two approaches have also been discussed in detail in the literature.

### 3.1 Discrete Models of Clonal Selection

The discrete variable that describes the populations of the cells in the discrete models is sometimes called an "automaton" and a system consisting of such mutually-interacting automata are referred to as "cellular automata"

(CA). The concept of CA was introduced by Von Neumann in the context of theories of evolution and, subsequently, analyzed in more detail by Wolfram [16]. The CA are known to exhibit a rich variety of spatio-temporal patterns depending on their rules of evolution. These have found practical applications in modelling, for example, fluid flow, etc.

Discrete models of cell population dynamics of the immune system can be formulated in terms of either "Threshold automata" or "Boolean automata" [17].

• **Threshold automata:** The population of the $i$-th type of cells is denoted by the symbol $S_i$, where each $S_i$ can take only two possible values: $S_i = 0$ corresponding to a low population and $S_i = 1$ corresponding to a high population. The population of the $i$-th type of cells at time $t+1$ is given by the dynamical map [18];

$$S_i(t+1) = \theta(h_i - \mu_i) \quad (i = 1, 2, ..., n) \tag{1}$$

where $\theta(y)$ is the step function, i.e., $\theta(y) = 0$ for $y < 0$ and $\theta(y) = 1$ for $y \geq 0$. Moreover, $h_i = \sum_j C_{ij} S_j$ is the total stimulus received by the cells of $i$-th type, where $C_{ij}$ is the interaction from cell type $j$ to the cell type $i$ and $\mu_i$ is a preassigned threshold at which $S_i$ switches from the state 0 to the state 1. The interactions $C_{ij}$ are allowed to take only a few integer values, for example, $-1, 0, 1$. A specific model is defined by the number $n$ of cell types, the set of values $\{C_{ij}\}$ for all the pairs $< ij >$ and the set of values $\{\mu_i\}$ for all $i$. If $S_i(t+1) = S_i(t)$ for all $i$ simultaneously then the corresponding values of the set $\{S_i\}$ is called a fixed point of the dynamics of the system. On the other hand, if $S_i(t+T) = S_i(t)$ for all $i$ simultaneously, then the system is said to have a limit cycle of period $T$. The fixed points and the limit cycles are referred to as the attractors of the dynamics.

The concept of *window automata* has also been used extensively in theoretical immunology[19,20]. Suppose, $S_i = 1$ only if $h_i$ falls within a certain window between two thresholds, i.e., if $\mu' < h_i < \mu''$, and $S_i = 0$ if $h_i$ falls outside this window; then $S_i$ is an example of window automaton.

• **Boolean Automata:** A Boolean automaton is a logical variable which can be only either "true" or "false", usually denoted by 1 and 0, respectively. Therefore, one can describe the cell populations in the discrete models by Boolean variables. However, one cannot carry out the standard algebraic operations, e.g., addition, multiplication, etc., with the Boolean variables. Therefore, if the discrete model is to be formulated in terms of Boolean automata, the dynamical maps will involve logical operations, viz., $OR$, $AND$, $NOT$, etc. For example, if $A, B$ and $C$ are Boolean automata, then

$$A = B.OR.C \quad is \quad 1 \quad if \quad either \quad B \quad or \quad C \quad or \quad both \quad are \quad 1$$

$$A = B.AND.C \quad is \quad 1 \quad if \quad and \quad only \quad if \quad both \quad B \; and \; C \; are \; 1$$

$$A = .NOT.B \quad is \quad 1 \quad if \quad B \quad is \quad 0 \; and \; vice - versa.$$

The attractors of the dynamics of a Boolean automata network can also be defined just as we did in the case of threshold automata networks.

We now present an illustrative example of a discrete model of NIR, within the framework of the clonal selection scenario, formulated using the language of Boolean automata; this model will be referred to as the e-KUT model as a model of this type was first considered by Kaufman, Urbain and Thomas [21] and extended later by Chowdhury and Stauffer [22,23] Suppose, $Ab, S, H, B$ and $Ag$ denote the populations of the antibodies, suppressor $T$-cells, helper $T$-cells, $B$-cells and the corresponding foreign antigen, respectively. In the e-KUT model the dynamical maps governing the population dynamics are given by

$$Ab(t+1) = Ag(t).AND.B(t).AND.H(t)$$

$$S(t+1) = H(t).OR.S(t)$$

$$H(t+1) = [Ag(t).AND.(.NOT.S(t))].OR.H(t)$$

$$B(t+1) = [Ag(t).OR.B(t)].AND.H(t)$$

$$Ag(t+1) = Ag(t).AND.(.NOT.Ab(t))$$

It is straightforward to check that this model has five fixed points each of which has a bio-medical interpretation. For example, the fixed point corresponding to $Ab = S = H = B = Ag = 0$ is the *virgin* or *tolerant* state whereas the fixed point corresponding to $Ag = Ab = 0$, $H = S = B = 1$ is interpreted as the immunized state where high populations of the lymphocytes carry the memory of the earlier encounter with the foreign antigen to which this clone responds specifically. Although the separate existence of suppressor $T$-cells is questionable, in the original model of Kaufman et al. [21] a different interpretation of the origin of this suppressing effect was proposed; however, that interpretation has been criticised by Hoffmann[24]. Not only the fixed points of the e-KUT model have interesting bio-medical interpretations, but the sequence of the intermediate states, through which the system evolves from an initial state before reaching the corresponding fixed point, have also been found to be consistent with experimentally known facts.

Chowdhury et al.[23] developed a "unified" model, by generalizing the e-KUT model, which also describes the population dynamics of the cells involved in NIR, AIR as well as NIR against non-HIV antigens in HIV-infected individuals and AIDS. Suppose, the concentrations of the "self-antigen" and HIV are denoted by the symbols $IO$ and $IV$, respectively, while the concentration of the killer or effector cells involved in the AIR is denoted by the symbol $IK$. The dynamical maps governing the population dynamics in this model are now postulated to be

$$Ab(t+1) = Ag(t).AND.B(t).AND.H(t)$$

$$S(t+1) = H(t).OR.S(t)$$

$$H(t+1) = [((Ag(t).OR.IO).AND.(.NOT.S(t)).OR.H(t)].AND.(.NOT.IV)$$

$$B(t+1) = [Ag(t).OR.B(t)].AND.H(t)$$

$$Ag(t+1) = Ag(t).AND.(.NOT.Ab(t))$$

$$IK(t+1) = (IO(t).AND.H(t)).AND.(.NOT.S)$$

Cellular-automata models for some other aspects of immune response have also been developed [25–27].

### 3.2 Continuum models of clonal selection

Starting from the discrete dynamical equations, written in terms of logical operations among boolean variables, it is possible to derive an analogous system of differential equations of the form

$$(dy_i/dt) = g_i(y_1, y_2, ..., y_N) - d_i y_i \tag{2}$$

for the $n$ types of cells where $y_i$ and $d_i$ represent, respectively, the concentration and the natural decay rate of the $i$-th type of cell. The functions $g_i$ involve combinations of sigmoid functions of $y_j$'s. Their functional forms can be derived from the form of the right hand side of the corresponding maps in the discrete theories following a well-defined prescription [21,28]. In order to derive the right-hand side of the differential equation for the concentration $y_i$ from the right-hand side of the corresponding discrete map for the discrete variable $S_i$: (i) each of the discrete variables $S_j$ is replaced by the corresponding sigmoid function

$$F_i^+(y_j) = y_j^m/(\theta_{ij}^m + y_j^m)$$

whereas each of the discrete variables $.NOT.S_j$ is replaced by the function

$$F_i^-(y_j) = 1 - F_i^+(y_j) = \theta_{ij}^m/(\theta_{ij}^m + y_j^m)$$

where the Hill number $m$ determines the steepness of the sigmoid functions $F^+$ and $F^-$ and $\theta_{ij}$ is the threshold for the regulation of the cell type $i$ by the cell type $j$; (ii) the logical operations $OR$ and $AND$ used in the discrete formulation are replaced by the arithmetic operations of addition (+) and multiplication (•), respectively, in the continuum formulation; (iii) an additional term of the form $-d_i y_i$ (with $d_i > 0$) is introduced to account for the natural decay of the populations of the cells of type $i$ with the passage of time. For example, the differential equation corresponding to the discrete equation

$$S_3 = (S_5.AND.(.NOT.S_2)).OR.S_3$$

is given by

$$(dy_3/dt) = k_3 F_3^+(y_5) \bullet F_3^-(y_2) + k_3' F_3^+(y_3) - d_3 y_3.$$

Following the prescriptions outlined above, Chowdhury [29] derived the differential equations corresponding to the discrete dynamical maps in the unified model and further simplified the differential equations.

An interesting feature of the NIR in this model is shown in fig.2. Note that a small amount of thc antigen is adequate to immunize the host so that it can mount a very strong secondary response against the same antigen even if the antigen dose is high; this captures the essential principle of immunization or vaccination.

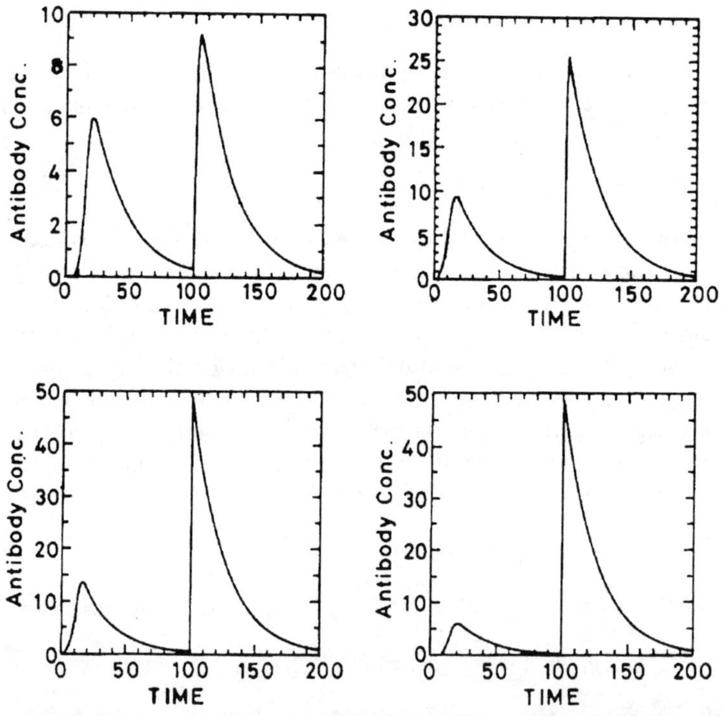


**Fig. 2.** The time-dependence of the population of the antibodies during the primary and secondary NIR for different antigen-dosages. The primary and secondary doses are given at $t = 0$ and $t = 100$, respectively. The strengths of the primary and secondary doses of antigen are both 1 (in (a)), 10 (in (b)), 100 (in (c)) whereas those of the antigen are, respectively, 1 and 100 (in (d))

Another interesting feature of this model is demonstrated in fig.3. If the host is infected with HIV but the concentration of HIV is low a secondary response to non-HIV antigens can take place despite depletion of the (memory-) $T_H$-cell populations. On the other hand, no secondary response to non-HIV antigen takes place if the concentration of HIV is sufficiently high. Thus, symptoms of AIDS (namely, lack of response to secondary antigens) would not be visible in an individual already infected by HIV, provided the level of HIV is low.

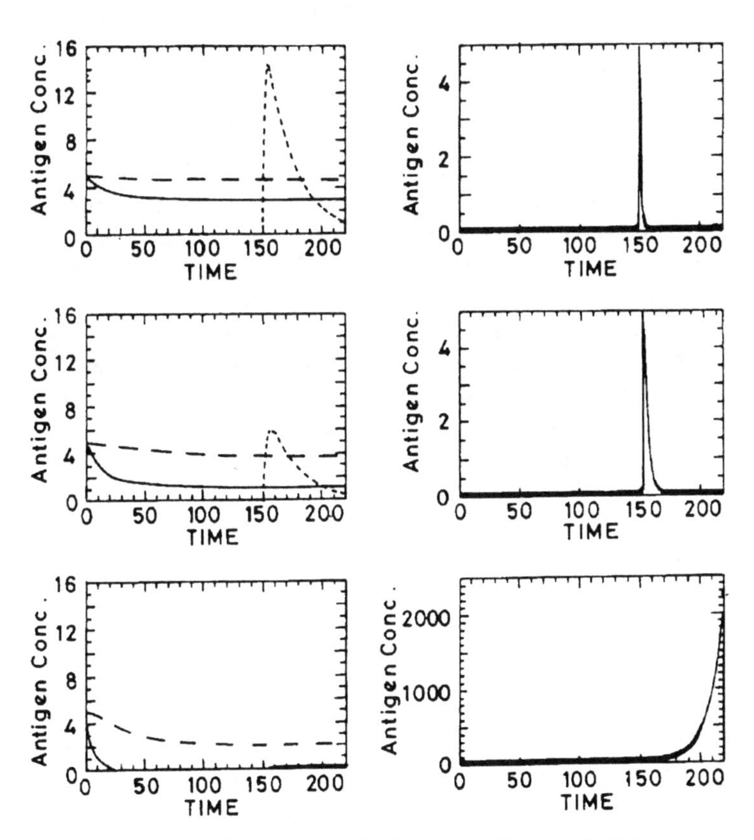


**Fig. 3.** The time-dependence of the helper-T cells (full line), suppressor-T cells (dashed line), the antibodies (dotted line) and the antigen (asterisk-marked line) of a host, which has been immunized first against a specific non-HIV antigen, during an infection by different levels of HIV dose and the subsequent secondary response. The HIV dose is given at $t = 0$ and the secondary dose of the non-HIV antigen is given at $t = 150$ where the strength of the secondary dose of the non-HIV antigen is 5. The levels of HIV doses are 0.5 (in (a)), 1.5 (in (b)) and 5.0 (in (c))

## 4 Beyond Clonal Selection; Immune Network

Clonal selection theory has been very successful in describing many aspects of immune response, but some crucial questions could not be answered so far within the framework of this theory. For example, what makes the memory cells retain their memory? One possibility is that some kind of stimulation of the immune system persists even after the antigen population falls below the tolerance level; in that case memory cells are nothing but cells which are perpetually in a stimulated state. But, if so, what keeps stimulating these cells so selectively and how [30,31]? Some experiments indicate that persistence of some traces of the foreign antigen after primary response can stimulate the "memory" $T-$ and $B-$cells [32,33]. But, although this mechanism may be sufficient, this may not always be necessary as demonstrated by more recent experiments [34,35].

A possible clue to this mystery of the identity of the specific stimulators, which keeps stimulating a clone so selectively long after the elimination of the foreign antigens, emerges from other sets of experiments. The clonal selection theory, in its classical form, assumed that all immune responses are triggered by antigens. But, it has been observed that in "germ-free" mice (i.e, mice kept for a few generations in environments free from foreign antigens) the number of activated lymphocytes is similar to the values measured in conventionally raised mice [36,37,45] This observation suggests the possibility of stimulating clones also through internal mechanisms. We shall now argue that such internal mechanisms of stimulation follow naturally by going beyond the classical clonal selection theory and invoking the concept of an immune network. This network theory may also explain more satisfactorily some other immunological phenomena, e.g., tolerance and self-nonself discrimination, etc.

Consider two clones $C_1$ and $C_2$. Suppose, the surface receptors of the lymphocytes and the free antibodies belonging to $C_1$ and $C_2$ "fit" with the epitopes of the foreign antigens $Ag_1$ and $Ag_2$, respectively. Therefore, according to the clonal selection theory, $C_1$ is expected to respond specifically to $Ag_1$ whereas $Ag_2$ is expected to stimulate $C_2$ selectively. It is quite natural to expect that the "molecular pattern" of the receptor molecules, which can recognize "molecular pattern" stored in the epitopes of foreign antigens, can themselves be recognized by others. For example, if the surface receptors of $C_1$ and $C_2$ "fit" with each other then $C_2$ would response to the proliferating lymphocytes of $C_1$ in exactly the same manner in which it responds against $Ag_2$. In other words, $C_2$ treats $C_1$ and $Ag_2$ on the same footing; therefore, $C_1$ may be regarded as an "internal image" of $Ag_2$. An epitope that is unique to the surface receptors and antibodies of a specific type is called an idiotope. Hence, a functional network formed on the basis of idiotope recognition is usually referred to as idiotypic network [38–40].

Proponents of the immune network theory [41–43] [44–46] maintain that the immune response to foreign antigens is offered by the entire immune system (or, at least, more than one clone) in a collective manner although the dominant role may be played by a single clone whose cell surface receptors "fit" best with the epitope of the specific invading antigen. However, the proliferating cells and antibodies of the responding clone (idiotype) trigger the response of the corresponding anti-idiotypes which, in turn, can stimulate their own anti-idiotypes, and so on. The detailed dynamics of the immune network, of course, would depend on the size and the nature of the connectivity.

•*Linear and cyclic networks:* Richter [47] introduced the earliest models of immune networks where a "chain-reaction" of the clones was postulated. Suppose, the clones are such that $C_1$ stimulates $C_2$, then $C_2$ stimulates $C_3$ which, in turn, stimulates $C_4$, etc. However, this chain reaction is limited by the fact that each clone suppresses the particular clone that was responsible for its stimulation, i.e., simultaneously, suppose, $C_4$ responds to suppress $C_3$, $C_3$ suppresses $C_2$ which, in turn, suppresses $C_1$. Hiernaux [48] converted the linear chain into a cyclic network and analyzed its properties. Hoffmann and coworkers [49–51] have made several improvements over the Richter model. Farmer et al.[52,53] introduced a similar model and compared its features with the other networks used in adaptive computation [54]. This work has been subsequently extended [55,56] by incorporating memory B-cells. The attractors of the dynamics of such networks can be a limit cycle, where the populations of the antibodies vary periodically and the immunological memory is stored through a combination of "static" elements (namely, long-lived memory cells) and a "dynamic" process, namely, a limit cycle. A discrete toy model of a cyclic immune network has been developed by Chowdhury et al. [57] and its continuum counterpart has been investigated [58].

•*Cayley-tree-like network:* A Cayley tree is a loop-less tree characterized by the coordination number $z$ which is the number of branches emerging from each node. In such a network, the clones are organized in a hierarchical manner; the total stimulus received by the $B$-cells belonging to each of the clones at the $i$-th level is [59]

$$h^i = x^{(i-1)} + (z-1)x^{(i+1)} \tag{3}$$

where $x$ denotes the concentration of the $B$-cells. The concentration of the $B$-cells of the clones at the $i$-th level are, then, assumed to be governed by window automata (in the discrete formulation) or their continuum counterparts (in the continuum formulation).

•*Generalized shape-space approach:* This formulation exploits the fact that the binding affinity of the surface receptors and free antibodies belonging to different clones is determined by the degree of complimentarity of their geometric shape, electric charge, etc. Therefore, if the generalized shape (includes $d$ different characteristics) of a clone is represented by a lattice site at $\boldsymbol{r}$ in a $d$-dimensional space then the location of its anti-idiotype should be $-\boldsymbol{r}$ on the same $d$- dimensional lattice (see fig.4). Thus the strength of the interaction between the clones at the lattice site $\boldsymbol{r}$ and $-\boldsymbol{r}$ is maximum. Moreover, since the clone at $\boldsymbol{r}$ has still significant amount of complimentarity in generalized shape with the nearest-neighbour sites of $-\boldsymbol{r}$ the clone at the site $\boldsymbol{r}$ is usually assumed to interact also with those at the sites $-\boldsymbol{r} \pm \boldsymbol{\delta}_x$ and $-\boldsymbol{r} \pm \boldsymbol{\delta}_y$, although these interactions are much weaker than that between $\boldsymbol{r}$ and $-\boldsymbol{r}$ [60–62,46,63,64]. It is desirable that if the virgin system is infected by a single specific antigen that the response activities should remain confined over a limited region of the generalized shape space in spite of the fact that the entire network is connected. After all, when a person gets infected by tuberculosis he is not expected to show large populations of antibodies against cholera! It has been found that the dimensionality of the generalized shape space determines whether the response activities remain localized or percolate over the entire network.

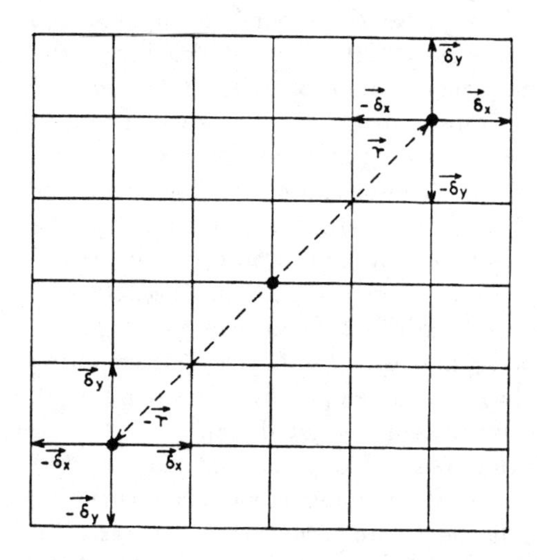


**Fig. 4.** A schematic representation of the two-dimensional generalized shape space

Chowdhury et al. [57] have extended the e-KUT model [22,23] of clonal selection so as to incorporate explicitly both intra-clonal and inter-clonal interactions. They postulated that the immune system in a host consists of several functional networks of various different sizes; clones belonging to different networks do not interact among themselves and only clones belonging to the same network can interact among themselves through inter-clonal interactions. For example, on a square lattice the dynamical maps governing the time evolution of the populations of the various cell types are given by

$$Ab(\boldsymbol{r}, t+1) = Ag(\boldsymbol{r}, t).AND.B(\boldsymbol{r}, t).AND.H(\boldsymbol{r}, t)$$

$$B(\boldsymbol{r},t+1) = [Ag(\boldsymbol{r},t).OR.H(-\boldsymbol{r},t).OR.H(-\boldsymbol{r}+\boldsymbol{\delta}_1,t)$$
$$.OR.H(-\boldsymbol{r}+\boldsymbol{\delta}_2,t).OR.H(-\boldsymbol{r}+\boldsymbol{\delta}_3,t)$$
$$.OR.H(-\boldsymbol{r}+\boldsymbol{\delta}_4,t)].AND.H(\boldsymbol{r},t)$$

$$H(\boldsymbol{r},t+1) = [Ag(\boldsymbol{r},t).OR.H(-\boldsymbol{r},t).OR.H(-\boldsymbol{r}+\boldsymbol{\delta}_1,t)$$
$$.OR.H(-\boldsymbol{r}+\boldsymbol{\delta}_2,t).OR.H(-\boldsymbol{r}+\boldsymbol{\delta}_3,t).OR.H(-\boldsymbol{r}+\boldsymbol{\delta}_4,t)]$$
$$.AND.[.NOT.[H(-\boldsymbol{r},t).AND.H(-\boldsymbol{r}+\boldsymbol{\delta}_1,t)$$
$$.AND.H(-\boldsymbol{r}+\boldsymbol{\delta}_2,t).AND.H(-\boldsymbol{r}+\boldsymbol{\delta}_3,t)$$
$$.AND.H(-\boldsymbol{r}+\boldsymbol{\delta}_4,t)]]$$

$$Ag(\boldsymbol{r},t+1) = Ag(\boldsymbol{r},t).AND.[.NOT.Ab(\boldsymbol{r},t)]$$

where $\boldsymbol{r}+\boldsymbol{\delta}_1, \boldsymbol{r}+\boldsymbol{\delta}_2, \boldsymbol{r}+\boldsymbol{\delta}_3, \boldsymbol{r}+\boldsymbol{\delta}_4$ denote the positions of the four nearest-neighbours of the site $\boldsymbol{r}$. Thus, every clone at $\boldsymbol{r}$ can stimulate not only the antiidiotype at $-\boldsymbol{r}$ but also those clones which are located at the nearest-neighbour sites of $-\boldsymbol{r}$. On the other hand, so far as suppression is concerned, the high population of the clone at $\boldsymbol{r}$ can be reduced to a low level if and only if the populations of the clone at $-\boldsymbol{r}$ and the clones at the latter's $2d$ neighbouring sites are high simultaneously. Therefore, on the one hand, mutual stimulation is symmetric in the sense that the clone at $\boldsymbol{r}$ excites the clone at $-\boldsymbol{r}$ and vice versa. On the other hand, mutual suppression is also symmetric in the sense that clones at $\boldsymbol{r}$ and its $2d$ neighbouring sites together can reduce the population of the clone at$-\boldsymbol{r}$ and, similarly, the clones at $-\boldsymbol{r}$ and its nearest-neighbours can reduce the high population of the clone at $\boldsymbol{r}$ to a low level. However, there is asymmetry between stimulation and suppression because suppression succeeds only if the entire neighbourhood of the antiidiotype, rather than the antiidiotype alone, is highly populated. Chowdhury et al.[57] observed that, in this model, once a site of the shape space is infected a pulse propagates and the pattern of the pulse keeps recurring for ever, thereby carrying the memory of the encounter with the foreign antigen through a dynamic mechanism.

## 5 Summary and Conclusion

The immune system is an example of complex adaptive systems. Other important adaptive systems include the brain (neural network) [65]. There are several striking similarities between the brain and the the immune system despite many crucial differences. Adaptive systems learn or adapt as living systems do. Different systems learn on widely different time scales; for example, brains learn in seconds to hours, immune systems in hours to days, species in days to centuries and ecosystems in centuries to millenia. In my opinion, there are at least two different aspects of the dynamics of the immune system: (a) the populations of the cells of a specific clone (and, perhaps, closely related clones) increase very rapidly following the recognition of any foreign antigen and, after the elimination of the antigen, decrease again; (b) because of the natural death of unstimulated lymphocytes and recruitment of fresh immunocompetent cells the immune network itself evolves with time and all its characteristic properties, e.g., size, connectivity, etc., may also keep changing with time. Both the processes (a) and (b) occur on comparable time scales. Therefore, inclusion of both these aspects in the same model is more desirable than studying the cell-population dynamics in a network of fixed size and connectivity. In fact, not only the later evolution but also the formation of the immune network in a newborn child is a challenging problem. Even the size and the connectivity of the immune system may be among its emergent collective properties [66]. It has been speculated [67] that immunologcal memory would be much more robust if it is distributed over many clones rather than a single one.

In this chapter we have not only explained some interesting methods of modelling in theoretical immunology but also presented some models as illustrative examples. Even if some of these models turn out to be inadequate to capture the complexities of the real immune system they may, nevertheless, find use in designing artificial immune systems for the protection of information systems (e.g., computer, internet, etc.) against the corresponding "antigens" (e.g., computer virus and internet worms, etc.).

### Acknowledgements

I thank D. Stauffer for enjoyable collaborations over almost a decade on the modelling of immune networks and for his comments on an earlier version of the manuscript.

## References

1. Silverstein A M, 1989, *A history of immunology* (Academic Press)
2. Alberts et al., 1989, *The Molecular Biology of the Cell*, 2nd ed. (Garland, New York)
3. Darnell et al., 1990, *Molecular Cell Biology* (Freeman/Scientific American, San Francisco)
4. Jaret P and Nilsson L, 1986, National Geographic (June) 702
5. Perelson A S and Weisbuch, 1997, Reviews of Modern Physics **69**, 1219
6. Chowdhury D and Stauffer D, 1992, Physica A **186**, 61
7. Perelson A S, 1988, (ed.) *Theoretical Immunology* parts I and II (Addison-Wesley)
8. Marchuk G I, 1983, *Mathematical Models in Immunology*, (Optimization Software Inc., New York)

9. Burnet F M, 1957, Australian Journal of Science **20**, 67; see more detailed account in *The Clonal Selection Theory of Acquired Immunity* (Cambridge University Press, 1959); see also Scientific American **204(1)**, 58 (1961)
10. Rennie J, 1990, Scientific American (12) 77; see also the special issue on "Frontiers in Biotechnology: Tolerance in the immune system" of Science, **248** (15th June) 1990.
11. Cohen I R, 1988, Scientific American **258**, 34; see also *Perspectives on Autoimmunity* (CRC press, Boca Raton, 1988)
12. Weber J N and Weiss R A, 1988, Scientific American (1) 81; see also the other articles in this special issue on AIDS
13. Bell G I, 1970, Journal of Theoretical Biology **29**, 191
14. Bell G I, 1971, Journal of Theoretical Biology **33**, 339
15. Atlan H, 1989, Bulletin of Mathematical Biology **51**, 247
16. Wolfram S, 1986, *Theory and Applications of Cellular Automata* (World Scientific)
17. Weisbuch G, 1991, *Complex Systems Dynamics: An Introduction to Automata Networks* (Addison-Wesley)
18. Weisbuch G and Atlan H, 1988, J. Phys. A **21**, L189; see also Cohen I R and Atlan H, 1989, J. Autoimmunity, **2**, 613
19. Neumann A U and Weisbuch G, 1992, Bulletin of Mathematical Biology. **54**, 21
20. Neumann A U and Weisbuch G, 1992, Bulletin of Mathematical Biology. **54**, 699
21. Kaufman M, Urbain J and Thomas R, 1985, Journal of Theoretical Biology **114**, 527
22. Chowdhury D and Stauffer D, 1990, Journal of Statistical Physics **59**, 1019
23. Chowdhury D, Stauffer D and Choudary P V, 1990, Journal of Theoretical Biology **145**, 207
24. Hoffmann G W, 1987, Journal of Theoretical Biology **129**, 355
25. Pandey R B, 1991, Physica A **179**, 442
26. Pandey R B and Stauffer D, 1990, J. Stat. Phys. **61**, 235
27. Celada F and Seiden P E, 1996, Eur. J. Immunol. **26**, 1350
28. Kaufman M and Thomas R, 1987, Journal of Theoretical Biology **129**, 141
29. Chowdhury D, 1993, Journal of Theoretical Biology **165**, 135
30. Vitetta E S, Berton M T, Burger C, Kepron M, Lee W T and Yin Xiao-Ming, 1991, Annual Reviews of Immunology **9**, 193
31. Sprent J, 1994, Cell **76**, 315
32. Gray D and Skarvall H, 1988, Nature **336**, 70
33. M.A. Fishman and A.S. Perelson, 1995, Journal of Theoretical Biology **173**, 241
34. Lau L L, Jamieson B D, Somasundaram T and Ahmed R, 1994, Nature **369**, 648
35. Hou S, Hyland L, Ryan K W, Portner A and Doherty P C, 1994, Nature **369**, 652
36. Hoykaas H, Benner R, Pleasants R and Wostmann B, 1984, European Journal of Immunology **14**, 1
37. Pereira P, Forni L, Larsson E L, Cooper M, Heisser C and Coutinho A, 1986, European Journal of Immunology **16**, 685
38. Jerne N K, 1973, Scientific American **229**, 52

39. Jerne N K, 1974, Ann. Immunol. (Inst. Pasteur) **125C**, 373
40. Jerne N K, 1984, Immunological Reviews **79**, 5
41. Perelson A S, 1989, Immunological Reviews **110**, 5
42. Atlan H and Cohen I R, 1989, (eds.) *Theories of Immune Networks* (Springer)
43. Stewart J and Varela F J, 1989, Immunological Reviews **110**, 37
44. Coutinho A, 1989, Immunological Reviews **110**, 63
45. Varela F J and Coutinho A, 1991, Immunology Today **12**, 159
46. De Boer R J, Neumann A U, Perelson A S, Segel L A and Weisbuch G, 1992a, in: Proc. of the first European Biomathematics Conference, eds. V. Capasso and P. Demongot (Springer)
47. Richter P H, 1975, European Journal of Immunology **5**, 350
48. Hiernaux J, 1977, Immunochemistry, **14**, 733
49. Hoffmann G W, 1975, European Journal Immunology **5**, 638
50. Hoffmann G W, Kion T A, Forsyth R B, Soga K G and Cooper-Willis,1988, in: *Theoretical Immunology*, part Two, ed. Perelson A S (Addison-Wesley)
51. S. Royer, 1994, Masters Thesis, Univ. of British Columbia.
52. Farmer J D, Packard N H and Perelson A S, 1986, Physica D **22**, 187
53. Farmer J D, Kaufman S A, Packard N H and Perelson A S, 1987, in: *Perspectives in Biological Dynamics and Theoretical Medicine*, eds. S.H. Koslow, A.J. Mandell and M.F. Schlesinger (New York Academy of Sciences, New York)
54. Farmer J D, 1990, Physica D **42**, 153
55. Behn U and Van Hemmen J L, 1989, Journal of Statistical Physics **56**, 533
56. Behn U, Van Hemmen J L and Sulzer B, 1993, Journal of Theoretical Biology **165**, 1; see also Lippert K and Van Hemmen J L, 1997, in: *Annual Reviews of Computational Physics*, ed. D. Stauffer, vol.V (Wold Scientific)
57. Chowdhury D, Deshpande V and Stauffer D, 1994, International Journal of Modern Physics **C5**, 1049
58. Chowdhury D, 1995, Indian Journal of Physics, **69B**, 539
59. Weisbuch G, De Boer R J and Perelson A S, 1990, Journal of Theoretical Biology **146**, 483
60. Perelson A S and Oster G F, 1979, Journal of Theoretical Biology **81**, 645
61. Segel L A and Perelson A S, 1989, in: *Theories of Immune Networks*, eds. Atlan H and Cohen I R (Springer)
62. De Boer R J, Segel L A and Perelson A S, 1992b, Journal of Theoretical Biology **155**, 295
63. Stauffer D and Weisbuch G, 1992, Physica A **180**, 42
64. Sahimi M and Stauffer D, 1993, Physical Review Letters **71**, 4271
65. Amit D J, 1989, *Modelling Brain Functions* (Cambridge University Press)
66. De Boer R J and Perelson A S, 1991, Journal of Theoretical Biology **149**, 381
67. Parisi G, 1988, in: *Chaos and Complexity*, eds. R. Livi, S. Ruffo, S. Ciliberto and M. Buiatti (World Scientific)

**Dr. Debashish Chowdhury** is a Professor of Physics at Indian Institute of Technology, Kanpur. He is author of a book titled "Spin Glasses and Other Frustrated Systems", published jointly by the Princeton university Press and World Scientific. He has also published about one hundred research papers. He has been studying the structure and dynamics of disordered and complex systems using the techniques of statistical physics.

# Immunological Memory is Associative*

Derek J. Smith[1], Stephanie Forrest[1], and Alan S. Perelson[2]

[1] Department of Computer Science
University of New Mexico
Albuquerque, NM 87131, USA
[2] Theoretical Division
Los Alamos National Laboratory
Los Alamos, NM 87545, USA

**Abstract.** This paper argues that immunological memory is in the same class of associative memories as Kanerva's *Sparse Distributed Memory*, Albus's *Cerebellar Model Arithmetic Computer*, and Marr's *Theory of the Cerebellar Cortex*. This class of memories derives its associative and robust nature from a sparse sampling of a huge input space by recognition units (B and T cells in the immune system) and a distribution of the memory among many independent units (B and T cells in the memory population in the immune system).

## 1 Introduction

Cowpox vaccination, used to protect humans from smallpox, was the first known deliberate use of associative recall in the immune response [1]. The modern investigation of associative recall began with the observation that antibodies induced during an influenza infection often have greater affinity to prior strains of influenza than to the infecting strain—suggesting that the antibodies were generated by memory cells to prior infections [2,3]. Others [4] and [5] continued the investigation by injecting laboratory animals with one antigen and then recalling the memory of that antigen by subsequent injection of a second, related, antigen. Some researchers considered associative recall "a degeneracy in the secondary immune response" [6]. However, as research continued, and associative recall was observed in many animal models with many types of antigen, it became clear that it was a general phenomenon of immunological memory [7–11]. Immunologists refer to associative recall as a cross-reactive secondary response, or as original antigenic sin [5].

The purpose of this paper is to show that immunological memory is an associative and robust memory that belongs to the class of sparse distributed memories. This class of memories derives its associative and robust nature by sparsely sampling the input space and distributing the data among many independent agents [12]. Other members of this class include a model of the

* This chapter was first presented at the workshop IMBS96 *Immunity-based systems* December 10, 1996, Kyoto Japan.

cerebellar cortex [13], the *Cerebellar Model Arithmetic Computer* (CMAC) [14], and *Sparse Distributed Memory* (SDM) [15]. First, we present a simplified account of the immune response and immunological memory. Next, we present SDM, and then we show the correlations between immunological memory and SDM. Finally, we show how associative recall in the immune response can be both beneficial and detrimental to the fitness of an individual.

## 2 Immunological Memory

The immune system must recognize a large number of cells and molecules (antigens) that it has never seen before, and it must decide how to respond to them. Some antigens, such as those that make up the individual's body, must not be attacked[1]. Other antigens, such as viruses, bacteria, parasites and toxins are responded to by mixtures of the T cell response and the different types of antibody responses. The immune system remembers antigens it has seen before and when it sees them again is often capable of eliminating them before disease occurs. This memory is the basis for vaccination, and the reason why we do not get most diseases more than once. The immune response and immunological memory are complex and not fully understood. This exposition is necessarily simplified and restricted.

*Recognition.* The human immune system uses a large number of highly specific B and T cells to recognize antigen. An individual has the genetic material and a combinatorial based randomizing mechanism to express $>10^{10}$ distinct B cell receptors [16]. At any time, the immune system expresses a subset of these consisting of the order of $10^7$ to $10^8$ distinct B cell receptors [17–19]. The number of possible distinct antigens is difficult to calculate, but it is thought to be in the range $10^{12}$ to $10^{16}$ [20]. B and T cell receptors are stimulated by antigen if their affinity for the antigen is above some threshold. Typically $10^{-5}$ to $10^{-4}$ of an individual's B cells are stimulated by an antigen [21–23]. B cells that are stimulated by an antigen are said to be in the *ball of stimulation* of that antigen [24] (Figure 1a).

*Response.* B and T cells that are stimulated by antigen divide. The B cell receptor sometimes mutates on cell division and this can increase the affinity of its daughter cells for the antigen. Towards the end of a response, when antigen becomes scarce, higher affinity B cells have a fitness advantage over lower affinity B cells and are preferentially selected in a process similar to natural evolution (Figure 1b) [25]. During the replication of cells in response to antigen, some B cells change into plasma cells and secrete antibodies which eliminate the antigen. In the case of a viral infection, some T cells change into cytotoxic T lymphocytes (CTLs), which can kill virus-infected cells.

[1] Diseases such as multiple sclerosis, rheumatiod arthritis and insulin-resistant diabetes are examples of autoimmune diseases where the immune system attacks the body it usually protects.

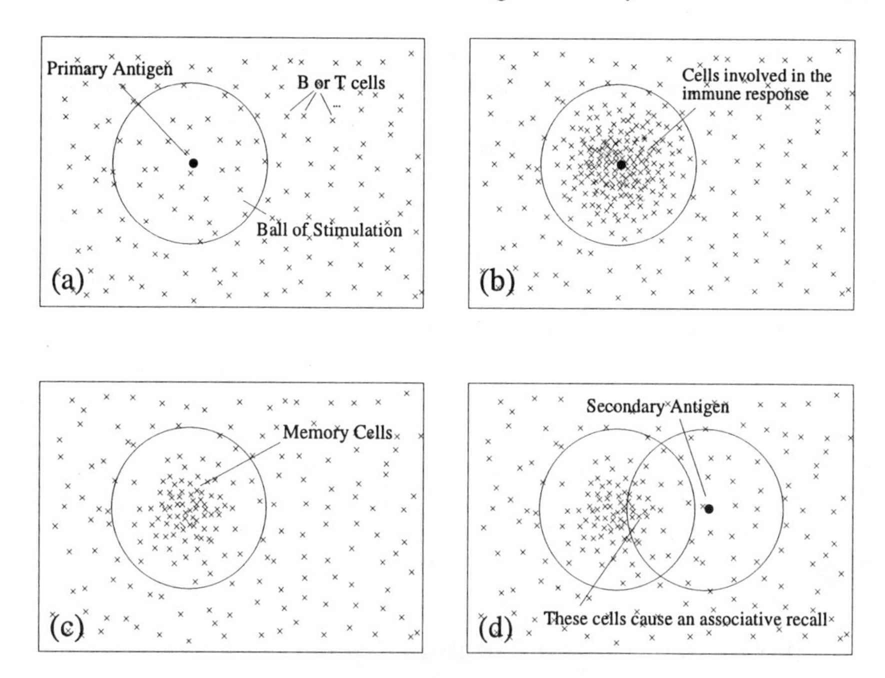


**Fig. 1.** (a) A two dimensional illustration of (a high dimensional) sparse distribution of B or T cell receptors in a space where distance is a measure of affinity for an antigen. B and T cells within some threshold affinity bind the antigen and become activated. The region the antigen activates is called the *ball of stimulation* of the antigen. (b) Activated B cells replicate and mutate and the higher affinity ones are selected. (c) After the antigen is cleared a memory population persists. (d) A second exposure to the same antigen, or here a related antigen, restimulates the memory population inducing an associative recall.

At the end of an immune response, when the antigen is cleared, the B cell population decreases, leaving a persistent sub-population of memory cells (Figure 1c). The mechanism(s) by which memory cells persist is not fully understood. One theory is that memory cells live for a long time [26]. Another is that memory cells are restimulated at some low level. A number of mechanisms for restimulation have been proposed. [27] proposed the idiotypic network theory in which cells co-stimulate each other in a way that mimics the presence of the antigen. Another theory is that small amounts of the antigen are retained in lymph nodes [28,29]. Another is that related environmental antigens provide cross-stimulation [30].

The idiotypic network theory has been proposed as a central aspect of the associative properties of immunological memory [31,32]. However, in this exposition, it is but one of the possible mechanisms that maintains the memory population and is key to neither the associative nor robust properties of immunological memory.

The persistent population of memory cells is the mechanism by which the immune system remembers. If the same antigen is seen again, the memory population quickly produces large quantities of antibodies (or CTLs) and often times the antigen is cleared before it causes disease. This is called a secondary immune response. If the secondary antigen is slightly different from the primary antigen, its ball of stimulation may overlap part of the memory population raised by the primary antigen (Figure 1d). Memory cells in the overlap bind the antigen and produce antibodies and/or CTLs. Immunologists call this a cross-reactive response, people who work with associative memories would call it associative recall. The strength of the secondary immune response is approximately proportional to the number of memory cells in the ball of stimulation of the antigen. If a subset of the memory population is stimulated, by a related antigen, then the response is weaker [33]. Thus, memory appears to be distributed among the cells in the memory population. Immunological memory is robust because, even when a portion of the memory population is lost, the remaining memory cells persist to produce a response.

## 3 Sparse Distributed Memory (SDM)

Kanerva's SDM is a member of the class of sparse and distributed associative memories to which we show immunological memory belongs. SDM, like random access memory (the memory in a computer), is written to by providing an address and data, and read from by providing an address and getting an output. Unlike random access memory, the address space of SDM is enormous, sometimes 1,000 bits, giving $2^{1,000}$ possible addresses. SDM cannot instantiate such a large number of address-data locations so it instantiates a subset, of say 1,000,000 address-data locations. These instantiated address-data locations are called hard locations and are said to sparsely cover the input space [15].

When an address is presented to the memory hard locations that are within some threshold Hamming distance of the address are activated. This subset of activated hard locations is called the access circle of the address (Figure 2a).

On a write, each bit of the input data is stored independently in a counter in each hard location in the access circle. If the $i$th data bit is a 1, the $i$th counter in each hard location is incremented by 1, if the $i$th data bit is a 0 the counter is decremented by 1 (Figure 2b). On a read, each bit of the output is composed independently of the other bits. The value of the $i$th counter of each of the hard locations in the access circle are summed. If the sum is positive the output for the $i$th bit is a 1, if the sum is negative the output is a 0 (Figure 2c).

The distribution of the data among many hard locations makes the memory robust to the loss of some hard locations, and it permits associative recall

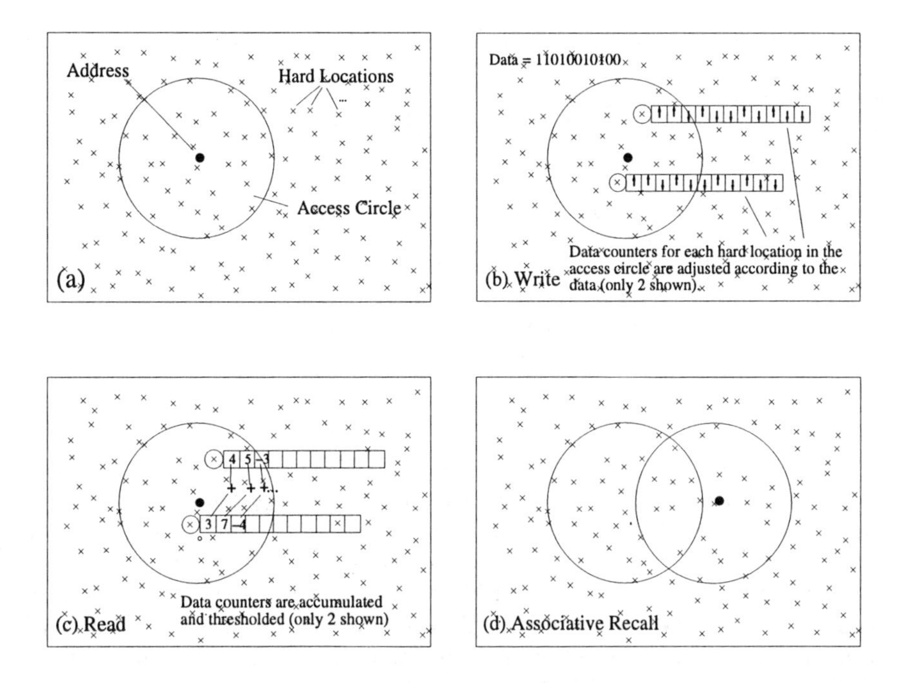


**Fig. 2.** (a) A two dimensional illustration of hard locations sparsely and randomly distributed in a high dimensional binary input space. Distance in the space represents Hamming distance between hard locations. Hard locations within some radius of an input address are activated and form an access circle. (b) Activated hard locations adjust their associated data counters on a write and (c) accumulate and threshold them on a read. (d) The access circle of a similar address might include some hard locations from the prior write and induce an associative recall.

of the data if a read address is slightly different from a prior write address. If the access circle of the read address overlaps the access circle of the write address, then hard locations that were written to by the write address are activated by the read address, and give an associative recall of the write data (Figure 2d).

## 4 Correspondence between Immunological Memory and SDM

The previous two sections showed that both immunological memory and SDM are sparse and distributed, and are thus associative and robust. The correspondence between the two memories is summarized in Table 1 and discussed below.

Both SDM and immunological memory use detectors to recognize input. In the case of SDM, hard locations recognize an address, in the case of im-

**Table 1.** Structural and functional correspondence between immunological memory and SDM.

| Immunological Memory | SDM |
|---|---|
| Antigen | Address |
| B/T Cell | Hard Location |
| Ball of Stimulation | Access Circle |
| Affinity | Hamming Distance |
| Response/Tolerance | Data |
| Primary Response | Write and Read |
| Secondary Response | Read |
| Cross-Reactive Response | Associative Recall |

munological memory, B and T cells recognize an antigen. In both systems the number of possible distinct inputs is huge and due to resource limitations, the number of detectors is much smaller than the number of possible inputs—both systems sparsely cover the input space. In order to respond to all possible inputs, detectors in both systems do not require an exact match with the input, but are activated if they are within some threshold distance of the input. In the case of SDM this is Hamming distance, in the case of immunological memory it is affinity. Thus, in both systems an input activates a subset of detectors. In SDM, this subset is called the access circle of the input address, in immunological memory, it is called the ball of stimulation of the antigen.

In both systems detectors store information associated with each input. In the case of SDM the information is a bit string and is supplied exogenously. In the case of immunological memory the information is determined by mechanisms within the immune system that determine whether to respond to an antigen and if so with what class of antibody and/or CTL response.

Both systems distribute all of the information to each activated detector. In the case of SDM the data is used to adjust counters, in the case of immunological memory a large number of memory cells are created which, in the case of B cells, have undergone genetic reconfigurations that determine the class of antibodies they will produce. Because all the information is stored in each detector, each detector can recall the information independently of the other detectors. The strength of the output, the signal, is an accumulation of the information in each activated detector. Thus, as detectors fail, the output signal degrades gracefully, and the signal strength is proportional to the number of activated detectors. Thus, the distributed nature of storing the information in both systems makes both systems robust to the failure of individual detectors.

In the case of SDM, the data is distributed to hard locations, each of which have different addresses, and in the case of immunological memory, to cells which have different receptors (although many copies of a cell with the same, or similar receptors also exist). If the activated subset of detectors of a related input (a noisy address in the case of SDM, or a mutant strain in the case of immunological memory) overlap the activated detectors of a prior input (Figures 1d and 2d), detectors from the prior input will contribute to the output. Such associative recall, and the graceful degradation of the signal as inputs differ, is due to the distribution of the data among the activated detectors.

# 5 Aspects of Associative Recall in the Immune Response

Prior exposure to one strain of a pathogen often protects against mutant strains. In influenza, for example, older individuals have greater immunity to new strains than younger individuals [2]. In this case associative recall is beneficial to the individual.

Associative recall can also be a disadvantage. If the ball of stimulation of a vaccine (secondary antigen) overlaps the memory to a prior infection (primary antigen), then the vaccine may be cleared by associative recall of the prior infection and fail to make highly specific memory to the vaccine strain. If the ball of stimulation of a subsequent challenge (tertiary antigen) also overlaps prior memory then all is well (Figure 3a). However, if there is no overlap, disease can ensue and the vaccine will have "failed" (Figure 3b).

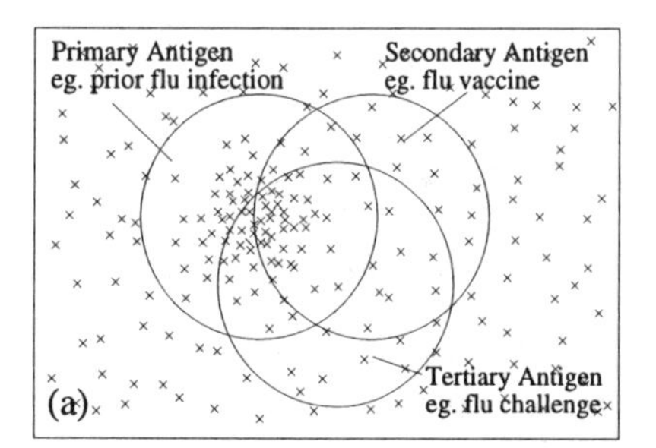


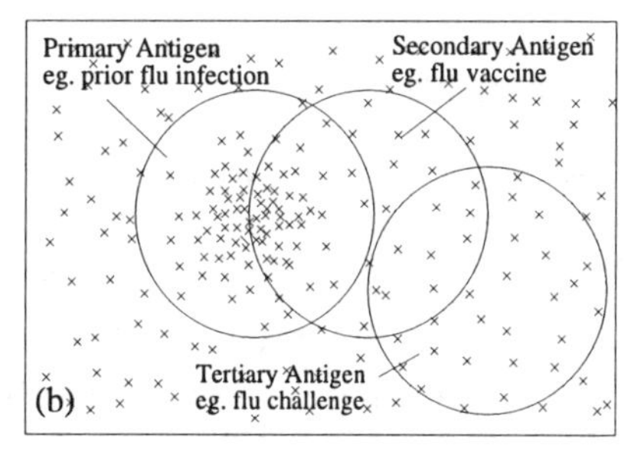


**Fig. 3.** Associative recall of prior infection (primary antigen) can cause a vaccine (secondary antigen) to fail. The prior infection might divert the vaccine and (a) also react with the challenge strain (tertiary antigen), or (b) be of no use against the challenge strain.

A potentially confusing situation for any associative memory is when two similar inputs require different outputs. In the case of immunological memory this would occur when an antigen requires one type of response and a related antigen a different type of response. Such a situation has been hypothesized in the case of some malaria infections, where prior exposure, to a related environmental antigen, is thought to divert the response [34].

## 6 Summary

We have shown the correspondence between B and T cells in the immune system and hard locations in a SDM. In particular B and T cells perform a sparse coverage of all possible antigens in the same way that hard locations perform a sparse coverage of all possible addresses in a SDM. Also, data are distributed among many independent B and T cells in immunological memory as they are among many independent hard locations in a SDM. Immunological memory is thus a member of the family of sparse distributed memories, and its associative and robust properties are due precisely to its sparse and distributed nature.

### Acknowledgments

DJS gratefully acknowledges the support of the Santa Fe Institute, the University of New Mexico Computer Science Department AI fellowship and Digital Equipment Fellowship. DJS also thanks David Ackley, Will Attfield, Ron Hightower, Terry Jones, Pentti Kanerva, Linda Cicarella, Ron Moore, Francesca Shrady and Paul Stanford for helpful comments on this work. Portions of this work were performed under the auspices of the U.S. Department of Energy. This work was supported by NIH (AI28433, RR06555), the Joseph P. and Jeanne M. Sullivan Foundation, ONR (N00014-95-1-0364), and NSF (IRI-9157644). The authors gratefully acknowledge the ongoing support of the Santa Fe Institute.

## References

1. E. Jenner. *An Inquiry into the Causes and Effects of the Variolae Vaccinae.* Low, London, 1798.
2. T. Francis. Influenza, the newe acquayantance. *Ann. Intern. Med.*, 39:203–221, 1953.
3. F. M. Davenport, A. V. Hennessy, and T. Francis. Epidemiologic and immunologic significance of age distribution of antibody to antigenic variants of influenza virus. *J. Exp. Med.*, 98:641–656, 1953.
4. R. V. Gilden. Antibody responses after successive injections of related antigen. *Immunology*, 6(30):30–36, 1963.
5. S. Fazekas de St. Groth and R. G. Webster. Disquisitions of original antigenic sin. II. Proof in lower creatures. *J. Exp. Med.*, 124:347–361, 1966.
6. H. N. Eisen, J. R. Little, L. A. Steiner, E. S. Simms, and W. Gray. Degeneracy in the secondary immune response: Stimulation of antibody formation by cross-reacting antigens. *Israel J. Med. Sci.*, 5:338–351, 1969.
7. J. Ivanyi. Recall of antibody synthesis to the primary antigen following successive immunization with heterologous albumins. A two-cell theory of the original antigenic sin. *Eur. J. Immunol.*, 2(4):354–359, 1972.
8. S. Deutsch and A. E. Bussard. Original antigenic sin at the cellular level. I. Antibodies produced by individual cells against cross-reacting haptens. *Eur. J. Immunol.*, 2:374–378, 1972.

9. S. Fish, E. Zenowich, M. Fleming, and T. Manser. Molecular analysis of original antigenic sin. I. Clonal selection, somatic mutation, and isotype switching during a memory B cell response. *J. Exp. Med.*, 170:1191–1209, 1989.
10. P. L. Nara and J. Goudsmit. Clonal dominance of the neutralizing response to the HIV-1 V3 epitope; evidence for original antigenic sin during vaccination and infection in animals including humans. In R. M. Chanock, editor, *Vaccines (Cold Spring Harbor Eighth Annual Meeting), Vol. 91, Modern Approaches to New Vaccines including Prevention of AIDS*. Cold Spring Harbor, NY, 1990.
11. D. J. Smith. A literature review of original antigenic sin. Technical Report TR 94–10, University of New Mexico, Albuquerque, NM, 1994.
12. P. Kanerva. Sparse distributed memory and related models. In H. M. Hassoun, editor, *Associative Neural Memories: Theory and Implementation*, chapter 3. Oxford University Press, 1992.
13. D. Marr. A theory of cerebellar cortex. *J. Physiology*, 202:437–470, 1969.
14. J. S. Albus. *Brains, Behavior, and Robotics*. Byte Books, Peterborough, NH, 1981.
15. P. Kanerva. *Sparse Distributed Memory*. MIT Press, Cambridge, MA, 1988.
16. C. Berek and C. Milstein. The dynamic nature of the antibody repertoire. *Immunol. Rev.*, 105:5–26, 1988.
17. G. Köhler. Frequency of precursor cells against the enzyme beta-galactosidase: An estimate of the BALB/c strain antibody repertoire. *Eur. J. Immunol.*, 6:340–347, 1976.
18. N. R. Klinman, J. L. Press, N. H. Sigal, and P. J. Gerhart. The acquisition of the B cell specificity repertoire: the germ-line theory of predetermined permutation of genetic information. In A. J. Cunningham, editor, *The Generation of Antibody Diversity*, pages 127–150. Academic Press, New York, 1976.
19. N. R. Klinman, N. H. Sigal, E. S. Metcalf, P. J. Gerhart, and S. K. Pierce. *Cold Spring Harbor Symp. Quant. Biol.*, 41:165, 1977.
20. J. K. Inman. In G. Bell, A. Perelson, and G. Pimberly, editors, *Immunology*, page 243. Marcel Decker, Inc., New York, 1978.
21. G. M. Edelman. Origins and mechanisms of specificity in clonal selection. In G. M. Edelman, editor, *Cellular Selection and Regulation in the Immune System*, pages 1–38. Raven Press, New York, 1974.
22. C. J. V. Nossal and G. L. Ada. *Antigens, Lymphoid Cells and The Immune Response*. Academic Press, New York, 1971.
23. N. K. Jerne. Clonal selection in a lymphocyte network. In G. M. Edelman, editor, *Cellular Selection and Regulation in the Immune System*, pages 39–48. Raven Press, New York, 1974.
24. A. S. Perelson and G. F. Oster. Theoretical studies of clonal selection: Minimal antibody repertoire size and reliability of self- non-self discrimination. *J. Theoret. Biol.*, 81:645–670, 1979.
25. F. M. Burnet. *The Clonal Selection Theory of Immunity*. Cambridge Univerity Press, London, 1959.
26. C. R. Mackay. Immunological memory. *Adv. Immunol.*, 53:217–265, 1993.
27. N. K. Jerne. Towards a network theory of the immune system. *Annals of Immunology (Institute Pasteur)*, 125C:373, 1974.
28. J. G. Tew and T. E. Mandel. Prolonged antigen half-life in the lymphoid follicules of antigen-specifically immunized mice. *Immunology*, 37:69–76, 1979.

29. J. G. Tew, P. R. Phipps, and T. E. Mandel. The maintenance and regulation of the humoral immune response. persisting antigen and the role of follicular antigen–binding dendritic cells. *Immunol. Rev.*, 53:175–211, 1980.
30. P. Matzinger. Immunological memories are made of this? *Nature*, 369:605–6, 1994.
31. J. D. Farmer, N. H. Packard, and A. S. Perelson. The immune system, adaptation, and machine learning. *Physica D*, 22:187–204, 1986.
32. C. J. Gibert and T. W. Routen. Associative memory in an immune-based system. In *Proceedings of the Twelfth National Conference on Artificial Intelligence*, pages 852–857, Cambridge, MA, 1994. AAAI Press/The MIT Press.
33. I. J. East, P. E. Todd, and S. J. Leach. Original antigenic sin: Experiments with a defined antigen. *Mol. Immunol.*, 17:1539–1544, 1980.
34. M. F. Good, Y. Zevering, J. Currier, and J. Bilsborough. "Original antigenic sin", T cell memory, and malaria sporozoite immunity: An hypothesis for immune evasion. *Parasitc Immunology*, 15(4):187–193, 1993.

**Dr. Derek Smith** is a postdoctoral fellow in the computer science department at the University of New Mexico. He received his Ph.D. in Computer Science from the University of New Mexico in 1997. He previously worked for 10 years in the research laboratories of Texas Instruments where he published in the areas of genetic algorithms, neural networks, computer aided design of integrated circuits, and computer architecture.

**Dr. Stephanie Forrest** is an Associate Professor of Computer Science at the University of New Mexico in Albuquerqe and a member of the External Faculty at the Santa Fe Institute. She received M.S. and Ph.D. degrees in Computer Science from the University of Michigan, Ann Arbor (1982,1985), and the B.A. degree from St. John's College, Annapolis MD and Santa Fe, NM (1977). She has edited two collections of scientific papers, is the author of a book on classifier systems, and has published numerous scientific papers in the area of parallel adaptive systems, including genetic algorithms, classifier systems, emergent computation, computational immunology, and computer security.

**Dr. Alan S. Perelson** is head of the Theoretical Biology and Biophysics Group at Los Alamos National Laboratory and director of the Theoretical Immunology Program at the Santa Fe Institute. His interests are in the application of mathematical modeling to problems in immunology and medicine.

# Estimating and Predicting the Number of Free HIV and T Cells by Nonlinear Kalman Filter

Wai-Yuan Tan and Zhihua Xiang

Department of Mathematical Sciences
The University of Memphis, Memphis, TN 38152, USA

**Abstract.** To estimate and to predict the number of free HIV and T cells in HIV-infected individuals, in this chapter we have developed some state space models for the HIV pathogenesis at the cellular level involving free HIV and different types of T cells. In these state space models, the stochastic system model is the stochastic model of the HIV pathogenesis expressed in terms of stochastic differential equations whereas the observation model is a statistic model based either on the observed RNA virus copies per unit volume of blood at different times or on the observed total numbers of $CD4^+$ T-cell counts per $mm^3$ at different times or on both of these observed numbers depending on which data sets are available. These are continuous time-discrete time Kalman filter models. Furthermore, the stochastic system equations are non-linear. For these models we have developed procedures for estimating and predicting the numbers of different types of T cells and free HIV through quadratic Kalman filter method and extended Kalman filter method. As an illustration, we have applied the methods of this chapter to a patient given in [1] treated by a protease inhibitor with observed RNA virus copies per unit volume of blood at 15 occasions within two weeks since treatment. For this patient, it is shown that in two weeks since treatment, most of the free HIV are non-infectious; further the Kalman filter estimates have revealed a much stronger effect within the first 10 days after treatment than that detected by the deterministic method.

## 1 Introduction

The HIV pathogenesis evolves by the infection of normal $CD4^+$ T cells by free HIV, leading to eventual depletion of $CD4^+$ T cells. As shown by Ho et al [2] and Wei et al [3], this is a highly dynamic process; the turnover of free HIV and HIV-infected $CD4^+$ T cells are both rapid and continuous since both the free HIV and the actively HIV-infected $CD4^+$ T cells are short lived. Thus, as shown by Ho [4], the $CD4^+$ T-cell depletion seen in AIDS is primarily a consequence of the destruction of these cells induced by HIV, not the lack of their production. Ho [4] has concluded that continuous, high-level replication of HIV is the engine that drives the pathogenesis of HIV infection. For better understanding and for monitoring the progression of the HIV pathogenesis, it is therefore important to estimate the number of free HIV and T cells over the time span in HIV-infected individuals. For this purpose, in this paper we will illustrate how to develop state space models for the HIV pathogenesis in HIV-infected individuals. The importance of estimating the number of free

HIV over time has further been underlined by studies in [5] and [6] who have confirmed that the number of free HIV can provide quite reasonable prediction of the status and severity of the disease.

In Section 2, we will describe how to derive stochastic models for the HIV pathogenesis at the cellular level in HIV-infected individuals by taking into account basic mechanisms of the HIV pathogenesis. Using results from Section 2, in Section 3 we will derive some state space models for HIV pathogenesis at the cellular level in HIV-infected individuals using data from RNA virus copies or from $CD4^+$ T cell counts . As an application of our models, in Section 4 we will apply the results of our model to a patient (patient No. 104) treated by a protease inhibitor given in [1]. In Section 5, we will generate some Monte Carlo studies to assess the efficiency and usefulness of the Kalman filter methods. Finally in Section 6, we will draw some conclusions and discuss some relevant issues regarding state space models.

## 2 A Stochastic Model of the HIV Pathogenesis

To model the HIV pathogenesis in HIV-infected individuals, let $T(t), T^{(*)}(t)$ and $V(t)$ be the numbers of normal $CD4^+$ T cells, actively HIV-infected $CD4^+$ T cells and free HIV at time t respectively. Under treatment by anti-viral drugs, then the free HIV is divided into non-infectious free HIV ($V_0$), sensitive infectious free HIV ($V_1$) and resistant free HIV ($V_2$) so that $V(t) = V_0(t) + V_1(t) + V_2(t)$, where $V_i(t)$ denotes the number of $V_i$ free HIV at time t respectively ($i = 0, 1, 2$). Further, the $T^{(*)}$ cells are divided into $\{T_j^{(*)}, j = 1, 2\}$ cells, where the $T_j^{(*)}$ cells are the actively infected $CD4^+$ T cells which were infected by the $V_j$ free HIV (j=1,2). Ignoring the latently infected T cells as it has little impacts on the total number of free HIV (see Remark 1 and [1]), in this section we will illustrate how to derive stochastic models for these processes.

For simplicity, in this preliminary research we will only consider the situation in which a protease inhibitor is applied, leaving the more general cases to our future research. To model development of drug resistance, we further let $V_1(a)$ denote the $V_1$ which have been exposed for a time period "$a$" to the drug treatment and let $V_1(t, a)$ be the number of free $V_1(a)$ at time t. Since the life span of free HIV is very short ( about 6 to 12 hours, see [1]), with no loss of generality we will assume that $a$ is less than 5 days. Let $\xi(t)$ be the minimum of $t - t_0$ and 5 days, where $t_0$ is the starting time of drug treatment. Then, $V_1(t) = \int_0^{\xi(t)} V_1(t, a)da$ for $t \geq t_0$.

### 2.1 Biological Consideration

To develop models of HIV pathogenesis in HIV-infected individuals, we refer to the biological studies in [7]-[10] and the papers by Kirschner, Perelson and their associates ([11]-[15]) and by Schenzle [16]. We give the following relevant biological observations for deriving these models and illustrate how to model the random variables of the process:

(a) New normal uninfected CD4$^+$ T cells ( referred to as T cells ) are produced by precursor stem cells in the bone marrow. These cells move to the thymus to mature before flowing into the blood stream or other sites. In the absence of HIV, these cells are produced at constant rates; however, in the presence of free HIV, these rates are decreasing functions of the number of free HIV since free HIV can also infect the precursor stem cells ([7],[12], [15]). We will model this by a Poisson process ( a pure birth process ) with rate $s(t)$ as a decreasing function of the numbers of free HIV; see [12] and [15]. Let $S(t)$ be the number of T cells generated by this avenue during $(t, t+\Delta t]$. Then, to order $o(\Delta t)$, $S(t)$ is distributed as a Poisson variable with mean $s(t)\Delta t$. That is, $S(t) \mid V(t) \sim$Poisson with mean $s(t)\Delta t$. Following [12] and [15], we will assume $s(t)$ as $s(t) = s\theta/\{\theta + V_1(t) + V_2(t)\}$, unless otherwise stated.

(b) As demonstrated in ([12],[15],[17]-[19]), HIV can infect actively ( dividing ) T cells and are integrated into the genome of the host cell to become provirus. These infected T cells are referred to as the actively infected T cells (referred to as $T^{(*)}$ cells); these cells will release free HIV and normally will die upon releasing free HIV. Let $k(t)$ be the infection rate of $T$ cells by free HIV at time t. Then, given $T(t)$ T cells at time t, to order $o(\Delta t)$ the probability that a free HIV will infect a T cell during $(t, t + \Delta t]$ is $k(t)T(t)dt + o(\Delta t)$. To specify $k(t)$, let $\delta(t)$ be the proportion of dividing T cells at time t, $N_I(t)$ the total number of cells which HIV can infect at time t other than dividing T cells and $\chi(t)$ the probability that the HIV will successfully infect the T cell given that the HIV has attached to this T cell. Then, under law of random mass interaction, the probability that a free HIV will infect a T cell during $(t, t+\Delta t]$ is, to order $o(\Delta t)$, $\chi(t)\frac{\delta(t)T(t)}{\delta(t)T(t)+N_I(t)}dt$ so that $k(t) = \chi(t)\frac{\delta(t)}{\delta(t)T(t)+N_I(t)}$. It follows that $k(t)$ is usually very small.

Remark 1: As demonstrated in [12], [15] and [17]-[19], HIV can also infect resting ( non-dividing ) T cells. However, when a free HIV infects a resting T cell, most of the viral DNA can not be integrated into the host genome and become extra chromosomal fragment in the cytoplasm of the cell [18]. These cells will not release HIV unless activated to become $T^{(*)}$ cells ([17]-[18]). However, since the extra chromosomal fragment will normally be lost, latently infected T cells will normally revert to normal T cells and will have little impact on the generation of free HIV ([1]). To model the HIV pathogenesis for estimating the number of free HIV, as in [1] we will thus ignore the pathway through the latently infected T cells.

(c) Because of the presence of antigen and HIV, $T$ cells are stimulated and activated to proliferate stochastically to generate new $T$ cells. On the other hand, the T cells have finite life span so that with positive probability they will die over the time span. Based on biological observations in [12] and [15] and studies in [20], we will model these processes by a stochastic birth and death process with a logistic birth rate $b_1(t) = \lambda(t)$ and with death rate $\mu_1(t)$, independently of the infection process, where $\lambda(t) = \gamma(t)\{1 - [T(t) + T^*(t)]/T_{Max}\}\frac{V(t)}{\theta_V + V(t)}$ with $T_{Max}$ being the maximum size for all $T$ and $T^{(*)}$ cells. Let $B_1(t)$ be the number of $T$ cells generated by proliferation through stimulation and activation by antigens and free HIV during $(t, t + \Delta t]$ and $D_1(t)$ the number of death of $T$ cells during $(t, t+\Delta t]$. Then, to order $o(\Delta t)$, $\{B_1(t), D_1(t)\} \mid [V(t), T(t), T^{(*)}(t)] \sim$Multinomial$\{T(t); \lambda(t)\Delta t, \mu_1(t)\Delta t\}$.

(d) One may assume that the $T^{(*)}$ cells would not proliferate by activation because the $T^{(*)}$ cells are short lived and will die upon activation ([1], [2], [12], [15]). On the other hand, as the $T$ cells, the $T^{(*)}$ cells and free HIV have finite life span so that with positive probability they will die over the time span. Because of cytopathic effects or apoptosis ( [12], [15], [17]-[19], [21] ), the $T^{(*)}$ cells are short lived with life span much shorter than that of the T cells. ( Or equivalently, the death rate of the $T^{(*)}$ cells is much greater than that of the $T$ cells (10 fold greater, see [1]-[3]).) Similarly, it has been documented that the free HIV are short lived and with life span shorter than that of the $T^{(*)}$ cells ( The average life span of free HIV is 0.3 days; see ([1]-[3]). Furthermore, the HIV viral clearance rate is not affected by disease status although advanced disease is associated with higher virus load ([2]-[4]).

(e) When a $T^{(*)}$ cell dies at time $t$, it will release $N(t)$ free HIV virus. In this preliminary study we will assume $N(t)$ as a deterministic function of $t$, ignoring possible random variation of this quantity. In our future work we will extend our model to general cases in which $N(t)$ will be assumed as a random variable following some probability distribution. We note from some Monte Carlo studies by Tan and Ye [22], however, that although randomness of $N(t)$ will increase the variance of the random noises, the trend, the dynamic and the conclusions are not affected by this assumption.

(f) At the current time, there are two categories of anti-viral drugs. One group attacks the virus by blocking the reverse transcription from RNA to DNA inside the $T_4$ cells to reduce the infection rate of T cells by free HIV. AZT, DDC and DDI are examples of this type of drugs. Another group attacks the HIV through its inhibition of protease to reduce the generation rate of infectious free HIV at the death of $T^{(*)}$ cells ( The newly generated free HIV become non-infectious. ). This latter group of drugs are called protease inhibitors. Thus, under treatment by Category 1 drugs, the attacked HIV are defective in reverse transcriptase so that they can not successfully infect the

$T$ cells; however, the damaged free HIV can still enter the $T$ cells so that they are removed from the pool of free HIV. On the other hand, under treatment by protease inhibitors, most of the released free HIV by the death of the $T^{(*)}$ cells are non-infectious. In this paper, for simplicity we will only consider the case in which a protease inhibitor is applied, leaving the general cases to our future work.

(g) Upon prolonged treatment, as observed by [23]-[27], $V_1$ HIV will mutate to become $V_2$ HIV through gene mutation but not vice versa. Further, the mutation rate from $V_1 \longrightarrow V_2$ depends on the time interval since exposure of $V_1$ to drug treatment. To model this, we let $m(a)$ be the mutation rate of $V_1(a) \longrightarrow V_2$. Then, during $(t, t+\Delta t]$, the probability that a free $V_1(a)$ HIV will mutate to a $V_2$ is, to order $o(\Delta t)$, $m(a)dt + o(\Delta t)$.

(h) Given $\boldsymbol{X}_t$, conditionally the above processes are assumed to be independently distributed of one another.

## 2.2 Derivation of Stochastic Differential Equations

To derive stochastic differential equations for the above model, consider the time interval $(t, t+\Delta t]$. Let $F_1(t,a)$ be the number of new $T_1^{(*)}$ cells generated by the infection of dividing $T$ cells by $V_1(a)$ free HIV during $(t, t+\Delta t]$ and $F_2(t)$ the number of new $T_2^{(*)}$ cells generated by the infection of dividing $T$ cells by $V_2$ free HIV during $(t, t+\Delta t]$ respectively. Let $M(t,a)$ be the number of new $V_2$ free HIV generated by mutation from $V_1(a)$ free HIV during $(t, t+\Delta t]$ and $\omega(t)$ the average proportion of $V_0$ free HIV ( non-infectious free HIV ) released by the death of a $T_1^{(*)}$ cell at time t. Let $D_{Vi}(t)$ be the number of death of $V_i$ free HIV (i=0, 2) during $(t, t+\Delta t]$, $D_{V1}(t,a)$ the number of death of $V_1(a)$ free HIV during $(t, t+\Delta t]$ and $D_2^{(j)}(t)$ the number of death of $T_j^{(*)}$ cells (j=1,2) during $(t, t+\Delta t]$ respectively. Then, the numbers of $\{T(t+\Delta t), T_j^{(*)}(t+\Delta t), j=1,2, V_i(t+\Delta t), i=0,2, V_1(t+\Delta t, 0), V_1(t+\Delta t, a+\Delta t), \xi(t) \geq a > 0\}$ can be expressed by the following stochastic equations:

$$T(t+\Delta t) = T(t) + S(t) + B_1(t) - F_1(t) - F_2(t) - D_1(t), \tag{1}$$

$$T_j^{(*)}(t+\Delta t) = T_j^{(*)}(t) + F_j(t) - D_2^{(j)}(t), \; (j=1,2), \tag{2}$$

$$V_0(t+\Delta t) = V_0(t) + \omega(t)N(t)D_2^{(1)}(t) - D_{V0}(t), \tag{3}$$

$$V_1(t+\Delta t, 0) = [1-\omega(t)]N(t)D_2^{(1)}(t), \tag{4}$$

$$V_1(t+\Delta t, a+\Delta t) = V_1(t,a) - F_1(t,a) - M(t,a) - D_{V1}(t,a), a > 0, \tag{5}$$

$$V_2(t+\Delta t) = V_2(t) + N(t)D_2^{(2)}(t) + M(t) - F_2(t) - D_{V2}(t), \tag{6}$$

where $\{S(t), B_1(t), D_1(t)\}$ are defined in the above subsection and where with $\xi(t)$ =minimum of $t - t_0$ and 5 days, $F_1(t) = \int_0^{\xi(t)} F_1(t,a)da$ and $M(t) = \int_0^{\xi(t)} M(t,a)da$.

In the above equations all quantities are assumed to be random variables. As discussed in the above subsection, the conditional probability distributions of these variables given $\boldsymbol{X}_t = \{T(t), T_j^{(*)}(t), j = 1,2, V_i(t), i = 0,2, V_1(t,0), V_1(t,a), \xi(t) \geq a > 0\}$ can be summarized as follows:

- $S(t) \mid V(t) \sim$Poisson with mean $s(t)\Delta t$;
- $M(t,a) \mid V_1(t,a) \sim$Binomial$[V_1(t,a); m(a)\Delta t], a > 0$;
- $\boldsymbol{G}(t,a) = \{F_1(t,a), D_{V1}(t,a)\} \mid \{V_1(t,a), T(t)\} \sim$Multinomial$[V_1(t,a); k(t)T(t)\Delta t, \mu_V(t)\Delta t], \xi(t) \geq a > 0$;
- $\boldsymbol{G}_2(t) = \{F_2(t), D_{V2}(t)\} \mid \{V_2(t), T(t)\} \sim$Multinomial$[V_2(t); k(t)T(t)\Delta t, \mu_V(t)\Delta t]$;
- $\boldsymbol{M}_1(t) = \{B_1(t), D_1(t)\} \mid T(t) \sim$Multinomial $[T(t), \lambda(t)\Delta t, \mu_1(t)\Delta t]$;
- $D_2^{(j)}(t) \mid T_j^{(*)}(t) \sim$Binomial$[T_j^{(*)}(t); \mu_2(t)\Delta t]$;
- $D_{V0}(t) \mid V_0(t) \sim$Binomial$[V_0(t), \mu_V(t)\Delta t]$;

where $\lambda(t) = \gamma(t)\{1 - [T(t) + \sum_{j=1}^{2} T_j^{(*)}(t)]/T_{\max}\}\frac{V(t)}{\theta_V + V(t)}$, $V(t) = V_0(t) + V_1(t) + V_2(t)$. Further, given $\boldsymbol{X}_t$, $S(t), M(t,a), \boldsymbol{G}(t,a), \boldsymbol{G}_2(t), \boldsymbol{M}_1(t), D_2^{(j)}(t)$, $j = 1,2$ and $D_{V0}(t)$ are independently distributed of one another.

Let $\boldsymbol{\varepsilon}_t = [\varepsilon_1(t), \varepsilon_2^{(j)}(t), j = 1,2, \varepsilon_3(t), \varepsilon_4(t,0), \varepsilon_4(t,a), \xi(t) \geq a > 0, \varepsilon_5(t)]^T$, where

$$\begin{aligned}\varepsilon_1(t)\Delta t = [S(t) - s(t)\Delta t] + [B_1(t) - \lambda(t)T(t)\Delta t] - \sum_{i=1}^{2}[F_i(t) \\ - k(t)T(t)V_i(t)\Delta t] - [D_1(t) - \mu_1(t)T(t)\Delta t];\end{aligned}$$

$$\varepsilon_2^{(j)}(t)\Delta t = [F_j(t) - k(t)V_j(t)T(t)\Delta t] - [D_2^{(j)}(t) - \mu_2(t)T_j^{(*)}(t)\Delta t];$$

$$\varepsilon_3(t)\Delta t = \omega(t)N(t)[D_2^{(1)}(t) - T_1^{(*)}(t)\mu_2(t)\Delta t] - [D_{V0}(t) - \mu_V(t)V_0(t)\Delta t];$$

$$\varepsilon_4(t,0)\Delta t = [1 - \omega(t)]N(t)[D_2^{(1)}(t) - T_1^{(*)}(t)\mu_2(t)\Delta t];$$

$$\begin{aligned}\varepsilon_4(t,a)\Delta t = -[F_1(t,a) - k(t)T(t)V_1(t,a)\Delta t] - [M(t,a) - m(a)V_1(t,a)\Delta t] \\ - [D_{V1}(t,a) - \mu_V(t)V_1(t,a)\Delta t], \xi(t) \geq a > 0;\end{aligned}$$

$$\begin{aligned}\varepsilon_5(t)\Delta t = N(t)[D_2^{(2)}(t) - T_2^{(*)}(t)\mu_2(t)\Delta t] + [M(t) - \int_0^{\xi(t)} m(a)V_1(t,a)da\Delta t] \\ - [F_2(t) - k(t)T(t)V_2(t)\Delta t] - [D_{V2}(t) - \mu_V(t)V_2(t)\Delta t].\end{aligned}$$

Then, denoting by $\frac{d}{dt}Z(t) = \lim_{\Delta t \longrightarrow 0} \frac{Z(t+\Delta t)-Z(t)}{\Delta t}$, equations (1)-(6) are equivalent to the following stochastic differential equations:

$$\frac{d}{dt}T(t) = s(t) + \lambda(t)T(t) - T(t)\{\mu_1(t) + k(t)[V_1(t) + V_2(t)]\} + \varepsilon_1(t), \quad (7)$$

$$\frac{d}{dt}T_j^{(*)}(t) = k(t)V_j(t)T(t) - T_j^{(*)}(t)\mu_2(t) + \varepsilon_2^{(j)}(t), j = 1, 2, \quad (8)$$

$$\frac{d}{dt}V_0(t) = \omega(t)N(t)T_1^{(*)}(t)\mu_2(t) - V_0(t)\mu_V(t) + \varepsilon_3(t), \quad (9)$$

$$\frac{d}{dt}V_1(t, 0) = [1 - \omega(t)]N(t)T_1^{(*)}\mu_2(t) + \varepsilon_4(t, 0), \quad (10)$$

$$\begin{aligned}(\frac{\partial}{\partial t} + \frac{\partial}{\partial a})V_1(t, a) &= -\{m(a) + k(t)T(t) + \mu_V(t)\}V_1(t, a) \\ &+ \varepsilon_4(t, a), \xi(t) \geq a > 0, \quad (11)\end{aligned}$$

$$\begin{aligned}\frac{d}{dt}V_2(t) &= N(t)\mu_2(t)T_2^{(*)}(t) + \int_0^{\xi(t)} m(a)V_1(t, a)da \\ &- k(t)V_2(t)T(t) - \mu_V(t)V_2(t) + \varepsilon_5(t), \quad (12)\end{aligned}$$

If drug resistance has not yet been developed by time $t_N$, then for $t \leq t_N$, $V_2(t) = 0$ and $T_2^{(*)}(t) = 0$. In the absence of drug resistance, we will write $T_1^{(*)}(t) = T^{(*)}(t)$ and let $m(a) = 0$. Then the above equations (7)-(12) reduce to:

$$\frac{d}{dt}T(t) = s(t) + \lambda(t)T(t) - T(t)[\mu_1(t) + k(t)V_1(t)] + \varepsilon_1(t), \quad (13)$$

$$\frac{d}{dt}T^{(*)}(t) = k(t)V_1(t)T(t) - T^{(*)}(t)\mu_2(t) + \varepsilon_2(t), \quad (14)$$

$$\frac{d}{dt}V_0(t) = \omega(t)N(t)T^{(*)}(t)\mu_2(t) - V_0(t)\mu_V(t) + \varepsilon_3, \quad (15)$$

$$\begin{aligned}\frac{d}{dt}V_1(t) &= [1 - \omega(t)]N(t)T^{(*)}(t)\mu_2(t) - \{k(t)T(t) \\ &+ \mu_V(t)\}V_1(t) + \varepsilon_4(t), \quad (16)\end{aligned}$$

In equations (7)-(12), given $\boldsymbol{X}_t$, the random noises $\boldsymbol{\varepsilon}_t = \{\varepsilon_1(t), \varepsilon_2^{(i)}(t), i = 1, 2, \varepsilon_3(t), \varepsilon_4(t, a), \xi(t) \geq a \geq 0, \varepsilon_5(t)\}$ have expectation zero. It follows that the expected value of $\boldsymbol{\varepsilon}_t$ is $\mathbf{0}$. Using the basic formulas $\text{Cov}(X, Y) = \text{E}\{\text{Cov}[(X, Y)|Z]\} + \text{Cov}[\text{E}(X|Z), \text{E}(Y|Z)]$, it is also obvious that elements of

$\boldsymbol{\varepsilon}_t$ are uncorrelated with elements of $\boldsymbol{X}_t$. Further, the variances and covariances of elements of $\boldsymbol{\varepsilon}_t$ are easily obtained as, to order $o(\Delta t)$:

$$
\begin{aligned}
&\mathrm{VAR}[\varepsilon_1(t)] = \mathrm{E}\{s(t) + \lambda(t)T(t) + [\mu_1(t) + k(t)(V_1(t) + V_2(t))]T(t)\}, \\
&\mathrm{COV}[\varepsilon_1(t), \varepsilon_2^{(j)}(t)] = -k(t)\mathrm{E}[V_j(t)T(t)] \ (j = 1, 2), \\
&\mathrm{COV}[\varepsilon_1(t), \varepsilon_3(t)] = \mathrm{COV}[\varepsilon_1(t), \varepsilon_4(0, t)] = 0, \\
&\mathrm{COV}[\varepsilon_1(t), \varepsilon_4(a, t)] = k(t)\mathrm{E}[V_1(a, t)T(t)](a > 0), \\
&\mathrm{COV}[\varepsilon_1(t), \varepsilon_5(t)] = k(t)\mathrm{E}[V_2(t)T(t)], \\
&\mathrm{VAR}[\varepsilon_2^{(j)}(t)] = \mathrm{E}[k(t)V_j(t)T(t) + \mu_2(t)T_2^{(*)}(t)] \ (j = 1, 2), \\
&\mathrm{COV}[\varepsilon_2^{(1)}(t), \varepsilon_3(t)] = -\omega(t)N(t)\mathrm{E}[T_1^{(*)}(t)], \\
&\mathrm{COV}[\varepsilon_2^{(1)}(t), \varepsilon_4(0, t)] = -[1 - \omega(t)]N(t)\mathrm{E}[T_1^{(*)}(t)], \\
&\mathrm{COV}[\varepsilon_2^{(1)}(t), \varepsilon_4(a, t)] = -k(t)\mathrm{E}[V_1(a, t)T(t)], \\
&\mathrm{COV}[\varepsilon_2^{(1)}(t), \varepsilon_2^{(2)}(t)] = \mathrm{COV}[\varepsilon_2^{(2)}(t), \varepsilon_3(t)] \\
&\qquad\qquad = \mathrm{COV}[\varepsilon_2^{(2)}(t), \varepsilon_4(b, t)] = 0 \ (b \geq 0), \\
&\mathrm{COV}[\varepsilon_2^{(1)}(t), \varepsilon_5(t)] = 0, \\
&\mathrm{COV}[\varepsilon_2^{(2)}(t), \varepsilon_5(t)] = -k(t)\mathrm{E}[V_2(t)T(t)] - N(t)\mu_2(t)ET_2^{(*)}(t), \\
&\mathrm{VAR}[\varepsilon_3(t)] = \omega^2(t)N^2(t)\mu_2(t)\mathrm{E}T_1^{(*)}(t), \\
&\mathrm{COV}[\varepsilon_4(0, t), \varepsilon_3(t)] = \omega(t)[1 - \omega(t)]N^2(t)\mu_2(t)\mathrm{E}[T_1^{(*)}(t)], \\
&\mathrm{COV}[\varepsilon_4(a, t), \varepsilon_3(t)] = \mathrm{COV}[\varepsilon_3(t), \varepsilon_5(t)] = 0(a > 0, \\
&\mathrm{VAR}[\varepsilon_4(0, t)] = [1 - \omega(t)]^2 N^2(t)\mu_2(t)\mathrm{E}T_1^{(*)}(t), \\
&\mathrm{VAR}[\varepsilon_4(a, t)] = \mathrm{E}\{[k(t)T(t) + \mu_V(t) + m(a)]V_1(a, t)\}(a > 0), \\
&\mathrm{COV}[\varepsilon_4(a_1, t), \varepsilon_4(a_2, t)] = \mathrm{COV}[\varepsilon_4(0, t), \varepsilon_5(t)] = 0(a_1 \neq a_2, a_j \geq 0), \\
&\mathrm{VAR}[\varepsilon_5(t)] = N^2(t)\mu_2(t)ET_2^{(*)}(t) + \int_0^{\xi(t)} m(a)\mathrm{E}[V_1(a, t)]da \\
&\qquad\qquad + \mathrm{E}\{[\mu_V(t) + k(t)T(t)]V_2(t)\}, \\
&\mathrm{COV}[\varepsilon_4(a, t), \varepsilon_5(t)] = -m(a)\mathrm{E}[V_1(a, t)] \ (a > 0).
\end{aligned}
$$

## 3 A State Space Model for the HIV Pathogenesis

The state space model (Kalman filter model) consists of the stochastic system model which is the stochastic model of the system and the observation model which is a statistical model based on available observed data from the system. Hence the state space model adds one more dimension to the stochastic system model and to the statistical model by combining both of these models into one model; it takes into account the basic mechanisms of the system and the random variation of the system through its stochastic system model and incorporate all these into the observed data from the system. Thus the state space model is superior to both the stochastic model and the statistic model since it combines information and advantages from both of these models. The major theme of the state space model is to derive optimal estimates of the sample path and the future trajectories of the stochastic process (i.e. the stochastic state variables) by combining information from the stochastic model with the observation model based on available observed data from the system.

For the state space model of the HIV pathogenesis in the HIV- infected individuals as described in Section 2, the stochastic system model is given by the stochastic differential equations given in equations (7)-(12) whereas the observation model is either based on the number of RNA virus copies per unit volume of blood over time or on the total number of $CD4^+$ T cell counts per $mm^3$ over time or on both depending on which data sets are available. To illustrate, suppose that the total number of RNA virus copies ( or $CD4^+$ T cell counts ) per $mm^3$ have been measured over the time span. Let $Y_j$ be the observed total number of RNA virus copies ( or $CD4^+$ T cell counts ) per $mm^3$ at time $t_j, j = 1, \ldots, n$. Then, based on the observed data of the number of RNA virus copies, the equations of the observation model of the Kalman Filter is given by:

$$Y_j = [\sum_{i=0}^{2} V_i(t_j)] + e_j = V(t_j) + e_j; j = 1, \ldots, n \tag{17}$$

where $e_j$ is the random measurement error associated with measuring $Y_j$. ( Replace $V(t_j) = \sum_{i=0}^{2} V_i(t_j)$ by $T(t_j) + \sum_{i=1}^{2} T_i^{(*)}(t_j)$ if $Y_j$ is the number of the observed data of $CD4^+$ T cell counts per $mm^3$.) As usual, $e_j$ is assumed as independently distributed normal variables with means 0 and variance $\sigma_j^2$. One may also assume that the $e_j$'s are independently distributed of the random noises $\varepsilon(l)$'s of the stochastic system equations.

The above state space model has continuous time stochastic system equations and discrete time observation equations. Further, while the observation equations are linear, the stochastic system equations are nonlinear. To make the problem even more complicated, the stochastic system equations involve a two dimensional stochastic partial differential equation. For such state space models, general theories are non-existent and remain to be developed. To derive some basic theories, one approach is to discretize the time and age variables to approximate the stochastic system equations by stochastic difference equations. This is the approach adopted by Tan and Zhang [28] to derive approximate results for some cases involving anti-viral treatment and drug resistance. When the time elapsed since treatment is not very long, however, one may expect that drug resistance has not yet been developed. This is the case with the studies in [1]. Since we will use as an illustrative example a case study in [1], in this preliminary report we will assume that during the time interval of study, drug resistance has not yet developed. Then the stochastic system equations in the state space model is given by equations (13)-(16). In what follows, we will thus assume these equations as the stochastic system equations, unless otherwise stated.

### 3.1 The Quadratic Kalman Filter Method

In the stochastic system equations given by (13)-(16), aside from the term involving $s(t)$ in equation (13), the equations are basically quadratic. Furthermore, since the number of free HIV for the time period since treatment is usually very large, $s(t)$ can be closely approximated by first order Taylor series approximation. In this section we will thus proceed to derive some basic results for state space models with quadratic stochastic system models and linear observation models.

To proceed, consider the state space model with system equations given by (A) and with observation equations given by (B).

(A) System Equations:

$$\frac{d}{dt}\underset{\sim}{X}(t) = \underset{\sim}{a}(t) + B(t)\underset{\sim}{X}(t) + \underset{\sim}{R}(\underset{\sim}{X}(t)\underset{\sim}{X}^T(t)) + \underset{\sim}{\epsilon}(t), \tag{18}$$

where $\underset{\sim}{a}(t)$ and $\underset{\sim}{B}(t)$ are non-stochastic and $\underset{\sim}{\epsilon}(t)$ is the vector of random noises and where $\underset{\sim}{R}(\underset{\sim}{X}(t)\underset{\sim}{X}^T(t))$ is a column vector with the $i$th element given by $\underset{\sim}{X}^T(t)\boldsymbol{R}_i\underset{\sim}{X}(t) = tr\{\boldsymbol{R}_i\underset{\sim}{X}(t)\underset{\sim}{X}^T(t)\}$ ($\boldsymbol{R}_i$ *symmetric*).

(B) Observation Equations:

$$\underset{\sim}{Y}(t_j) = \underset{\sim}{Y}(j) = H(j)\underset{\sim}{X}(t_j) + \underset{\sim}{e}(j) \tag{19}$$

where $H(j)$ is non-stochastic and $\underset{\sim}{e}(j)$ the vector of random disturbances from measurement errors associated with measuring $Y(t_j)$.

In the above equations, it is assumed that $E\underset{\sim}{\epsilon}(t) = \underset{\sim}{0}$, $E\underset{\sim}{e}(j) = \underset{\sim}{0}$, $Var[\underset{\sim}{\epsilon}(t)] = V_X(t)$, $Var[\underset{\sim}{e}(j)] = \Sigma_j$, $Cov[\underset{\sim}{\epsilon}(t), \underset{\sim}{e}(j)] = 0$ and $\underset{\sim}{\epsilon}(t)$ and $\underset{\sim}{e}(j)$ are uncorrelated with $\underset{\sim}{X}(\tau)$ for all $t, j, \tau$.

Given the above setup, in this section we proceed to derive the estimator or predictor of $\underset{\sim}{X}(t)$ and the covariance matrix of the residuals by assuming Gaussian distributions for $\underset{\sim}{\epsilon}(t)$ and $\underset{\sim}{e}(j)$. The Gaussian assumption for the random noises is justified by results in [29] which showed that under steady state conditions, the random noises can be closely approximated by Gaussian distributions. Note that under Gaussian distributions, the maximum likelihood estimators are identical to nonlinear least square estimators. To derive these estimators, put:

- For $t_j \le t < t_{j+1}, j = 0, 1, \ldots,$
  $\hat{\underset{\sim}{X}}(t|t_j)$ =The L.S. estimator ( or predictor ) of $\underset{\sim}{X}(t)$ given data $\{\underset{\sim}{Y}(l), l = 1, \ldots, j\}$,
- $\hat{\underset{\sim}{\epsilon}}(t|j) = \hat{\underset{\sim}{X}}(t|t_j) - \underset{\sim}{X}(t)$ and $\hat{\underset{\sim}{e}}(j|j) = \hat{\underset{\sim}{X}}(t_j|t_j) - \underset{\sim}{X}(t_j)$ with $Var[\hat{\underset{\sim}{\epsilon}}(t|j)] = Q(t|j)$ and $Var[\hat{\underset{\sim}{e}}(j|j)] = P(j|j)$,
- At time $t_0 = 0$, let $\hat{\underset{\sim}{X}}(0) = \hat{\underset{\sim}{X}}(0|0)$ be an estimator of $\underset{\sim}{X}(0)$ satisfying $E\hat{\underset{\sim}{X}}(0|0) = E\underset{\sim}{X}(0)$ and $Var[\hat{\underset{\sim}{e}}(0|0)|\underset{\sim}{X}(0)] = P(0) = P(0|0)$.

To derive the L.S. estimator of $\underset{\sim}{X}(t)$, approximate the system equations by:

$$\underset{\sim}{X}(t+dt) \approx \underset{\sim}{a}(t)dt + [I + B(t)dt]\underset{\sim}{X}(t) + \underset{\sim}{R}(\underset{\sim}{X}(t)\underset{\sim}{X}^T(t))dt + \int_t^{t+dt} \underset{\sim}{\epsilon}(u)du \tag{20}$$

Since the random noises are Gaussian, given data $\{\underset{\sim}{Y}(l), l = 1, \ldots, j,\}$, $\underset{\sim}{X}(t+dt)$ is then Gaussian with conditional mean $\hat{\underset{\sim}{X}}(t+dt|t_j) \approx \underset{\sim}{a}(t)dt + [I + B(t)dt]\hat{\underset{\sim}{X}}(t|t_j) + \underset{\sim}{R}(\hat{\underset{\sim}{X}}(t|t_j)\hat{\underset{\sim}{X}}^T(t|t_j))dt + \underset{\sim}{R}(Q(t|t_j))dt$. The conditional covariance matrix of $\hat{\underset{\sim}{X}}(t+dt|t_j)$ given data $\{\underset{\sim}{Y}(l), l = 1, \ldots, j,\}$ and given $\underset{\sim}{X}(t+dt)$ is $Q(t|t_j)$. It follows that the L.S. estimator $\hat{\underset{\sim}{X}}(t|t_j)$ of $\underset{\sim}{X}(t)$ given data $\{\underset{\sim}{Y}(l), l = 1, \ldots, j,\}$ satisfies the equation

$$\frac{d}{dt}\hat{\underset{\sim}{X}}(t|t_j) = \underset{\sim}{a}(t) + B(t)\hat{\underset{\sim}{X}}(t|t_j) + \underset{\sim}{R}(\hat{\underset{\sim}{X}}(t|t_j)\hat{\underset{\sim}{X}}^T(t|t_j)) + \underset{\sim}{R}(Q(t|t_j)) \tag{21}$$

with boundary condition $\lim_{t \longrightarrow t_{j+1}} \hat{\underset{\sim}{X}}(t|t_j) = \hat{\underset{\sim}{X}}(t_{j+1}|t_j) = \hat{\underset{\sim}{u}}(j+1|j)$ Furthermore, for $t_{j+1} - t_j = ndt$ and $0 \leq i < n$, $\hat{\underset{\sim}{X}}(t + (i+1)dt|t_j) \approx \underset{\sim}{a}(t + i\,dt)dt + [I + B(t + i\,dt)dt]\hat{\underset{\sim}{X}}(t + i\,dt|t_j) + \underset{\sim}{R}(\hat{\underset{\sim}{X}}(t + i\,dt|t_j)\hat{\underset{\sim}{X}}^T(t + i\,dt|t_j))dt + \underset{\sim}{R}(Q(t + i\,dt|t_j))dt$.

To derive formula for $Q(t|t_j)$, observe that the conditional residuals at time $t+\Delta t$ are given by $\hat{\underset{\sim}{\epsilon}}(t+\Delta t|j) = \hat{\underset{\sim}{X}}(t+\Delta t|t_j) - \underset{\sim}{X}(t+\Delta t) \approx \{I + [B(t) + 2C(t)]\Delta t\}\hat{\underset{\sim}{\epsilon}}(t|j) + \underset{\sim}{R}(Q(t|t_j))\Delta t + \underset{\sim}{R}(\hat{\underset{\sim}{\epsilon}}(t|j)\hat{\underset{\sim}{\epsilon}}^T(t|j))\Delta t - \int_t^{t+\Delta t} \underset{\sim}{\epsilon}(x)dx$, where $C(t)$ is a symmetric matrix with $i$th row being given by $\hat{\underset{\sim}{X}}^T(t|t_j)\boldsymbol{R}_i$. Since the random noises are Gaussian, we have:

$$
\begin{aligned}
Q(t + \Delta t|t_j) \approx \{I + [B(t) + 2C(t)]\Delta t\}Q(t|t_j)\{I + [B(t) + 2C(t)]\Delta t\}^T \\
+ 2\Omega(t)\Delta t + \int_t^{t+\Delta t} V_X(u)du
\end{aligned}
$$

where $\Omega(t)$ is a symmetric matrix with the $(u, v)$th element being given by $tr\{\boldsymbol{R}_u Q(t|t_j)\boldsymbol{R}_v Q(t|t_j)\}$.

It follows that $Q(t|t_j)$ satisfies the equation

$$
\begin{aligned}
\frac{d}{dt}Q(t|t_j) &= \{I + [B(t) + 2C(t)]\}Q(t|t_j) \\
&+ Q(t|t_j)\{I + [B(t) + 2C(t)]\}^T + 2\Omega(t) + V_X(t), \qquad (22)
\end{aligned}
$$

with boundary condition $\lim_{t \longrightarrow t_{j+1}} Q(t|t_j) = Q(t_{j+1}|t_j) = P(j+1|j)$. Furthermore, for $t_{j+1} - t_j = ndt$ and $0 \leq i < n$, $Q(t + (i+1)\Delta t|t_j) \approx \{I + [B(t + i\,\Delta t) + 2C(t + i\,\Delta t)]\Delta t\}Q(t + i\,\Delta t|t_j)\{I + [B(t + i\,\Delta t) + 2C(t + i\,\Delta t)]\Delta t\}^T + 2\Omega(t + i\,\Delta t)\Delta t + \int_{t+i\,\Delta t}^{t+(i+1)\Delta t} V_X(u)du$.

From the above formula, given $\hat{\underset{\sim}{X}}(t_j|t_j) = \hat{\underset{\sim}{u}}(j|j)$ and $Q(t_j|t_j) = P(j|j)$, one may readily derive the L.S. forward estimator ( or predictor ) of $\underset{\sim}{X}(t)$ and $Q(t|t_j)$. To derive formula for computing $\hat{\underset{\sim}{u}}(j|j)$ and $P(j|j)$, let $\hat{\underset{\sim}{X}}(t_{j+1}|t_j) = \hat{\underset{\sim}{u}}(j+1|j)$ and $Q(t_{j+1}|t_j) = P(j+1|j)$. Since $\underset{\sim}{e}(j)$ is Gaussian, the conditional distribution of $\underset{\sim}{Y}(j+1)$ given data $\{\underset{\sim}{Y}(l), l = 1, \ldots, j\}$ is Gaussian with conditional mean $H(j+1)\hat{\underset{\sim}{u}}(j+1|j)$. The conditional covariance matrix of $\underset{\sim}{Y}(j+1)$ given data $\{\underset{\sim}{Y}(l), l = 1, \ldots, j\}$ and given $\underset{\sim}{X}(t_{j+1})$ is $H(j+1)P(j+$

$1|j)H^T(j+1)+\Sigma_{j+1}$. It follows that the conditional mean of $\underset{\sim}{X}(t_{j+1})$ given data $\{\underset{\sim}{Y}(l), l=1,\ldots,j+1\}$ is

$$\underset{\sim}{\hat{u}}(j+1|j+1) = \underset{\sim}{\hat{u}}(j+1|j) + K_{j+1}\{\underset{\sim}{Y}(j+1) - H(j+1)\underset{\sim}{\hat{u}}(j+1|j)\}$$

where

$$K_{j+1} = P(j+1|j)H^T(j+1)\{H(j+1)P(j+1|j)H^T(j+1)+\Sigma_{j+1}\}^{-1}$$

Furthermore, it can readily be shown that the covariance matrix of the residual $\underset{\sim}{\hat{e}}(j+1|j+1) = \underset{\sim}{\hat{X}}(t_{j+1}|t_{j+1}) - \underset{\sim}{X}(t_{j+1})$ is $\{I-K_{j+1}H(j+1)\}P(j+1|j)$ ( See [30] ).

The above formula for computing $\underset{\sim}{\hat{X}}(t|t_j)$ and $Q(t|t_j)$ are extensions of formula given in [30]. These are the forward filter procedures. For quadratic state space models, backward filtering and smoothing methods are not yet available and remain to be developed.

## 3.2 Extended Kalman Filter

In the system equations given by (13)-(16), the quadratic terms are mainly associated with $k(t)T(t)\triangle t$. Since $k(t)$ is usually very small, it is expected that these equations can be closely approximated by an extended Kalman filter model through first order Taylor series expansion. For the model given in Section 2, this is confirmed by some Monte Carlo studies given in Section 5.

To proceed, write the system model equations (13)-(16) and the observation model in (17) with $V_2(t)=0$ respectively as:

$$\frac{d}{dt}\underset{\sim}{X}(t) = \underset{\sim}{f}[\underset{\sim}{X}(t)] + \underset{\sim}{\epsilon}(t)$$

for $t_j \le t < t_{j+1}, j=0,1,\cdots,n$;

$$Y_j = H_j \underset{\sim}{X}(t_j) + e_j, \quad j=1,\cdots,n.$$

where $H_j = \{0,0,1,1\}$

Define the estimator (or predictor) $\underset{\sim}{\hat{X}}(t)$ as an unbiased estimator ( or predictor ) of $\underset{\sim}{X}(t)$ if $E\underset{\sim}{\hat{\epsilon}}(t) = 0$, where $\underset{\sim}{\hat{\epsilon}}(t) = \underset{\sim}{\hat{X}}(t) - \underset{\sim}{X}(t)$. Suppose that $\underset{\sim}{\hat{X}}(0)$ is unbiased for $\underset{\sim}{X}(0)$ and has covariance matrix $P(0)=P(0|0)$. Then, starting with $\underset{\sim}{\hat{X}}(0) = \underset{\sim}{\hat{X}}(0|0)$, the procedures given in the following two theorems provide close approximations to some optimal methods for estimating and predicting $\underset{\sim}{X}(t)$. The proof of these procedures is sketched in the appendix.

**Theorem (3.1):**

Assume the notations as in Section 3.1. Then, starting with $\hat{\underset{\sim}{X}}(0) = \hat{\underset{\sim}{u}}(0|0)$ with $P(0) = P(0|0)$, the linear, unbiased and minimum varianced estimators of $\underset{\sim}{X}(t)$ given data $(Y_u, u = 1, \cdots, j)$ $(j \leq n)$ are closely approximated by the following recursive equations:
(i) For $t_j \leq t < t_{j+1}$, $j = 0, 1, \cdots, n$ $(t_0 = 0, t_{n+1} = \infty)$, $\hat{\underset{\sim}{X}}(t|t_j)$ satisfies the following equations with boundary conditions

$$\lim_{t \to t_j} \hat{\underset{\sim}{X}}(t|t_j) = \hat{\underset{\sim}{X}}(t_j|t_j) = \hat{\underset{\sim}{u}}(j|j)$$

where $\hat{\underset{\sim}{u}}(j|j)$ is given in (iii):

$$\frac{d}{dt}\hat{\underset{\sim}{X}}(t|t_j) = \underset{\sim}{f}[\hat{\underset{\sim}{X}}(t|t_j)] \qquad t_j \leq t < t_{j+1}, j = 0, 1, \cdots, n;$$

(ii) For $t_j \leq t < t_{j+1}$, $j = 0, 1, \cdots, n$, the covariance matrix $Q(t|t_j)$ satisfies the following equations with boundary conditions

$$\lim_{t \to t_j} Q(t|t_j) = Q(t_j|t_j) = P(j|j)$$

where $P(j|j)$ is given in (iii):

$$\frac{d}{dt}Q(t|t_j) = F_j(t)Q(t|t_j) + Q(t|t_j)F_j^T(t) + V_X(t),$$

for $t_j \leq t < t_{j+1}, j = 0, 1, \cdots, n,$ where $F_j(t) = (\frac{\partial}{\partial \underset{\sim}{X}^T}\underset{\sim}{f}(\underset{\sim}{X}))_{\underset{\sim}{X} = \hat{\underset{\sim}{X}}(t|t_j)}$. and where $V_X(t)$ is the variance and covariance matrix of the random noises in the stochastic system equations.

(iii) Denote by $\hat{\underset{\sim}{u}}(j+1|j) = \lim_{t \to t_{j+1}} \hat{\underset{\sim}{X}}(t|t_j)$ from (i) and $P(j+1|j) = \lim_{t \to t_{j+1}} Q(t|t_j)$ from (ii). Then $\hat{\underset{\sim}{u}}(j+1\,|\,j+1)$ and $P(j+1|j+1)$ are given respectively by:

$$\hat{\underset{\sim}{u}}(j+1\,|\,j+1) = \hat{\underset{\sim}{u}}(j+1\,|\,j) + K_{j+1}\{Y_{j+1} - h[\hat{\underset{\sim}{u}}(j+1|j)]\},$$

and

$$P(j+1|j+1) = [I - K_{j+1}H_{j+1}]P(j+1\,|\,j),$$

where,

$$K_{j+1} = P(j+1\,|\,j)\,\underset{\sim}{H}_{j+1}[\underset{\sim}{H}^T_{j+1}P(j+1|\,j)\,\underset{\sim}{H}_{j+1} + \sigma_j^2]^{-1}$$

with $\sigma_j^2$ being the variance of $e_j$.

To implement the above procedure, one starts with $\hat{\underset{\sim}{X}}(0) = \hat{\underset{\sim}{u}}(0|0)$ and $P(0) = P(0|0)$. Then by (i) and (ii), one derives $\hat{X}(t|t_0)$ and $Q(t|t_0)$ for $t_0 \le t \le t_1$ and derives $\hat{\underset{\sim}{u}}(1\,|1)$ and $P(1|1)$ by (iii). Repeating these procedures one may derive $\hat{X}(t|t_j)$ and $Q(t|t_j)$ for $t_j \le t < t_{j+1}$, $j = 0, 1, \cdots, n$. These procedures are referred to as forward filtering procedures.

**Theorem (3.2):**

Let $\hat{\underset{\sim}{X}}(t|n)$ be an estimator of $\underset{\sim}{X}(t)$ given data $(Y_j, j = 1, \cdots, n)$. Let $Q(t|n)$ be the covariance matrix of $\hat{\underset{\sim}{\epsilon}}(t|n) = \hat{\underset{\sim}{X}}(t|n) - \underset{\sim}{X}(t)$. Denote by $\hat{\underset{\sim}{u}}(j\,|n) = \hat{\underset{\sim}{X}}(t_j|n)$ and $P(j|n) = Q(t_j|n)$. Then, starting with $\hat{\underset{\sim}{X}}(0) = \hat{\underset{\sim}{u}}(0|0)$ and $P(0) = P(0|0)$, the linear, unbiased and minimum varianced estimators of $\underset{\sim}{X}(t)$ given data $(Y_j, j = 1, \cdots, n)$ are closely approximated by the following recursive equations:

(i) For $t_j \le t < t_{j+1}$, $j = 0, 1, \cdots, n$ $\hat{\underset{\sim}{X}}(t|n)$ satisfies the following equations with boundary conditions $\lim_{t \to t_j} \hat{\underset{\sim}{X}}(t|n) = \hat{\underset{\sim}{u}}(j|n)$, where $\hat{\underset{\sim}{u}}(j|n)$ is given in (iii):

$$\frac{d}{dt}\hat{\underset{\sim}{X}}(t|n) = \underset{\sim}{f}\,[\hat{\underset{\sim}{X}}(t|n)]$$

for $t_j \le t < t_{j+1}, j = 0, 1, \cdots, n$.

(ii) For $t_j \le t < t_{j+1}$, $j = 0, 1, \cdots, n$, $Q(t|n)$ satisfies the following equations with boundary condition

$$\lim_{t \to t_j} Q(t|n) = P(j|n),$$

where $P(j|n)$ is given in (iii):

$$\frac{d}{dt}Q(t|n) = F_j(n)Q(t|n) + Q(t|n)F_j^T(n) + V_X(t),$$

for $t_j \le t < t_{j+1}, j = 0, 1, \cdots, n$, where $F_j(n) = (\frac{\partial}{\partial \underset{\sim}{X}^T}\underset{\sim}{f}(\underset{\sim}{X}))_{\underset{\sim}{X} = \hat{\underset{\sim}{X}}(t|n)}$.

(iii) $\hat{\underset{\sim}{u}}(j|n)$ and $P(j|n)$ for $j = 1, \cdots, n-1$ are given by the following recursive equations:

$$\hat{\underset{\sim}{u}}(j\,|n) = \hat{\underset{\sim}{u}}(j\,|\,j) + A_j\{\hat{u}(j+1\,|n) - \hat{\underset{\sim}{u}}(j\,+1|j)\}$$

and

$$P(j|n) = P(j|j) - A_j\{P(j+1|j) - P(j+1\,|\,n)\}A_j^T,$$

where

$$A_j = P(j|j)F_j^T(j+1)P^{-1}(j+1|j).$$

To implement the above procedure to derive $\hat{\underset{\sim}{X}}(t|n)$ for given initial distribution of $\hat{\underset{\sim}{X}}(t)$ at $t_0$, one first derive results by using formulas in Theorem (3.1) (forward filtering). Then one goes backward from $n$ to 1 by using formulas in Theorem (3.2) (backward filtering).

# 4 An Illustrative Example

As an illustration, in this section we apply the theories of Section 3 to a patient ( Patient No. 104 ) in [1] treated by a protease inhibitor. For this patient, RNA virus copies per $mm^3$ blood have been taken at 15 occasions in two weeks after treatment (Data given in Table 1 were extrapolated from Figure 1 of Perelson et al [1]). Because of the short time period after treatment, for this patient, drug resistance has not yet been developed; further as in [1] one may assume that the patient is in the pseudo-steady state condition and that $N(t) = N_0$ is independent of $t$.

**Table 1.** Number of Observed RNA Virus Copies per $mm^3$ for Patient N0. 104

| Time (hours) | RNA Copies $mm^3$ | Time (hours) | RNA Copies $mm^3$ |
|---|---|---|---|
| 0 | 52000 | 36 | 57000 |
| 2 | 94000 | 42 | 60000 |
| 4 | 180000 | 48 | 55000 |
| 6 | 175000 | 72 | 34000 |
| 12 | 110000 | 96 | 22000 |
| 18 | 110000 | 120 | 20000 |
| 24 | 100000 | 144 | 18000 |
| 30 | 110000 | 168 | 3000 |

The estimates of the parameters for this patient are ($s(t) = s = 20$/day $/mm^3$, $\theta(t) = \theta = 0.4571 \times 10^{-3}$/day$/mm^3$, $\gamma = 0.023757$/day, $\mu_1(t) = \mu_1 = 0.02$/day, $\mu_2(t) = \mu_2 = 0.5$/day, $\mu_V(t) = \mu_V = 3.6792$/day, $N_0 = 618374$/day, $k(t) = k = 5.1989 \times 10^{-5}$/day$/mm^3$. In these estimates $(s, \mu_i, i = 1, 2, \mu_V)$ were taken from literature ([1]-[3], [12], [15]) but $(\gamma, k, \theta, N_0)$ were estimated by nonlinear least square procedures (see [29]). Further, $\{V_0(0) = 0, V_1(0) = 9.8 \times 10^4/mm^3, T(0) + T^*(0) = 2/mm^3\}$.

Using these estimates and the methods given in the previous sections, we have estimated the numbers of infectious as well as non-infectious free HIV, the total number of the T cells and the $T^{(*)}$ cells at different times by both the quadratic Kalman filter method and the extended Kalman filter method. It appeared that the results obtained by the quadratic Kalman filter method were almost identical to the corresponding results by the extended Kalman filter method, indicating that results by the extended Kalman filter method have provided very close approximations to results of quadratic Kalman filter method. To illustrate the main features of the Kalman filter estimates, we will thus only use results from the extended Kalman filter method.

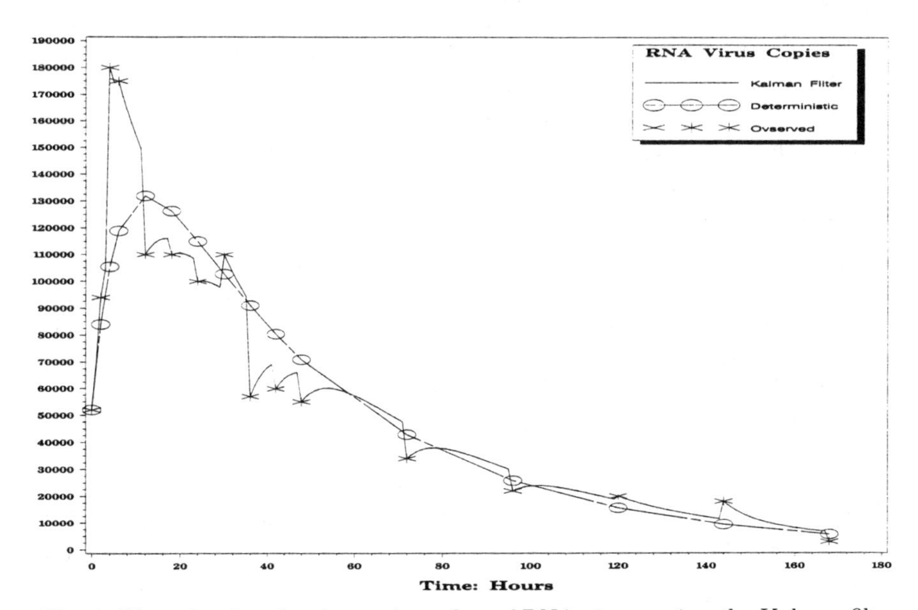


**Fig. 1.** Plots showing the observed number of RNA virus copies, the Kalman filter estimates and the estimates by the deterministic model for patient No. 104

Given in Figure 1 are the fitted curves plotted against the observed numbers of RNA virus copies. Given in Figure 2 are the curves of the estimated numbers of un-infected T cells and actively infected T cells. Given in Figure 3 are the curves of the estimated total numbers of infectious free HIV and non-infectious free HIV. The following results have been observed.

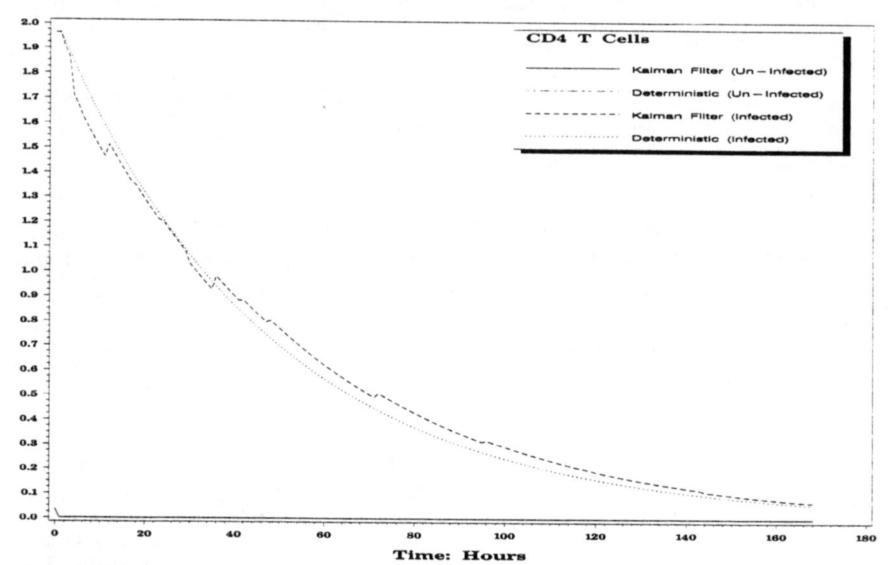


**Fig. 2.** Plots showing the Kalman filter estimates of the total number of CD4 T cells and the estimates by the deterministic model for the patient No. 104

(i) From Figure 1, it appeared that the Kalman filter estimates fitted to the observed data much better than the estimates by the deterministic model which is obtained by ignoring the random noises in the system model. The Kalman filter estimates of the total numbers of HIV have traced the observed numbers closely; on the other hand, the estimated numbers by the deterministic model appeared to draw a smooth line across the observed numbers.

(ii) Results from Figure 3 indicated that for the infectious HIV, there were little differences between Kalman filter estimates and estimates by the deterministic model, due presumably to the relative small numbers. On the other hand, for the non-infectious HIV, significant differences between the Kalman filter estimates and the estimates by the deterministic model have been observed, especial before 60 hours since treatment began. It appeared that for patient No. 104, the Kalman filter estimates were considerably larger than the corresponding estimates by the deterministic model before 10 hours since treatment, but the opposite is true during the period 15-50 hours since treatment. Thus, for patient No. 104, the Kalman filter estimates have revealed a much stronger effect of treatment within the first 10 hours than that by using the deterministic model.

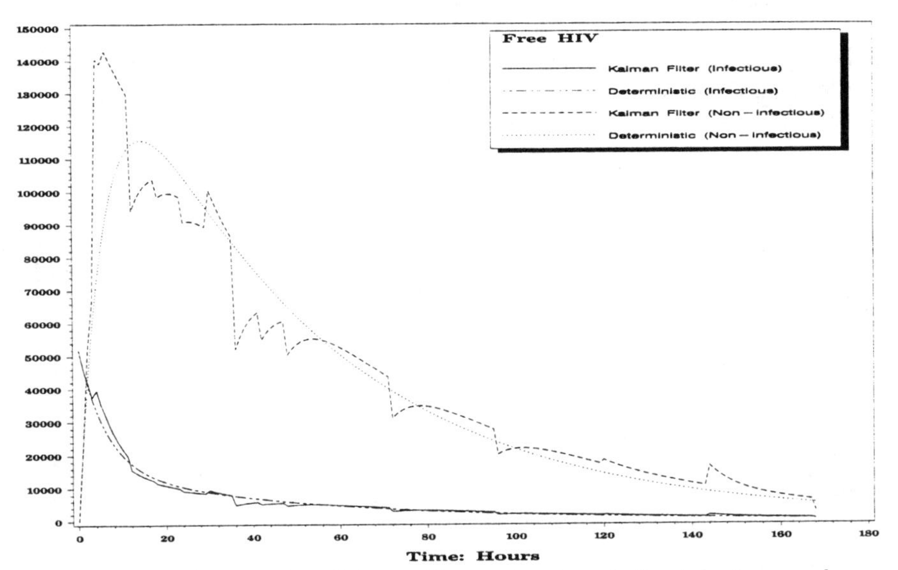


**Fig. 3.** Plots showing the Kalman filter estimates of the infectious and non-infectious free HIV and the estimates by the deterministic model for the patient No. 104

## 5 Some Monte Carlo Studies

To justify and confirm the usefulness of the Kalman filter methods for the state space model with stochastic system equations (13)-(16) and with observation equation (17), in this section we generate some Monte Carlo studies through computer by using this state space model. The parameter values of this model were taken from those of the estimates of the numerical example in Section 4 but with $T(0) = 1$ and $T^{(*)}(0) = 20$.

To generate the numbers of $T$ cells, $T^{(*)}$ cells and the numbers of $V_0$ and $V_1$ free HIV for the above state space model, we use the distribution theories given in Section 2, which involve basically Poisson variables, binomial variables and multinomial variables. For these variables, random generators are available from the IMSL [31] library functions. We generate these variables using 2.4 hours (0.1 day) as the time unit. To generate the observation model, we add some Gaussian noises to the generated total number of free HIV to produce $Y_j = Y(t_j)$ at 16 different times as given in the example of Section 4. That is, we generate $Y_j$ by the equation

$$Y_j = V_0(t_j) + V_1(t_j) + e_j = V(t) + e_j, j = 1, \ldots, n \tag{23}$$

where $e_j$ is assumed as independently distributed normal random variables with mean 0 and variance $V(t_j)\sigma^2$ with $\sigma^2 = 4$ and where $V(t_j) = V_0(t_j) + V_1(t_j)$ were generated as described above.

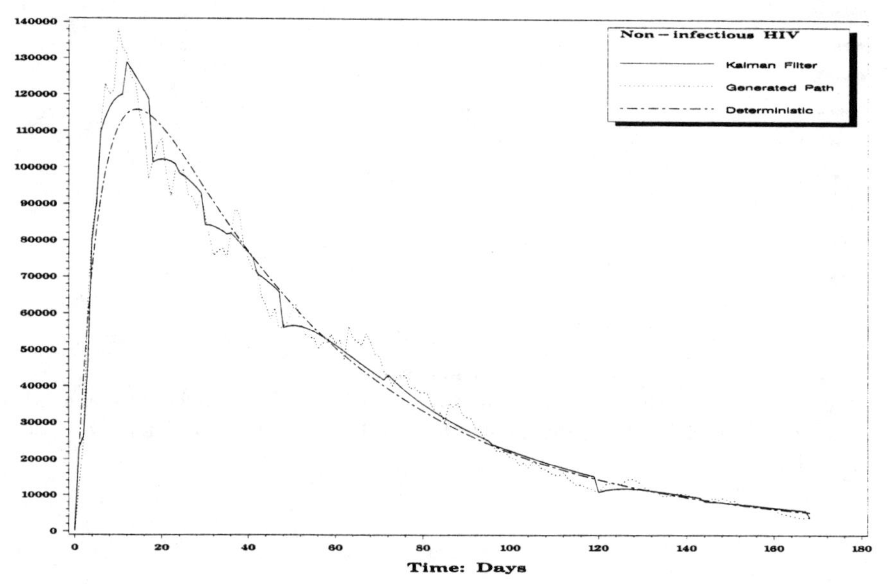


**Fig. 4.** Plots showing the Kalman filter estimates of the total of non-infectious free HIV and the estimates number by the deterministic model

Given in Table 2 are one set of the generated $Y_j = Y(t_j)$. We have repeated the experiments 200 times. Using these generated data on the RNA virus copies, we have derived estimates of the state variables for the above state space model by both the quadratic Kalman filter method and the extended Kalman filter method. These estimates are compared with the computer generated numbers respectively. Given in Table 3 are the generated numbers, the Kalman filter estimates and the estimates by the deterministic model for the $T$ cells, the $T^{(*)}$ cells, the $V_0$ free HIV and the $V_1$ free HIV based on data in Table 2. ( Because the numbers of $T$ cells are very small, the differences can not be revealed in pictures so that we present them in table.) For illustration, the results for the $V_0$ free HIV were plotted in Figure 4. The following observations have been made:

**Table 2.** Generated Numbers of RNA Virus Copies at 16 Time Points

| Time (hours) | RNA Copies $mm^3$ | Time (hours) | RNA Copies $mm^3$ |
|---|---|---|---|
| 0 | 52000 | 36 | 95320 |
| 2 | 79742 | 42 | 77322 |
| 4 | 94515 | 48 | 74642 |
| 6 | 124585 | 72 | 45710 |
| 12 | 148138 | 96 | 22906 |
| 18 | 131254 | 120 | 14273 |
| 24 | 111024 | 144 | 10726 |
| 30 | 99262 | 168 | 5155 |

(1) There are little differences between results by the quadratic Kalman filter method and results by the extended Kalman filter method. Furthermore, the estimates by the Kalman filter methods appear to trace the generated numbers very closely. These results indicate that in estimating the numbers of T cells and free HIV, one may in fact use the extended Kalman filter method as described in Section 3.

(2) As shown in Table 3, for the numbers of $T$ cells and $V_1$ free HIV, there are little differences between the Kalman filter estimates and the estimates by the deterministic model. As shown in Figure 4, for the non-infectious free HIV (i.e. $V_0$), however, there are significant differences between the Kalman filter estimates and the estimates by using the deterministic model. It appears that the Kalman filter estimates have revealed a much stronger effect of the treatment at early times (before 10 hours) than that detected by the deterministic model.

## 6 Conclusion and Discussion

In this chapter we have developed a state space model for the HIV pathogenesis at the cellular level in HIV-infected individuals. In this state space model, the stochastic system model is the stochastic model of HIV pathogenesis expressed in terms of stochastic differential equations whereas the observation model is a statistical model based on the numbers of RNA virus copies per unit volume of blood measured at different times or on the total number of CD4$^+$ T cell counts per $mm^3$ at different times. As discussed in Section 3, such models are advantageous over both stochastic models and statistical models since it combines information from both of these models.

**Table 3.** Estimates of the Numbers of T Cells, $T^*$ Cells, $V_O$, and V Free HIV (Per $mm^3$)

| $t=$ | Uninfected T Cell | | | | Infected $T^*$ Cells | | | |
|---|---|---|---|---|---|---|---|---|
| | (1) | (2) | (3) | (4) | (1) | (2) | (3) | (4) |
| 0 | 3.632E-01 | 3.632E-01 | 3.632E-01 | 3.632E-01 | 1.964E+01 | 1.964E+01 | 1.964E+01 | 1.964E+01 |
| 2 | 4.291E-03 | 4.079E-03 | 4.549E-03 | 2.812E-03 | 1.960E+01 | 1.960E+01 | 1.934E+01 | 1.926E+01 |
| 4 | 3.044E-04 | 2.481E-04 | 3.057E-04 | 1.585E-04 | 1.840E+01 | 1.843E+01 | 1.869E+01 | 1.847E+01 |
| 6 | 4.720E-05 | 3.583E-05 | 5.208E-05 | 2.527E-05 | 1.742E+01 | 1.743E+01 | 1.769E+01 | 1.771E+01 |
| 12 | 1.781E-06 | 1.231E-06 | 2.121E-06 | 1.112E-06 | 1.509E+01 | 1.516E+01 | 1.529E+01 | 1.561E+01 |
| 18 | 3.550E-07 | 1.772E-07 | 2.995E-07 | 2.080E-07 | 1.370E+01 | 1.372E+01 | 1.346E+01 | 1.375E+01 |
| 24 | 1.333E-07 | 6.542E-08 | 6.922E-08 | 6.987E-08 | 1.212E+01 | 1.213E+01 | 1.195E+01 | 1.212E+01 |
| 30 | 9.977E-08 | 2.673E-08 | 1.807E-08 | 3.236E-08 | 1.087E+01 | 1.086E+01 | 1.057E+01 | 1.068E+01 |
| 36 | 7.526E-08 | 1.770E-08 | 6.311E-09 | 1.876E-08 | 9.656E+00 | 9.542E+00 | 9.194E+00 | 9.416E+00 |
| 42 | 4.092E-08 | 1.099E-08 | 0.000E+00 | 1.306E-08 | 8.545E+00 | 8.476E+00 | 8.169E+00 | 8.298E+00 |
| 48 | 3.286E-08 | 5.216E-09 | 2.980E-09 | 1.065E-08 | 7.790E+00 | 7.657E+00 | 7.094E+00 | 7.314E+00 |
| 72 | 2.281E-08 | 1.216E-08 | 3.343E-09 | 1.404E-08 | 4.577E+00 | 4.570E+00 | 4.198E+00 | 4.412E+00 |
| 96 | 4.527E-08 | 3.352E-08 | 0.000E+00 | 4.220E-08 | 2.621E+00 | 2.766E+00 | 2.556E+00 | 2.662E+00 |
| 120 | 1.866E-07 | 7.063E-09 | 0.000E+00 | 1.738E-07 | 1.721E+00 | 1.707E+00 | 1.547E+00 | 1.606E+00 |
| 144 | 8.584E-07 | 5.186E-08 | 3.410E-07 | 8.705E-07 | 1.011E+00 | 1.036E+00 | 9.249E-01 | 9.691E-01 |
| 168 | 3.395E-06 | 2.044E-07 | 0.000E+00 | 5.036E-06 | 6.467E-01 | 6.318E-01 | 5.589E-01 | 5.847E-01 |

| $t=$ | Infectious HIV | | | | Uninfectious HIV | | | |
|---|---|---|---|---|---|---|---|---|
| | (1) | (2) | (3) | (4) | (1) | (2) | (3) | (4) |
| 0 | 5.200E+04 | 5.200E+04 | 5.200E+04 | 5.200E+04 | 0.000E+00 | 0.000E+00 | 0.000E+00 | 0.000E+00 |
| 2 | 4.064E+04 | 3.963E+04 | 4.079E+04 | 4.115E+04 | 2.482E+04 | 2.602E+04 | 3.882E+04 | 4.284E+04 |
| 4 | 3.198E+04 | 3.399E+04 | 3.232E+04 | 3.326E+04 | 8.259E+04 | 8.034E+04 | 6.193E+04 | 7.226E+04 |
| 6 | 2.791E+04 | 2.909E+04 | 2.791E+04 | 2.744E+04 | 1.112E+05 | 1.098E+05 | 9.683E+04 | 9.164E+04 |
| 12 | 1.651E+04 | 1.871E+04 | 1.876E+04 | 1.743E+04 | 1.312E+05 | 1.288E+05 | 1.294E+05 | 1.147E+05 |
| 18 | 1.111E+04 | 1.177E+04 | 1.331E+04 | 1.288E+04 | 1.020E+05 | 1.014E+05 | 1.184E+05 | 1.136E+05 |
| 24 | 9.109E+03 | 9.867E+03 | 1.011E+04 | 1.043E+04 | 9.905E+04 | 9.851E+04 | 1.012E+05 | 1.048E+05 |
| 30 | 5.864E+03 | 7.978E+03 | 8.519E+03 | 8.858E+03 | 8.632E+04 | 8.431E+04 | 9.029E+04 | 9.404E+04 |
| 36 | 7.221E+03 | 7.546E+03 | 8.005E+03 | 7.682E+03 | 8.228E+04 | 8.200E+04 | 8.708E+04 | 8.350E+04 |
| 42 | 5.706E+03 | 6.454E+03 | 6.481E+03 | 6.725E+03 | 7.159E+04 | 7.084E+04 | 7.113E+04 | 7.383E+04 |
| 48 | 4.547E+03 | 5.098E+03 | 6.213E+03 | 5.910E+03 | 5.671E+04 | 5.617E+04 | 6.850E+04 | 6.515E+04 |
| 72 | 4.478E+03 | 3.910E+03 | 3.802E+03 | 3.559E+03 | 4.266E+04 | 4.322E+04 | 4.203E+04 | 3.934E+04 |
| 96 | 2.315E+03 | 2.173E+03 | 1.910E+03 | 2.147E+03 | 2.378E+04 | 2.402E+04 | 2.111E+04 | 2.374E+04 |
| 120 | 1.088E+03 | 9.848E+02 | 1.193E+03 | 1.295E+03 | 1.081E+04 | 1.089E+04 | 1.319E+04 | 1.432E+04 |
| 144 | 6.750E+02 | 7.434E+02 | 8.754E+02 | 7.815E+02 | 8.280E+03 | 8.220E+03 | 9.679E+03 | 8.641E+03 |
| 168 | 4.165E+02 | 3.526E+02 | 4.327E+02 | 4.715E+02 | 3.879E+03 | 3.899E+03 | 4.785E+03 | 5.213E+03 |

(1)= Generated Number, (2)=Extended Kalman Filter Estimates, (3)Quadratic Kalman Filter Estimates, (4)=Deterministic Model.

The state space model we have developed in Section 3 is a state space model with continuous-time system equations and discrete-time observation equations. For the system equations, aside from the term involving $s(t)$, the equations are basically quadratic. Under the assumption of no drug resistance, in Section 3 we have thus developed some general theories for the estimation and prediction of the state variables by using non-linear least square procedures. Alternatively, we note that since the HIV infection rates are usually very small, the model of Section 3 can be closely approximated by an extended Kalman filter model. By using extended Kalman filter approximation, in this paper we have also developed some approximately optimal procedures to estimate the numbers of different T cells and the numbers of non-infectious free HIV and infectious free HIV over the time course under the assumption of no drug resistance. For the numerical example in Section 4, we have shown that the results by using the extended Kalman filter approximations are in fact very close to the results by using the quadratic Kalman filter method.

To illustrate the application of the state space model given in Section 3, we have applied the model to the data set of a patient ( No. 104) given in [1] under treatment by a protease inhibitor.

For this patient, the data consist of the numbers of RNA virus copies per unit volume of blood of these patients at 15 occasions within two weeks since treatment. By using this data set we have developed a state space model for this patient under the assumption of no drug resistance and have obtained Kalman filter estimates of the numbers of $V_0$ and $V_1$ free HIV and the numbers of different types of T cells over the time course. We have found that the estimates by the extended Kalman filter methods are almost identical to the corresponding estimates by the quadratic non-linear least square methods, indicating the closeness of the approximation by an extended Kalman filter method. However, it appeared that for the $V_0$ free HIV, there are significant differences between estimates by Kalman filter methods and the corresponding estimates by using deterministic models. Furthermore, for this patient, the Kalman filter methods have also revealed a much stronger effect of the drug before 10 days since treatment than that by using the deterministic model.

To assess the efficiency and usefulness of the Kalman filter methods, in Section 5 we have also generated some Monte Carlo studies by using the state space model of Section 3 under the assumption of no drug resistance. Our numerical results have shown clearly that the estimates by the Kalman filter methods can trace the generated numbers very closely in most of the cases. Furthermore, the estimates by the quadratic Kalman filter method are almost identical to those by the extended Kalman filter method. These results suggest that the extended Kalman filter estimates would provide very close approximation to the true numbers, due presumably to the fact that the HIV infection rate is usually very small. On the other hand, it appeared that for the $V_0$ free HIV, there are significant differences between estimates by the Kalman filter methods and the corresponding estimates by using the deterministic model. These results suggest the usefulness of the Kalman filter methods.

From the above analysis, it is obvious that the state space models as given in Section 3 are useful for monitoring the dynamic behavior of the HIV process at the cellular level in HIV-infected individuals and for assessing the efficiencies and usefulness of the anti-viral treatment. To make the model more useful, of course, it is necessary to extend the model to more general situations involving the development of drug resistance of HIV to these drugs. Further work in this direction and other extensions are definitely needed.

### Acknowledgment

The research of this paper was partially supported by a research grant from National Institute of Allergy and Infections Diseases / NIH, Grant Nō: R21 AI31869.

## References

1. Perelson, A.S., Neumann, A.U., Markowitz, M., Leonard, J.M. and Ho, D.D., *HIV-1 dynamics in vivo: Virion clearance rate, infected cell life-span,and viral generation time*, Science, **271**, 1582-1586 (1996).
2. Ho, D.D., Neumann, A.U., Perelson, A.S., Chen, W., Leonard, J.M. and Markowitz, M., *Rapid turnover of plasma virus and CD4 lymphocytes in HIV-1 infection*, Nature, **373**, 123-126 (1995).
3. Wei,X., Ghosh, S.K., Taylor, M.E., Johnson, V.A., Emini, E.A., Deutsch, P., Lifson, J.D., Bonhoeffer,S., Nowak,M.A., Hahn,B.H., Saag,M.S. and Shaw,G.M., *Viral dynamics in human immunodeficiency virus type 1 infection.* Nature, **373**, 117-122 (1995).
4. Ho, D.D., *Pathogenesis of HIV infection*, New York Meeting, Aaron Diamond AIDS Research Center and New York University, New York, 1996.
5. Ioannidis, J.P.A., Cappelleri, J.C., Lau, J., Sacks,H.S.,and Skolnik, P.R., *Predictive value of viral load measurements in asymptomatic untreated HIV-1 infection: A mathematical models* AIDS, **10**, 225-262 (1996).
6. Mellors, J.W., Rinaldo, C.R. Jr.,Gupta, P., White, R.M., Todd, J.A., Kingsley, L.A., *Prognosis in HIV-1 infection prediced by the quantity of virus inplasma*, Science, **272**, 1167-1170 (1996).

7. Fauci, A.S., *Immunopathogenic mechanisms in human immunodeficiency virus (HIV)*, Annals of Internal Medicine, **114**, 678-693 (1993).
8. Haseltine, W.A.,*Replication and pathogenesis of the AIDS virus, Jour. AIDS*,**1**, 217-240 (1988).
9. Levy, J.A., *HIV research: a need to focus on the right target*, Lancet, **345**, 1619-1621 (1995).
10. Pantaleo, G., Graziosi, C. And Fauci, A.S., *The immunopathogenesis of human immunodeficiency virus infection*, New England Journal of Medicine, **328**, 327-335 (1993).
11. Kirschner, D., *AZT chemotherapy of HIV infection: Scheduling and resistance*, Fourth International Conference on Mathematical Population Dynamics, Rice University, Houston, TX, May 23-27, 1995.
12. Kirschner, D. and Perelson, A.S., *A model for the immune system response to HIV: AZT treatment studies.* In: "Mathematical population Dynamics 3 ,Chapter 18",O.Arino, D.E. Axelrod and M. Kimmel eds., Wuerz Publishing Ltd., Winnipeg, Manitoba, Canada, 1993.
13. Kirschner,D. and Webb, G.F., *A model for treatment strategy in the chemotherapy of AIDS.* To appear in Bulletin of Math. Biology, 1997.
14. Perelson, A.S., *Modeling HIV infection*, Fourth International Conference on Mathematical Poplylation Dynamics, Rice University, Houston, TX, May 23-27, 1995.
15. Perelson, A.S., Kirschner, D. and Boer, R.D., *Dynamics of HIV infection of* $CD4^{+}$ *T cells*, Math. Biosciences, **114**, 81-125 (1993).
16. Schenzle, D., *A model for AIDS pathogenesis*, Statisitcs in Medicine,**13**, 2067-2069 (1994).
17. Essunger, P. and Perelson,A.S., Modeling HIV infection of CD4+ T-cell subpopulations. J. Theor. Biol.,**170**, 367-391 (1994).
18. Stevenson,M., Stanwick, T.L., Dempsey,M.P. and Lamonica,C.A., *HIV-1 replication is controlled at the level of T-cell activation and proviral integration*, EMBO J., **9**, 1551-1560 (1990).
19. Philips, A.N., *Reduction of HIV concentration during acute infection: Independence from specific immune response.* Science, **271**, 497-499 (1996).
20. Tan, W.Y. and Piantadosi, S.(1991).*On stochastic growth process with application to stochastic logistic growth*, Statistica Sinica, **1**, 527-540 (1991).
21. Levy, J.A., *HIV research: a need to focus on the right target*, Lancet, **345**, 1619-1621 (1995).
22. Tan, W.Y. and Ye, Zhengzheng (1997) *Assessing effects of different types of free HIV and macrophage on HIV pathogenesis by a stochastic model*, invited paper at the International Statistic Symposium, August 11-15, 1998, Taipei, Taiwan.

23. Demeter, L.M., Nawaz, T., Morse, G., Dolin, R., Dexter, A.,Gerondelis,P., and Reichman, R.C., Development of zidovudine resistance mutations in patients receiving prolonged didanosine monotherapy. The Jour. Infect. Diseases,**172**, 1480-1485 (1995).
24. Erice, A. and Balfour, H. H., Resistance of HIV-1 to anti-retroviral agents: A review. Clin. Infect. Diseases,**18**, 149-156 (1995).
25. Kozal, M.J., Kroodsma,K., Winters, M.A., Shafer, R.W., Efron, B., Katzenstein, D.A., and Merigan, T.C., *Didanosine resistance in HIV-infected patients switched from zidovudine to didanosine monotherapy*, Ann. Intern. Med., **121**, 263-268 (1994).
26. Schininazi, R.F., Lloyd, R.M. Jr., Ramanathan, C.S. and Taylor, E.W., *Antiviral drug resistance mutations in human immunodeficiency virus type 1 reverse transcriptase occur in specific RNA structural regions*, Antimicrob. Agents Chemother.,**38**, 268-274 (1994).
27. Zhang, D.,Galiendo, A.M., Eron, J.J., DeVore, K.M.,Kaplan, J.C., Hirsch, M.S. and D'aquila, R.T.,. Resistance to 2',3'-dideoxycytidine conferred by a mutation in codon 65 of the human immunodeficiency virus type 1 reverse transcriptase. Antimicrobial Agents and Chemotherapy,**38**, 282-287 (1994).
28. Tan, W.Y. and Zhang, D.Z., *Modeling effects of drug resistance in HIV-infected individuals*, paper in preparation.
29. Tan, W.Y. and Wu, H., *Stochastic modeling of the dynamic of $CD4^+$ T cell infection by HIV and some monte carlo studies.* Math. Biosciences, 147, 173-205 (1998).
30. Catlin, D.E., *Estimation, Control and Discrete Kalman Filter*, Springer-Verlag, New York, 1989.
31. IMSL, *MATH/LIBRARY User's Manual*, IMSL, Houston, Texas, 1989.
32. Gelb, A., *Applied Optimal Estimation*, M.I.T. Press, Cambridge, MA., 1974.
33. Sage, A.P. and Melsa, J.L., *Estimation Theory With Applications to Communications and Control*, McGraw-Hill Book Com.,New York, NY., 1971.

## Appendix: Proof of Theorem (3.1) and (3.2)

Since the extended Kalman filter model is linear, it suffice to prove the results for the following linear state space model:

$$\frac{d}{dt}\underset{\sim}{X}(t) = F(t)\underset{\sim}{X}(t) + \underset{\sim}{\epsilon}(t) \tag{24}$$

for $t_0 \leq t$;

$$Y_j = H_j\underset{\sim}{X}(t_j) + \underset{\sim j}{e}, \quad j = 1, \cdots, n. \tag{25}$$

where $Cov(\underset{\sim}{\epsilon}(t), \underset{\sim j}{e}) = 0, Cov(\underset{\sim}{\epsilon}(t), \underset{\sim}{\epsilon}(\tau)) = \delta(t-\tau)V_X(t)$, $Cov(\underset{\sim j}{e}, \underset{\sim u}{e}) = \delta_{ju}\Sigma_j$, $Cov(\underset{\sim}{\epsilon}(t), \underset{\sim}{X}(t)) = 0$ and $Cov(\underset{\sim}{X}(t), \underset{\sim j}{e}) = 0$ with $\delta(t)$ being the Dirac's $\delta$ function and with $\delta_{ju}$ being the Kronecter's $\delta$.

Then the results in (i) of Theorems (3.1) and (3.2) can be restated respectively as:

(ia) For $t_j \le t < t_{j+1}$, $j = 0, 1, \cdots, n$ $(t_0 = 0, t_{n+1} = \infty)$, $\underset{\sim}{\hat{X}}(t|t_j)$ satisfies the following equations with boundary conditions

$$\lim_{t \to t_j} \underset{\sim}{\hat{X}}(t|t_j) = \underset{\sim}{\hat{X}}(t_j|t_j) = \underset{\sim}{\hat{u}}(j|j)$$

where $\underset{\sim}{\hat{u}}(j|j)$ is given in (iii):

$$\frac{d}{dt}\underset{\sim}{\hat{X}}(t|t_j) = F(t)\underset{\sim}{\hat{X}}(t|t_j) \qquad t_j \le t < t_{j+1}, j = 0, 1, \cdots, n;$$

(ib) For $t < t_n$ $\underset{\sim}{\hat{X}}(t|n)$ satisfies the following equations with boundary conditions $\lim_{t\to t_n} \underset{\sim}{\hat{X}}(t|n) = \underset{\sim}{\hat{u}}(n|n)$, where $\underset{\sim}{\hat{u}}(n|n)$ is given in Theorem (3.1):

$$\frac{d}{dt}\underset{\sim}{\hat{X}}(t|n) = F(t)\underset{\sim}{\hat{X}}(t|n)$$

To prove the results for the above linear state space model, define $R(t, t_j) = \lim_{\Delta t \to 0} \prod_{i=1}^{n} [I_p + F(t_j + (i-1)\Delta t)\Delta t]$ for $t = t_j + n\Delta t$ . Then $R(t, t) = I_p$ and $\frac{d}{dt}R(t, t_j) = F(t)R(t, t_j)$ for $t \ge t_j$. Further, for $t \ge t_j$, the solution of equation (24) is given by:

$$\underset{\sim}{X}(t) = R(t, t_j)\underset{\sim}{X}(t_j) + \underset{\sim j}{\epsilon}(t)$$

where $\underset{\sim j}{\epsilon}(t) = \int_{t_j}^{t} R(t, x)\underset{\sim}{\epsilon}(x)\, dx$.

Obviously, $E\underset{\sim j}{\epsilon}(t) = \underset{\sim}{0}$ , Cov$[\underset{\sim j}{\epsilon}(t), \underset{\sim}{e}(l)] = 0$ for all $j, l$, and $t \ge t_j$, and the covariance matrix of $\underset{\sim j}{\epsilon}(t)$ is

$$Var(\underset{\sim j}{\epsilon}(t)) = \int_{t_j}^{t} R(t, x)V_X(x)R^T(t, x)\, dx.$$

Put $\underset{\sim}{u}(j) = \underset{\sim}{X}(t_j)$, $G(j) = R(t_{j+1}, t_j)$ and $\underset{\sim j}{\epsilon}(t_{j+1}) = \underset{\sim}{\zeta}(j+1)$. Then

$$\underset{\sim}{u}(j+1) = G(j)\underset{\sim}{u}(j) + \underset{\sim}{\zeta}(j+1) \tag{26}$$

$$\underset{\sim}{Y}_{j+1} = H_{j+1}\underset{\sim}{u}(j+1) + \underset{\sim}{e}(j+1) \tag{27}$$

Thus, the state space model for $\underset{\sim}{u}(j)$ is discrete and linear. For this type of model, the linear, unbiased and minimal varianced estimator of $\underset{\sim}{u}(i)$ given data $(\underset{\sim}{Y}_u, u = 1, \cdots, j)$, are given respectively by (iii) of Theorem (3.1) if $i = j$ and by (iii) of Theorem (3.2) if $0 < j \leq n$. The proof can be found in [30] and [32]-[33]. This proves (iii) of Theorems (3.1) and (3.2).

Now for $t_j \leq t$, the conditional mean of $\underset{\sim}{X}(t)$ and the associated residual given data $\{\underset{\sim}{Y}_l, l = 1, \ldots, j\}$ are given respectively by $\hat{\underset{\sim}{X}}(t|t_j) = R(t, t_j)\hat{\underset{\sim}{u}}(j|j)$ and $\hat{\underset{\sim}{\epsilon}}(t|t_j) = \hat{\underset{\sim}{X}}(t|t_j) - \underset{\sim}{X}(t) = R(t, t_j)\hat{\underset{\sim}{\epsilon}}(t_j|t_j) - \underset{\sim}{\epsilon}_j(t)$. The covariance matrix of the residual $\hat{\underset{\sim}{\epsilon}}(t|t_j)$ is

$$Q(t|t_j) = R(t, t_j)P(j|j)R^T(t, t_j) + \int_{t_j}^{t} R(t, x)V_X(x)R^T(t, x)\, dx.$$

Obviously, the above $\hat{\underset{\sim}{X}}(t|t_j)$ and $Q(t|t_j)$ satisfy respectively the following equations with boundary conditions $\lim_{t \longrightarrow t_j} \hat{\underset{\sim}{X}}(t|t_j) = \hat{\underset{\sim}{u}}(j|j)$ and $\lim_{t \longrightarrow t_j} Q(t|t_j) = P(j|j)$:

$$\frac{d}{dt}\hat{\underset{\sim}{X}}(t|t_j) = F(t)R(t, t_j)\hat{\underset{\sim}{u}}(j|j) = F(t)\hat{\underset{\sim}{X}}(t|t_j)$$

and

$$\begin{aligned}\frac{d}{dt}Q(t|t_j) &= F(t)R(t, t_j)P(j|j)R^T(t, t_j) + R(t, t_j)P(j|j)R^T(t, t_j)F^T(t) \\ &\quad + R(t, t)V_X(t)R^T(t, t) + F(t)\int_{t_j}^{t} R(t, u)V_X(u)R^T(t, u)\, du \\ &\quad + \int_{t_j}^{t} R(t, u)V_X(u)R^T(t, u)\, du\, F^T(t) \\ &= F(t)Q(t|t_j) + Q(t|t_j)F^T(t) + V_X(t).\end{aligned}$$

Since $\hat{\underset{\sim}{u}}(j|j)$ is the linear, unbiased and minimum varianced estimator of $\underset{\sim}{u}(j)$ given data $\{\underset{\sim}{Y}_l, l = 1, \ldots, j\}$, so does $\hat{\underset{\sim}{X}}(t|t_j)$ as an estimator for $\underset{\sim}{X}(t)$ given data $\{\underset{\sim}{Y}_l, l = 1, \ldots, j\}$ for $t_j \leq t$. This proves (i) and (ii) of Theorem (3.1). Similarly one proves (i) and (ii) of Theorem (3.2).

**Dr. Wai-Yuan Tan** has three MS degree (Agronomy, Statistics and Mathematics) and a Ph.D in Mathematical Statistics. He is currently a Research Professor in the Department of Mathematical Sciences at the University of Memphis, USA. He has published 4 books and over 160 papers in refereed journals and book chapters. He is an ASA fellow of the American Statistical Association. His current research are in Cancer, AIDS and Risk

Assessment of environmental agents. In the past, he has made important contributions in many different areas in Statistics including Bayesian inferences, robust inferences, linear models, special functions and sampling distributions, multivariate analysis, biostatistics, mathematical genetics, applied stochastic processes, stochastic models of cancer, AIDS and biomedical systems as well as regression analysis and analysis of variances.

**Dr. Zhihua Xiang** has two MS degrees in Statistics and a Ph.D in Applied Statistics. He has published 14 papers in Bayesian inferences and AIDS modeling.

# Modeling the Effects of Prior Infection on Vaccine Efficacy*

Derek J. Smith[1], Stephanie Forrest[1]
David H. Ackley[1], and Alan S. Perelson[2]

[1] Department of Computer Science
University of New Mexico
Albuquerque, NM 87131 USA
[2] Theoretical Division
Los Alamos National Laboratory
Los Alamos, NM 87545 USA

**Abstract.** We performed computer simulations to study the effects of prior infection on vaccine efficacy. We injected three antigens sequentially. The first antigen, designated the *prior*, represented a prior infection or vaccination. The second antigen, the *vaccine*, represented a single component of the trivalent influenza vaccine. The third antigen, the *epidemic*, represented challenge by an epidemic strain. For a fixed vaccine to epidemic strain cross-reactivity, we generated prior strains over a full range of cross-reactivities to the vaccine and to the epidemic strains. We found that, for many cross-reactivities, vaccination, when it had been preceded by a prior infection, provided more protection than vaccination alone. However, at some cross-reactivities, the prior infection reduced protection by clearing the vaccine before it had the chance to produce protective memory. The cross-reactivities between the prior, vaccine and epidemic strains played a major role in determining vaccine efficacy. This work has applications to understanding vaccination against viruses such as influenza that are continually mutating.

## 1 Introduction

Continual and rapid antigenic change is a property of many viruses, including influenza virus, human immunodeficiency virus, and hepatitis C virus. As a result of their high mutation rate, thousands of strains of these viruses coexist in a *species swarm* (or *quasispecies*) [1]. Vaccination against species swarms is difficult because of the need to provide broad immunity to the many strains, and because new strains are constantly emerging. In the case of influenza,

* Reprinted, with permission from Proceedings of the IEEE International Conference on Systems, Man, and Cybernetics, Orlando, Florida, October 12-15, 1997, pp363-368.

for example, a worldwide network of surveillance centers identifies hundreds of influenza strains each year. Current public heath practice uses a trivalent vaccine against the three major influenza species swarms currently circulating. Year to year it is typically necessary to change at least one component of the vaccine to keep up with the evolution of the species swarm. Influenza vaccine efficacy and virus virulence varies; in a bad flu season it is not unheard of for 20% of the residents of an elderly persons nursing home to die from the effects of influenza, despite yearly vaccination. In part this is due to the effects of the species swarm and, as we investigate below, possibly due to the effects of prior infection (or vaccination) interfering with the current vaccination.

The effect of prior infection (or vaccination) on vaccine efficacy has not been throughly investigated. [2] and [3] established that the immune response to influenza was dominated by recall of immunological memory to prior influenza infections. Most of the experiments that followed this work were performed with two antigens [4,5]. However, to study the effect of prior infection on vaccine efficacy, at least three responses need to be studied—the prior infection, the vaccination, and the epidemic challenge [6]. In the case of three antigens, and considering say only eight degrees of cross-reactivity between any two antigens, there are hundreds of combinations of the cross-reactivities between the three antigens. The hundreds of combinations, and the necessity to have sufficient replicates of each experiment, necessitates thousands of experiments for a comprehensive survey.

Because of the difficulty of conducting this many experiments *in vivo*, we have built a computer model to perform the experiments *in machina*. An advantage of *in machina* experiments is that a large number can be performed and analyzed relatively cheaply and quickly. A disadvantage is that the computer model might not faithfully represent important aspects of the immune system and thus give misleading results. The model has been validated by replicating existing experiments and has shown good, *qualitative*, agreement. Parameters of the model have also been chosen to match immunological data important for modeling the cross-reactive immune response [7]. All the experiments reported here were done *in machina*. The predictions from the experiments are testable with a much smaller number of *in vivo* experiments.

## 2 Materials and Methods

The computer simulation is a simplified model of the vertebrate humoral immune system. It consists of B cells, plasma cells, antibodies, memory B cells, and antigens. T cell help is modeled implicitly by assuming that it is available whenever necessary. Each B cell, plasma cell and memory B cell is modeled as a separate entity within the simulation. In this way the model is *agent based* and similar to that of [8]. Because of the large number of antibodies in a real immune system, each antibody in the model corresponds to a large number of real antibodies, similarly each antigen in the model corresponds to a large number of real antigens. B cell, antibody, and antigen receptors are modeled as strings of symbols that can loosely be thought of as the amino acids of a binding site. When antigens are introduced into the simulation, B cells have a chance to bind the antigens depending on their affinity. B cells with antigen bound are stimulated to divide, and on division have some chance of mutation in their antibody receptor, and some chance to differentiate into a memory or plasma cell. Plasma cells secrete antibodies, which have a chance to bind antigens. If antigens have above a threshold number of antibodies bound they are removed from the simulation.

B cell, antibody and antigen receptors are made up of 20 symbols, where each symbol corresponds to one of four equivalence classes of amino acids. In the model, receptor sequence and shape are equivalent, and affinity is a function of the number of symbols that are complementary between receptors. We choose an affinity cut-off for clonal selection when receptors have less than 15 complementary symbols. This parameter selection was chosen to correspond to immunological data [7] and gives the following properties: a potential repertoire of $10^{12}$ B cells, a 1 in $10^5$ chance of a B cell responding to a particular antigen [9–11], and with an expressed repertoire of $10^7$ B cells [12–14] two antigens cease being cross-reactive when they have more than about 35% sequence difference [15,16]. Instead of referring to the percentage sequence difference between antigens, we refer to the *antigenic distance* between antigens which we define as the number of symbols in which the antigen's receptors differ. Thus, for receptors of length 20, there are 21 possible antigenic distances between antigens and any two antigens that are separated by an antigenic distance greater than or equal to seven (35% sequence difference) are not cross-reactive. Thus, effectively, there are eight degrees of cross-reactivity in our model corresponding to antigenic distances zero through seven.

To study the effect of a prior infection on vaccine efficacy we held the cross-reactivity between the vaccine and epidemic strains constant and varied the cross-reactivities of the prior to the vaccine and epidemic strains (Figure 1). The epidemic dose and replication rate were chosen (500 units of epidemic strain, replicating every six hours) so that, with high probability, an unvaccinated simulated organism would become diseased when challenged. The vaccine dose and strain were chosen (1,000 units of inactivated vaccine, antigenic distance two from the epidemic strain) to have about 50% efficacy against the epidemic challenge. Antigens at all combinations of antigenic distances to the vaccine and epidemic were generated for use as *prior* strains. In total 31 different prior strains were generated.

Ten control groups and 31 experimental groups were injected with combinations of prior, vaccine and epidemic strains according to Table 1. The timing of the injections of the prior, vaccine and epidemic strains was such that antibody titers were close to pre-injection levels before the next injection.

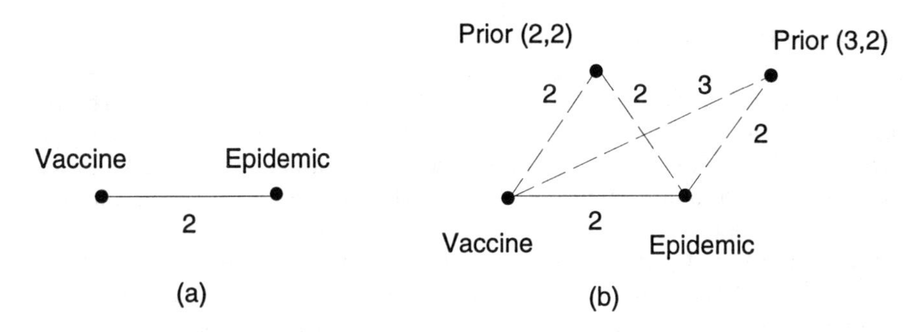


**Fig. 1.** (a) The antigenic distance between the vaccine and epidemic strains was fixed for all the experiment at two units. (b) 31 different prior strains were generated at different antigenic distances to the vaccine and epidemic strains (two shown).

For the controls (groups 1-10) 120 replications were performed, and for the experiments (groups 11-41) 250 replications were performed in each group. A "disease threshold" was set at 2,500 units and if the viral load exceeded it the simulation was stopped. During each experiment the viral load, and antibody titers and affinities for each antigen, were measured every six hours. In addition, prior to each injection, and at the peak of each response, the number, affinity for each antigen, and clonal history of each B cell involved in the response were recorded.

| Group | Purpose | Prior infection (replicating) (dose on day 5) | Vaccine (non replicating) (dose on day 75) | Epidemic infection (replicating) (dose on day 145) |
|---|---|---|---|---|
| 1 | control | | | 500 |
| 2 | control | | 1,000 | 500 |
| 3-10 | control | 200* | | 500 |
| 11-41 | experiment | 200† | 1,000 | 500 |

**Table 1.** The timing and dosage of the prior infection, vaccination , and epidemic infection is shown for the 41 groups. *Groups 3-10 received a prior infection at antigenic distances zero through seven respectively from the epidemic strain. †Groups 11-41 received a prior infection with different combinations of antigenic distances between zero and seven from the vaccine and epidemic strains. The correspondence between group and antigenic distances is shown in Figure 2.

## 3 Results and Discussion

The model exhibited classical behavior of cross-reactive memory in the response to the vaccine after the prior infection, and in response to the epidemic challenge after the prior infection and vaccination: the strength of each cross-reactive response increased as the antigenic distance between antigens decreased (Figure 2c, [16]), the number of cross-reactive memory cells increased as the antigenic distance between the antigens decreased (Table 2 and [17]), and the number of new memory cells produced in response to a cross-reactive antigen was reduced by the cross-reactive memory to previous antigens (Table 2 and [4]). This last phenomenon is sometimes called *original antigenic sin* [4].

Protection against epidemic challenge decreased as the antigenic distance between the prior and epidemic strains increased, for a constant antigenic distance between the prior and vaccine strains (columns of Figure 2d). This was because memory of the prior infection was more cross-reactive with the epidemic strain when the prior and epidemic strains were closer, while the effect of original antigenic sin between the prior and vaccine strains was constant.

Protection against epidemic challenge was lowest when the antigenic distance between the prior and vaccine strains was lowest, for a constant antigenic distance between the prior and epidemic strains (rows of Figure 2d). This was because the closer the prior strain was to the vaccine, the greater the effect of original antigenic sin in reducing the number of memory cells produced by the vaccination, and thus reducing the protection provided by the vaccination (Figure 3 and Table 2). This suggests that given a choice of strains to use as a vaccine, the one that is farthest from the prior strain will be least affected by original antigenic sin, and would thus be a good choice (assuming it is also a good choice because it is expected to be close to the epidemic strain).

Prior infection sometimes decreased vaccine efficacy below the situation when there was vaccination without prior infection (groups 24, 29, and 34, on the upper diagonal of Figure 2d). This occurred because the prior infection was far enough from the epidemic strain to provide little protection, but close enough to the vaccine strain to cause original antigenic sin and reduce the effectiveness of the vaccination (Figure 3 and Table 2). These situations occurred when the differences between the vaccine and epidemic strains were at different locations in the receptor than the differences between the prior and vaccine strains—so called *accumulative* mutations [18], and when the prior and epidemic strains were only moderately cross-reactive. Although only five of the 31 experimental groups have only accumulative mutations between the prior, vaccine and epidemic strains, these groups are more likely to occur in practice because, early in the evolutionary history of a subspecies, there are more residues that have not been mutated than ones that have, and thus more chance that a mutation at a random residue will be accumulative rather

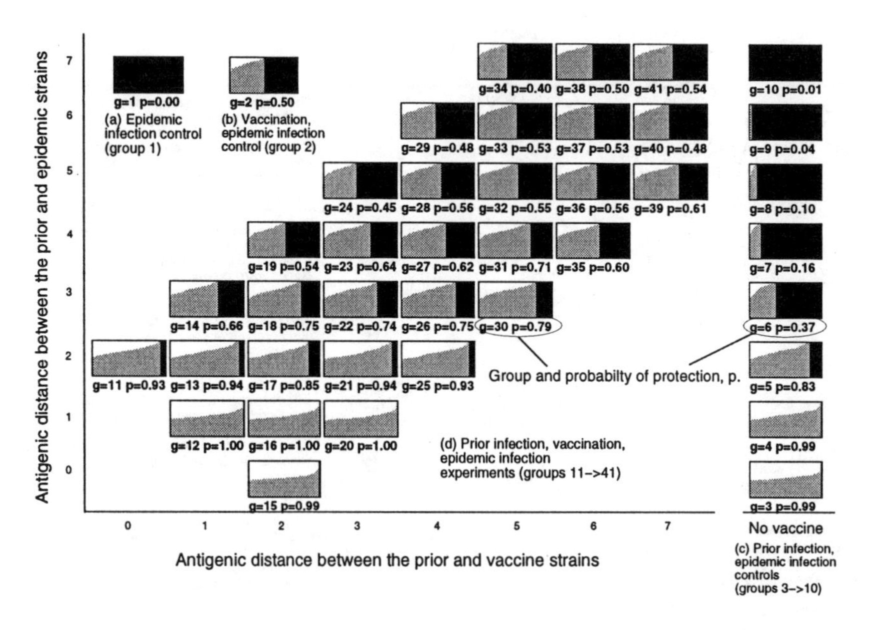


**Fig. 2.** A summary of the maximum viral load of the epidemic strain in each experiment. Each subplot is comprised of 250 vertical lines (120 for the control groups), the height of each vertical line indicates the maximum viral load during an experiment. The 250 experiments in each group (120 in the control groups) are plotted in order of increasing maximum viral load. Viral loads above the disease threshold are plotted in black, thus, the width of the black region indicates the frequency of disease in each group. (a) Exposure to the epidemic challenge, without prior infection or vaccination, caused disease in all cases. (b) Vaccine efficacy was, by design, 50% against the epidemic infection when there was no prior infection. (c) The frequency of disease due to a epidemic challenge after there had been a prior infection was proportional to the antigenic distance between the prior and epidemic strains. (d) The vaccine efficacy against the epidemic challenge, after there had been a prior infection, varied from 40 to 100% depending on the antigenic distances between the prior strain and the vaccine and epidemic strains. The timing of the injections of the prior, vaccine and epidemic strains was such that antibody titers had returned to pre-injection levels before the next injection.

than sequential. For example, the major epidemic strains of H3N2 influenza, from its emergence in 1968 until 1980, had only accumulative mutations from the A/Hong Kong/8/68 reference strain [18], although this might also be due to other factors.

Vaccination always increased protection against the epidemic challenge, because even if the vaccine was close to the prior strain, and was reduced

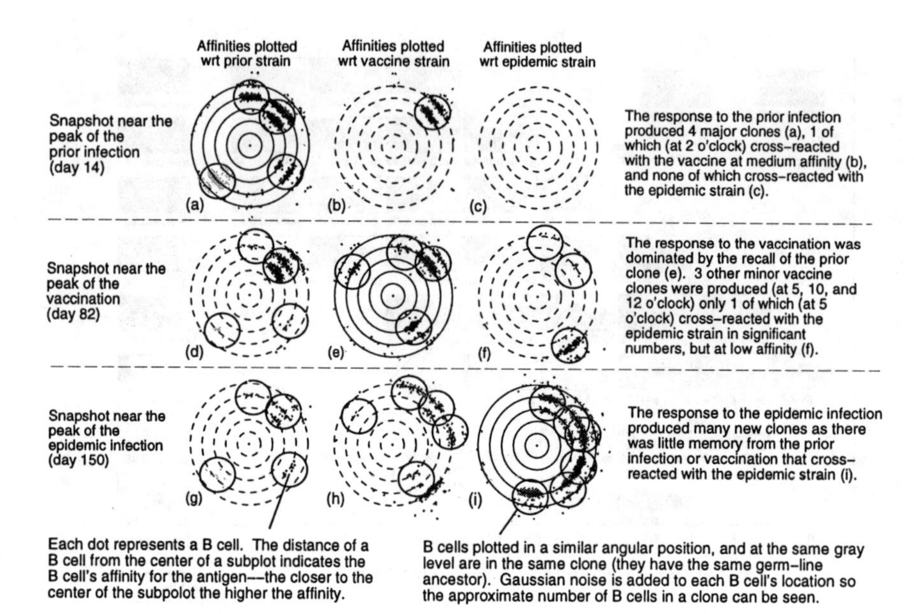


**Fig. 3.** An example of original antigenic sin causing vaccine failure. Experiment 81 of group 24 is shown, in which the prior strain was distance five from the epidemic strain and distance three from the vaccine strain. The major prior clone, that cross-reacted with the vaccine, dominated the vaccine response and prohibited the generation of new clones by the vaccine that might have been cross-reactive with the epidemic strain. Because there were few memory clones from the prior infection or vaccination that cross-reacted with the epidemic strain, the response to the epidemic infection was like a primary response and the maximum viral load exceeded the disease threshold.

in effectiveness by original antigenic sin, it still generated some new memory cells that potentially cross-reacted with the epidemic strain. The vaccination also increased protection by boosting the memory cells, produced by the prior infection, that cross-reacted with the vaccine and epidemic strains.

Among the memory cells that cross-reacted with the epidemic strain, there were a greater proportion originally generated by the prior infection than by the vaccination, when there was at least moderate cross-reactivity between the prior and epidemic strains (data not shown). This was because of original antigenic sin reducing the number of new memory cells produced by the vaccine, and because the vaccination boosted the memory cells, produced by the prior infection, that cross-reacted with the vaccine and epidemic strains. This is in partial agreement with the report by [19] that responses to influenza were dominated recall of prior infections. In our model however, once the prior

| Prior to vaccine distance | % prior x-reacts w/ vaccine | % vaccine generated (vs control) | Probability of protection |
|---|---|---|---|
| 3 | 12% | 66% | 45% |
| 4 | 5% | 79% | 56% |
| 5 | 1% | 94% | 55% |
| 6 | 0% | 96% | 56% |
| 7 | 0% | 100% | 61% |

**Table 2.** A cellular analysis of the row of Figure 2d in which the antigenic distance of the prior to epidemic strains was five, and the antigenic distance between the prior and vaccine strains varied between three and seven. When the prior was closest to the vaccine, a larger percentage of memory B cells, that were generated by the prior infection, cross-reacted with the vaccine. This led to a lower percentage of new memory cells generated by the vaccination compared to a control that had no prior infection. This lower number of new memory cells reduced the protection against the epidemic challenge.

and epidemic strains had little or no cross-reactivity, antibodies specific to the vaccine dominated the response to the epidemic infection.

We have shown the effects of cross-reactive memory and original antigenic sin in the context of three antigens, and investigated how they can lead to vaccine failure. Vaccine efficacy in the absence of prior infection was designed to be 50%. In the presence of prior infection, vaccine efficacy ranged from 40 to 100% depending on the antigenic distances between the prior strain and the vaccine and epidemic strains (for a fixed vaccine to epidemic strain antigenic distance). Even though the prior infection sometimes decreased the effectiveness of the vaccination, protection against an epidemic challenge was always increased by the vaccination. Extrapolating these results to the case where the prior infection is a prior vaccination, we can say that in the model, vaccination improves protection against the next challenge, but depending on antigenic distances between the antigens, might reduce the effectiveness of subsequent vaccination. Performing these experiments *in machina* was useful because of the large number of experiments necessary, however the predictions now need to be checked by a smaller number of *in vivo* experiments. Knowledge of the effects of different antigenic distances between the antigens might lead to more effective influenza vaccines by allowing prior infection or prior vaccination to be taken into account in the vaccine strain selection process.

**Acknowledgments**

The authors gratefully acknowledge the ongoing support of the Santa Fe Institute and its Joseph P. and Jeanne M. Sullivan program in theoretical immunology. DJS also acknowledges the University of New Mexico Computer Science Department AI fellowship and Digital Equipment Fellowship, and the help of Patrik D'haeseleer, Ron Hightower, Terry Jones, Andrew Kosoresow, Stan Lee, Wendell Miller, Ronald Moore, Mihaela Oprea, Francesca Shrady, Paul Stanford, Jason Stewart, Bernhard Sulzer, and Carla Wofsy. Portions of this work were performed under the auspices of the U.S. Department of Energy. This work was also supported by ONR (N00014-95-1-0364), NSF (IRI-9157644), and the Los Alamos National Laboratory LDRD program.

## References

1. M. Eigen. Viral quasispecies. *Scientific American*, 269(1):32–39, 1993.
2. T. Francis. Influenza, the newe acquayantance. *Ann. Intern. Med.*, 39:203–221, 1953.
3. F. M. Davenport, A. V. Hennessy, and T. Francis. Epidemiologic and immunologic significance of age distribution of antibody to antigenic variants of influenza virus. *J. Exp. Med.*, 98:641–656, 1953.
4. S. Fazekas de St. Groth and R. G. Webster. Disquisitions of original antigenic sin. II. Proof in lower creatures. *J. Exp. Med.*, 124:347–361, 1966.
5. S. Deutsch and A. E. Bussard. Original antigenic sin at the cellular level. I. Antibodies produced by individual cells against cross-reacting haptens. *Eur. J. Immunol.*, 2:374–378, 1972.
6. L. A. Angelova and Shvartsman. Original antigenic sin to influenza in rats. *Immunology*, 46:183–188, 1982.
7. D. J. Smith, S. Forrest, R. R. Hightower, and A. S. Perelson. Deriving shape space parameters from immunological data. *J. Theoret. Biol.*, 189:141–150, 1997.
8. P. E. Seiden and F. Celada. A model for simulating cognate recognition and response in the immune system. *J. Theoret. Biol.*, 158:329–357, 1992.
9. G. M. Edelman. Origins and mechanisms of specificity in clonal selection. In G. M. Edelman, editor, *Cellular Selection and Regulation in the Immune System*, pages 1–38. Raven Press, New York, 1974.
10. C. J. V. Nossal and G. L. Ada. *Antigens, Lymphoid Cells and The Immune Response*. Academic Press, New York, 1971.
11. N. K. Jerne. Clonal selection in a lymphocyte network. In G. M. Edelman, editor, *Cellular Selection and Regulation in the Immune System*, pages 39–48. Raven Press, New York, 1974.

12. G. Köhler. Frequency of precursor cells against the enzyme beta-galactosidase: an estimate of the BALB/c strain antibody repertoire. *Eur. J. Immunol.*, 6:340–347, 1976.
13. N. R. Klinman, J. L. Press, N. H. Sigal, and P. J. Gerhart. The acquisition of the B cell specificity repertoire: the germ-line theory of predetermined permutation of genetic information. In A. J. Cunningham, editor, *The Generation of Antibody Diversity*, pages 127–150. Academic Press, New York, 1976.
14. N. R. Klinman, N. H. Sigal, E. S. Metcalf, P. J. Gerhart, and S. K. Pierce. *Cold Spring Harbor Symp. Quant. Biol.*, 41:165, 1977.
15. A. B. Champion, K. L. Soderberg, A. C. Wilson, and R. P. Ambler. Immunological comparison of azurins of known amino acid sequence: Dependence of cross-reactivity upon sequence resemblance. *J. Mol. Evol.*, 5:291–305, 1975.
16. I. J. East, P. E. Todd, and S. J. Leach. Original antigenic sin: Experiments with a defined antigen. *Mol. Immunol.*, 17:1539–1544, 1980.
17. W. Gerhard. The analysis of the monoclonal immune response to influenza virus. III. The relationship between stimulation of virus-primed precursor B cells by heterologous viruses and reactivity of secreted antibodies. *J. Immunol.*, 120:1164–1168, 1978.
18. G. W. Both, M. J. Sleigh, N. J. Cox, and A. P. Kendal. Antigenic drift in influenza virus H3 hemagglutinin from 1968 to 1980: Multiple evolutionary pathways and sequential amino acid changes at key antigenic sites. *J. Virol.*, 48:52–60, 1983.
19. T. Francis, F. M. Davenport, and A. V. Hennessy. A serological recapitulation of human infection with different strains of influenza virus. *T. Assoc. Am. Physicians*, 66:231–239, 1953.

# Part III
# Artificial Immune Systems: Applications

# Jisys: The Development of an Artificial Immune System for Real World Applications

John Hunt, Jon Timmis, Denise Cooke, Mark Neal, and Clive King

Department of Computer Science
University of Wales, Aberystwyth
Penglais, Aberystwyth
Ceredigion, SY23 3DB, UK

**Abstract.** This chapter describes a machine learning system based on metaphors taken from the human immune system. This learning system, known as an Artificial Immune System (AIS), has been developed over the past 3 years. The current implementation, *Jisys*, embodies the results of this research. However, the Jisys implementation requires further development as well as application to complex real world problems. This chapter describes future developments of *Jisys* as well as consideration of how it can be applied to a complex problem in the domain of mortgage fraud detection. It should not be read as a design document, although it contains elements of such a document, rather it should be read as an indication of the directions which need to be followed, the issues which need to be addressed and some suggested solutions.

## 1 Introduction

The ISYS project is an UK government funded research project exploring the application of metaphors taken from the human immune system to machine learning systems. In particular it takes as its basis one particular theory describing how the immune system behaves [Perelson 1989]. It should be noted that the approach on which the ISYS project is based is controversial and is held by only some of the theoretical immunologists. This is not a problem for ISYS, as we are not attempting to model the immune system directly (as one might be within the Artificial Life community) rather we are attempting to exploit the basic theory and to employ other approaches as and where necessary. This is exemplified in our use of techniques developed in other areas such as nearest neighbour matching [Kolodner 1993], trigram string matching etc.

In the remainder of this chapter we first discuss the background to the ISYS project and outline the results of the first stage of the research work. We then consider our current research using the *Jisys* implementation of the AIS approach. Having done this we consider its application to the identification of patterns in mortgage fraud data. We then discuss the results we have obtained for *Jisys* with reference to both this application and the development of artificial immune systems. Finally we compare our work with other approaches.

## 2 Research into ISYS

The human immune system is a remarkable natural defense mechanism that continually learns about the foreign substances against which it must protect us. However, the immune system has not attracted the same kind of interest from the computing field as the neural operation of the brain or the evolutionary forces used in learning classifier systems. Machine learning systems based on the immune system, however, have a great deal of potential. For example, the immune system:

- possesses a content addressable memory which is accessed via a sophisticated pattern matching mechanism,
- dynamically learns about new substances when it encounters them,
- is a decentralised self organisation with no central controller (i.e. you cannot point to the central processing unit of the immune system),
- avoids becoming too specialized (i.e. you do not become immune to only one disease if you encounter large amounts of it),
- can forget little used information (this is why we need to get regular immunizations for diseases such as tetanus).

In the context of our work, an Artificial Immune System (AIS) implements some form of a learning technique inspired by the natural immune system. Within the ISYS project this has meant that our initial work attempted to provide a relatively close mapping between our AIS model and the human immune system [Cooke and Hunt 1995, Hunt and Cooke 1996, Hunt and Cooke 1995]. In particular we exploited some of the latest theories relating to how the immune system functions [Perelson 1989]. This resulted in an AIS model that inherited similar characteristics to the natural immune system. For example, it could not be over taught and was capable of forgetting little used information. This implementation is now known as *Pisys*[1].

### 2.1 How it worked

*Pisys* was comprised of a root object, a network of nodes, a teaching data set and a test data set (see Figure 1). Each node in the network possessed a

[1] The name *Pisys* is derived from the environment within which it was developed. This environment is called POPLOG and is a British AI environment that integrates CLOS, PROLOG and a Pascal like language called POP11. Thus *Pisys* is actually short for POPLOG-ISYS.

pattern-matching element that was generated randomly. These nodes evolved over time to recognize patterns in the input data set. This happened during the first phase of the system: the *learning phase*. The second phase represents a pattern recognition process during which *Pisys* attempted to classify new data relative to the data it had seen before.

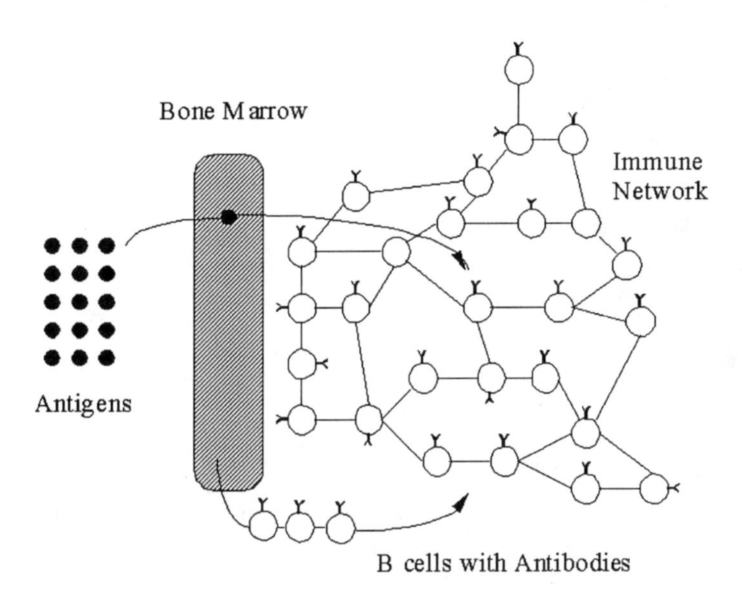


**Fig. 1.** The structure of the pisys system

During the learning phase, input data was inserted randomly into the node network. A circular, region-matching algorithm was then used to establish the match between the data and the node. This matching algorithm was designed so that continuous match would attract an additional weighting. It also attempted to find such regions at any point within the two data patterns being compared. This algorithm is described in detail in [Hunt and Cooke, 1996]. This matching process then produced a "match value" for the node.

If the match value exceeded the *match threshold*, then the node became stimulated. If the node's stimulation threshold rose above a specific point (the *clonal selection threshold*) then the node was sufficiently stimulated to clone itself. During this cloning process, the patterns held by the nodes could be mutated, thereby introducing variation and the potential to produce better matches for the input data. If these nodes are good enough they were then added to the network. Finding the $n$ nodes that were most similar to the new node and creating links between them did this. Each node could have up to $m$ links. If a node already possessed $m$ links then the link to the least similar node was deleted and a link to the new node added. This resulted in the emergence of regions that could solve similar problems. Between these regions bridges often occurred which indicated similarities between these problems. This is illustrated in Figure 2.

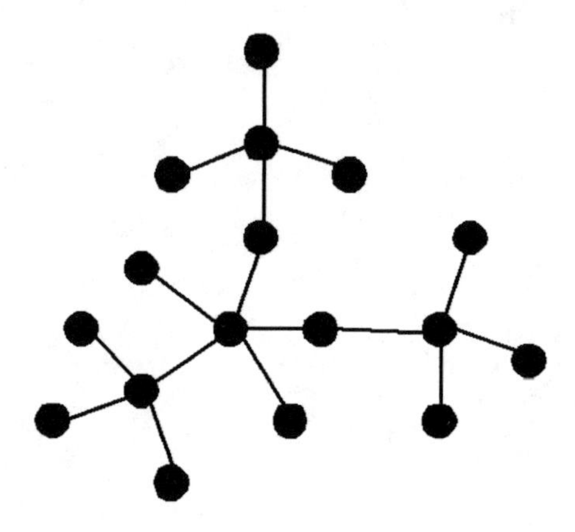

**Fig. 2.** The emerging immune network

In turn the network acted to reinforce the stimulation level of the better nodes and repress poorer nodes via a feedback mechanism. This feedback mechanism ensured that nodes with lots of similar neighbours generated higher stimulation levels than similar nodes without neighbours. The size of the network and the links within the network were dynamically generated by the interaction of the nodes. The effect of the network as well as matching data items on the nodes is illustrated in Figure 3.

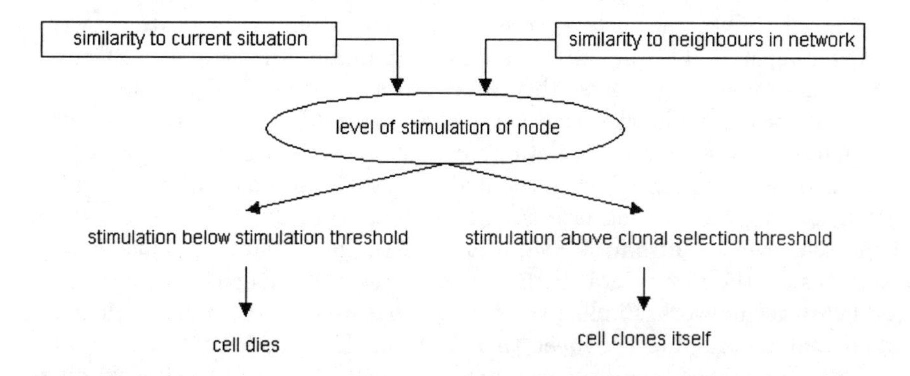


**Fig. 3.** Influences on the stimulation level of a node

Once each data item was presented to the network, those nodes whose stimulation levels were below the *stimulation threshold* were deleted from the network and destroyed. Thus over time the nodes in the network changed to reflect the improved performance of the network. In addition the actual structure of the network was continuously changing as new nodes were added, old nodes were deleted and the links between nodes were created and destroyed.

Note that when a node was inserted into the network, if the node matched the data item, then the nodes that were linked to that matched node, were also tested to see if they matched the data item. This matching process was performed using a reducing window. That is, initially 75% of the linked nodes considered the data item, then 50%, and finally 25%, before the matching process was terminated. This is illustrated in Figure 4.

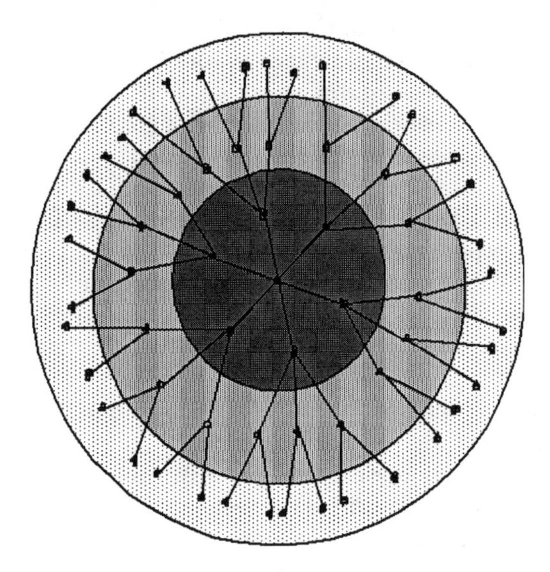

**Fig. 4.** Spreading consideration of data item

On completing the analysis of the data item the various thresholds were adjusted to take into account the improved (or not) performance of the whole system. In this way the thresholds were responsive to the way in which the network was learning the data presented to it.

Following the learning phase, the nodes are presented with test data. The system then tries to find any common features in the test set with those in the teaching set. This can indicate that the new data is similar to a particular class of teaching data, or that the new input contains a pattern similar to that present in some of the teaching data.

### 2.2 Problems with this approach

This approach worked acceptably for a number of (relatively small) tests nodes, see [Hunt and Cooke 1996] for further details regarding the experiments performed and the results obtained. However, for larger, more complex, real world applications this approach had a number of significant limitations that needed to be addressed. These included:

- **Node representation**: The representation used for nodes was very basic. In general each node possessed a string-based pattern, a match score and a stimulation level. Such a representation was insufficient for learning tasks with a variety of distinct fields.
- **Network initialization**: When the network was randomly initialized, it took a long time for the network to start to build useful patterns within the nodes and meaningful structures within the links.
- **Insertion overheads**: As the size of the immune network grew (due to the amount of data being stored) the performance of the node insertion algorithm degraded rapidly. This was because the insertion algorithm was required to compare the new node with every single node already in the network memory. This was necessary because the network memory was dynamically constructed from a network of interconnected nodes. The links between nodes in this network represented *similarity*. The algorithm therefore had to find the n most similar nodes, which would then be linked to the new node. The idea was that this would result in a structured self-organizing memory in which a retrieval algorithm could take advantage of the *similarity* links.
- **Too simplistic a matching algorithm**: We had also adopted a matching algorithm that mimicked the way in which matching is performed in the human immune system. This matcher attempted to find stable matches between continuous sequences of fields in the node. However, it relied on one fields' position, relative to another, being significant. While this approach was interesting and worked for simple binary and DNA sequences, the type of nearest neighbour matching normally found in CBR systems has proved more generally useful.
- **Node comparisons**: In the original system, locations within the network were selected randomly. This meant that the performance of the system was not only random, it could actually miss useful nodes altogether. For example, an ideal match for a new data item could exist within the network, however, because the node was not located near to one of the random locations, it may not be considered. Thus reducing the performance of the system as a whole.
- **Node deletion**: We also introduced the concept of node forgetting. Node forgetting allows little used information to be deleted. However, this was structured around the support (or not) of the surrounding nodes linked to a given node. However, as has already been stated, the network presented

undesirable overheads on the insertion algorithm. Therefore the ability of the system to forget little used nodes needed to be reconsidered.
- **Stimulation lead cloning**: In some situations a node would be a poor match for the current data but would be highly supported by its neighbours (who were often its clones). This resulted in high stimulation levels. This could result in a node being subsequently cloned even though it did not match the data. However, the stimulation level is extremely important in determining which nodes should be deleted and which should be retained. We therefore need to separate the stimulation from the cloning function[2].

However, there were a number of aspects to this previous work that we did not wish to lose. For example:

- The ability to forget little used information.
- The self-organizing nature of the immune node memory.
- The benefits of the immune network, within the retrieval algorithm.

We also wished to introduce new features, such as the benefits of the generality present in the immune system. That is, its ability to deal with infections which are similar, but not identical to ones it has seen before. The *Jisys* system was therefore developed to address the above issues.

## 3 The *JISYS* System

As a result of the limitations and problems identified with the original version various different avenues were explored. Much of the experimental research work carried out is reported in [Hunt and Fellows 1996] and [Hunt et al. 1995]. This research has been rationalized into a design for the *Jisys* system that is described in detail below.

The current version of the *Jisys* system is actually implemented in Java using a relational database for storing node information and the links between nodes[3]. The actual implementation will be outlined in section 4. Figure 5 illustrates the logical structure of the *Jisys* system.

The operation of *Jisys* is broken into four distinct stages. The first stage acts to initialize an immune memory, the second stage restructures the memory into an immune network, the next stage generalizes this memory (stages one and three use *different* training data sets) and the fourth stage acts as a classifier for new (unseen) data. Each of these stages and supporting operations, are considered below.

---

[2] Note that at present the *Jisys* implementation uses the stimulation as the indicator for cloning.

[3] Just as *Pisys* stood for POPLOG Isys, *Jisys* stands for Java Isys. Java was selected due to its object-oriented nature, its lack of pointers and the need for explicit memory management and for its portability.

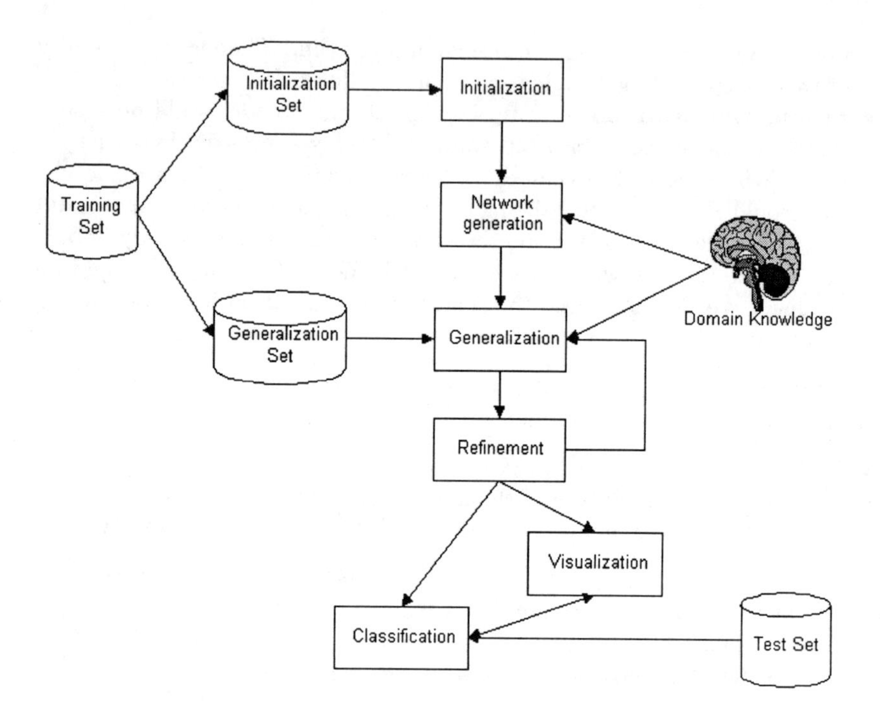


**Fig. 5.** The structure of the Jisys system

### 3.1 The node

In the *Jisys* system, a cell within the network is referred to as a node. This choice of term is intended to indicate that each network element represents one possible scenario. Each node has the structure illustrated in Figure 6. Note that the fields presented are those used for the application described later in this chapter. They are thus application dependent. It is interesting to note that the structure of this node is similar to that found in many CBR systems with the addition of the field labeled *stimulation level.* This field is modified by the *Jisys* system and will be discussed below.

### 3.2 The network memory: Initialization

During the initialization phase, when new data is being presented to the Jisys system, a linear node memory is used. A linear (or flat) node memory is one that does not impose any organizational structure on the nodes. Each node is considered to be as potentially significant as all the other nodes. The nodes are therefore held (conceptually at least) in a list. New nodes may then be added to the front, back or the middle of the list. In our system new nodes are added to the end of the list. This is a performance enhancement over the

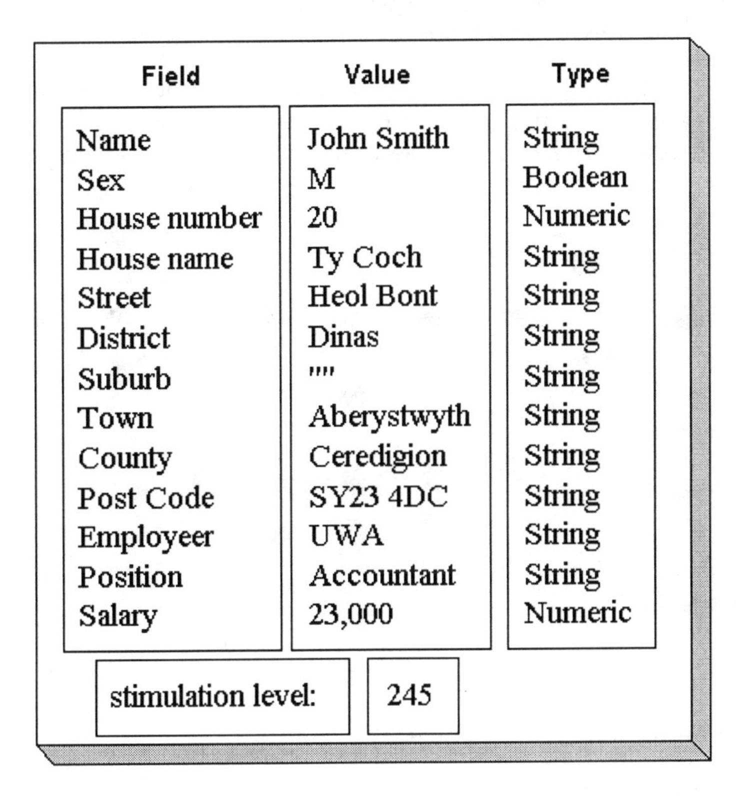

| Field | Value | Type |
|---|---|---|
| Name | John Smith | String |
| Sex | M | Boolean |
| House number | 20 | Numeric |
| House name | Ty Coch | String |
| Street | Heol Bont | String |
| District | Dinas | String |
| Suburb | "" | String |
| Town | Aberystwyth | String |
| County | Ceredigion | String |
| Post Code | SY23 4DC | String |
| Employeer | UWA | String |
| Position | Accountant | String |
| Salary | 23,000 | Numeric |

stimulation level: 245

**Fig. 6.** Structure of a node

original pisys system in which the network was being restructured each time a new node was added. The network is only restructured after all the nodes in the initialization phase have been added.

### 3.3 Restructuring

Next the node memory is transformed into a the immune network (this is illustrated in Figure 7). The immune network is a self-organizing structure (a feature particularly useful in data mining applications that often lack the domain knowledge required for the imposition of a predefined memory structure). Linking each node to n other nodes with which it has a "similarity" forms the immune network. The insertion algorithm is based on the algorithm described below.

Note that within the network:

- The nodes hold patterns which represent past data,
- Links represent similarity between nodes,
- Groups of linked nodes represent similar common features.

Figure 7 illustrates that in this particular network there are probably three distinct types of pattern that have a couple of common features. This diagram is actually taken from one of the network structures that were evolved.

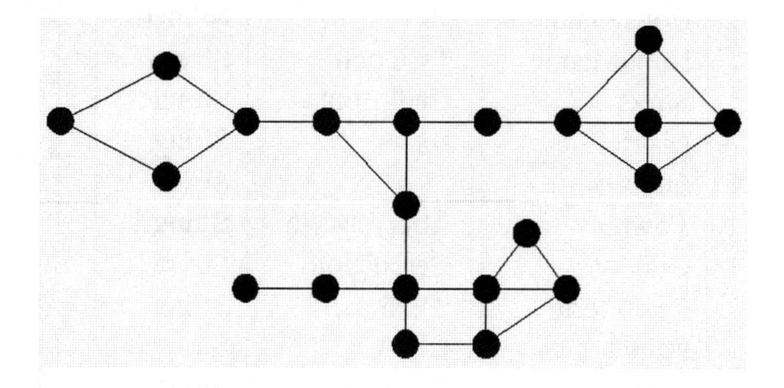

**Fig. 7.** The structure of the node network

### 3.4 The insertion algorithms

The insertion algorithm is based on the algorithm described in [Hunt et al 1995]. However, it is now only used once we have already obtained all the nodes we wish to use in the final system. Figure 8 illustrates the algorithm.

This algorithm illustrates how, when a node is inserted into the immune network, the system first finds the nodes that are most similar to the new node and links it to those. Over time this enables the emergence of regions within the network, which contain nodes which can deal with similar problems. Between these regions, bridges exist which indicate common characteristics between different problems.

Figure 7 is a schematic representation of the structure of the immune network. The emergence of such regions can itself, be a useful aid in the data mining process. We have now integrated the system with a tool, known as *JavaSpace*, that simplifies the viewing of, and interaction with, the immune network. The *JavaSpace* network viewer is illustrated in Figure 9.

### 3.5 The matching process

Figure 10 illustrates the structure of the node matching process within *Jisys*. The matcher uses three basic techniques during matching, these are:

```
For node in linear node memory do
      Search through nodes in immune network list and
                                               find n most similar
      For existing nodes in n most similar list do
             If node already has m links then
                  If least most similar link has lower
                                                  match value then
                  Delete least most similar link
                      Link node to existing nodes
                      Link existing nodes to node
                      Add node to immune network list
                  Endfor
      Endfor
Endfor
```

**Fig. 8.** The insertion algorithm

- circular region matching;
- trigram matching;
- number matching.

These techniques are described in detail in the remainder of this section. The three methods are used to obtain two different match scores.

The first score is obtained by performing circular region and trigram matching on all text fields and number matching on number fields. A match score is therefore obtained for each field. Nearest neighbour weighting is defined for each field, which is used to calculate a match for the entire structure.

The second match score is obtained by concatenating all the text fields of the node structure and performing both circular region and trigram matching on the resulting string. Number fields are excluded from this, and are compared using the number matcher.

Both the match scores are converted to a percentage of the maximum score that could be obtained. The highest of the nearest neighbour and concatenated match scores is then selected as the match score for the overall node. Note that in all matching algorithms we need to include the possibility of matching against a wild card value (indicated by a '*' below). Such a match should have 50% weighting (of whatever category is being used) to ensure that we don't learn that a node full of wild cards will match anything!

**Circular region matching** The top level of the algorithm checks for empty strings as shown below:

```
if at least one string empty then
```

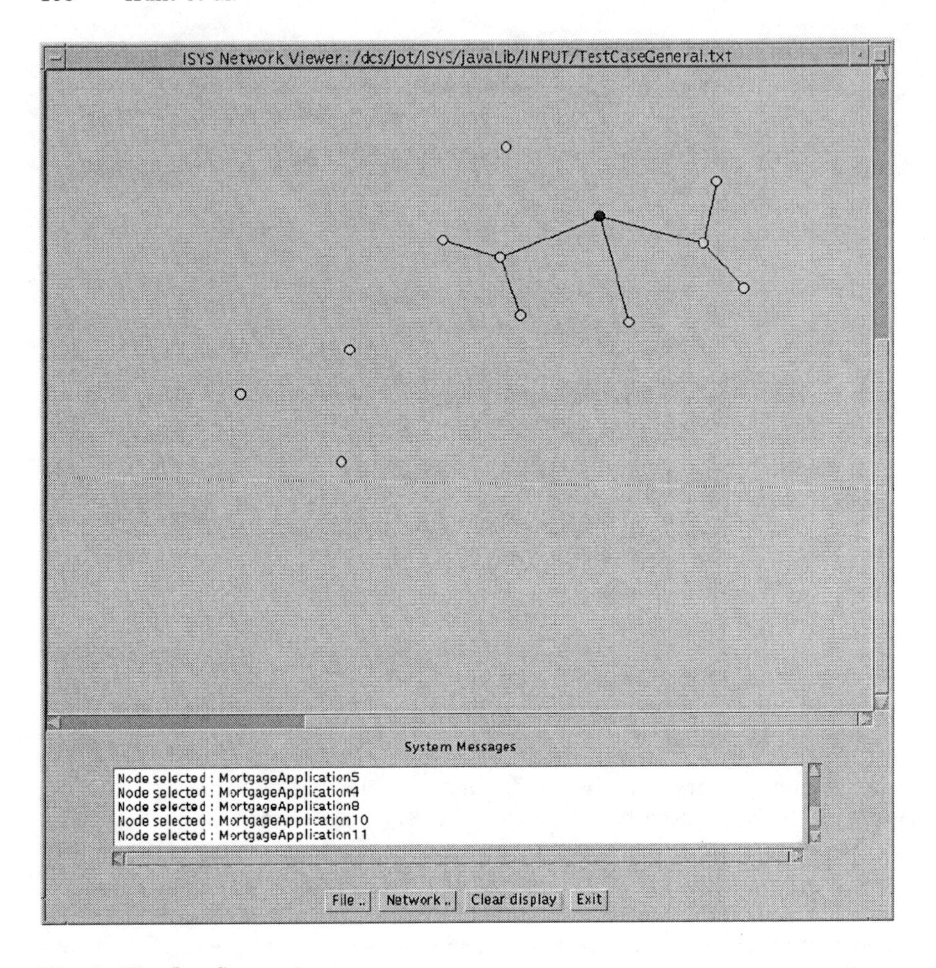


**Fig. 9.** The JavaSpace viewer

```
        percentage match is 0
    else
        perform circular region match on strings
    endif
```

This ensures that the circular region match will only be performed on two non-empty strings. The next step is to convert both strings to uppercase as the matcher is not case sensitive. The actual circular region match algorithm is then applied. This algorithm can be summarized as comparing two strings. Initially, the first string is compared directly with the second string. Subsequently, the second string is then logically shifted by one character. These strings are then compared until the second string returns to

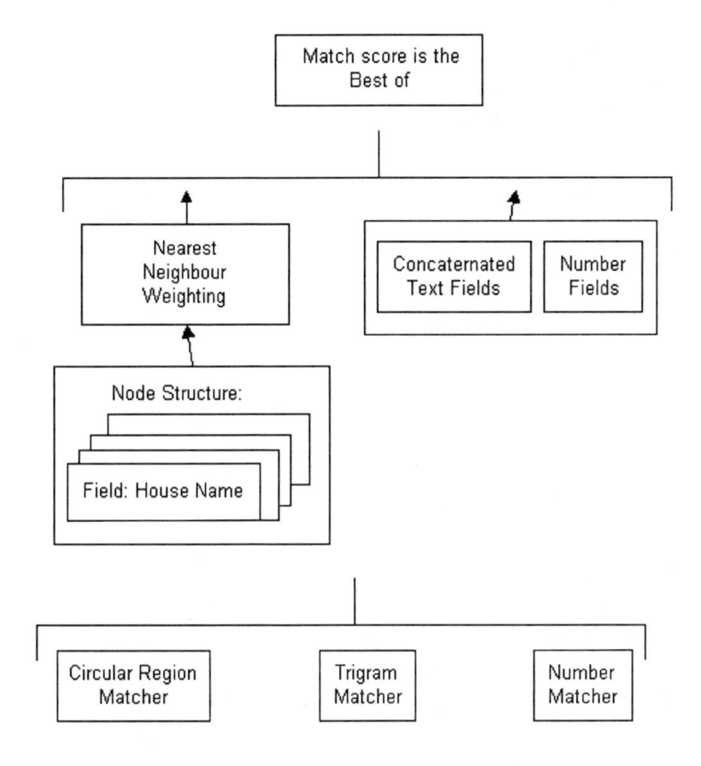


**Fig. 10.** The matching process in *Jisys*

its original pattern. For example, comparing the two strings "Monday" and "Tuesday" would result in the comparisons presented in Table 1.

**Table 1.** Comparing two strings using a circular matcher

| | Number matched | Length of region | Weighting of region | Total score |
|---|---|---|---|---|
| MONDAY $\Longleftrightarrow$ TUESDAY | 3 | 3 | *2 | 9 |
| MONDAY $\Longleftrightarrow$ UESDAYT | 0 | 0 | *2 | 0 |
| MONDAY $\Longleftrightarrow$ ESDAYTU | 0 | 0 | *2 | 0 |
| MONDAY $\Longleftrightarrow$ SDAYTUE | 0 | 0 | *2 | 0 |
| MONDAY $\Longleftrightarrow$ DAYTUES | 0 | 0 | *2 | 0 |
| MONDAY $\Longleftrightarrow$ AYTUESD | 0 | 0 | *2 | 0 |
| MONDAY $\Longleftrightarrow$ YTUESDA | 0 | 0 | *2 | 0 |

A match score for a single comparison is calculated by giving a score for the number of characters which match and keeping a region score that increases for the length of continuous regions which match. These two scores are added together for the final result. The highest score of any of the matches is chosen as the final match score.

**Trigram matching.** The trigram matcher starts by identifying individual words within the two strings to be compared. It does this by firstly converting all letters to uppercase, it then removes all punctuation etc., and finally it creates a list of words for each string. A trigram list is then created for each word. A trigram list is a list of all the possible trigrams for a word. Using the name John as an example, Table 2 illustrates the list of trigrams that would be produced.

**Table 2.** The trigrams for the string John

| - - J | - J O | J O H |
|---|---|---|
| O H N | H N - | N - - |

The trigram lists for the words in the two strings are then compared with each other. A score is given to each comparison based on the following:

- For each character in the same location add 6 to current score[4]
- For each character that is correct but in the wrong local add 2 to current score.

Each trigram is compared with each trigram from the second word. The resulting score is the highest score obtained for that trigram. The overall score for the string match is the percentage of the total of these scores from the possible maximum.

For example, using the name Malcolm and the mis-spelling Malcom the best comparisons found for each trigram in the first string are illustrated in Table 3.

This would result in a match score of 106 out of 126, or 85% indicating that the two strings are very similar.

**Number matching.** Using either of the methods described previously to compare number fields, for example the house number field, would result in a match score representing how closely the characters of one number matched the characters of another. A better way to compare a number field is to compare the values of the numbers themselves. The number matcher does this, comparing the number values of two fields. If the numbers are equal then the fields match completely. A close, but not exact match, is introduced by the concept of a range. If the numbers do not match exactly, but the

[4] The values 6 and 2 are illustrative. In *Jisys* these are desinable parameters in the configurartion file.

**Table 3.** Comparing two trigrams

| | | |
|---|---|---|
| - - M | - - M | 6 |
| - M A | - M A | 12 |
| M A L | M A L | 18 |
| A L C | A L C | 18 |
| L C O | L C O | 18 |
| C O L | C O M | 14 |
| O L M | C O M (or O M -) | 8 |
| L M - | O M - | 6 |
| M - - | M - - | 6 |

difference between them is less than or equal to the specified range, then they are said to match partially. In the following algorithm this results in an 80% match. If the numbers are outside this range then the percentage difference between the two numbers is calculated and used to determine the match score of the two numbers.

**Nearest neighbour matching.** Having found a match for each field of the node structure, using either circular region or trigram matching or both, a match score for the whole node is found using a nearest neighbour weighting system.

Each field has a weighting that reflects its importance. For example, the house number field may be more important than the post town field, the first having a weighting of 15 and the second 5. The match score for each field is multiplied by its weighting. The nearest neighbour score is then obtained by adding together the weighted match scores for each field. This is then turned into a percentage of the maximum nearest neighbour score. In this way a percentage figure is obtained for two entries.

The example below shows the scores for each field; followed by their weightings and the final scores this gives them.

This results in a final score of 4775 out of a possible 6600, giving a percentage of 72%.

### 3.6 The network memory: Generalization

The aim of this stage is to generalize the node memory such that it captures knowledge about the trends or patterns in the data rather than just the data itself. During this stage a second set of data items are presented to the system. However, this time all the nodes in the system are scanned in order to find ones that are similar to the new data. Having obtained the best n nodes, the system adds the match value obtained by comparing the new node and

**Table 4.** Calculating the nearest neighbour score

| Field | Score | Weighting | Weighted score |
|---|---|---|---|
| Name | 20 | 5 | 100 |
| Hse. Name | 45 | 5 | 225 |
| Hse. No. | 80 | 15 | 1200 |
| Street | 75 | 10 | 750 |
| Suburb | 0 | 10 | 0 |
| Town | 100 | 5 | 500 |
| County | 100 | 5 | 500 |
| Postcode | 100 | 15 | 1500 |
| | Nearest neighbor Score | | 4775 |

the existing nodes, to each of the existing nodes' stimulation levels. We are therefore using the following algorithm:

```
for existingNode in bestNNodes do
    matchValue := match(newNode, existingNode);
    existingNode.stimulationLevel :=
              existingNode.stimulationLevel +  matchValue;
```

When the match value obtained is above the *match selection threshold* the node is duplicated (or cloned)[5]. The number of clones generated is related to the difference between the average stimulation threshold of all nodes and the node's stimulation threshold. A clone is an exact copy of the original node.

Next one of three things can happen to a clone. The actual selection is made randomly and is one of[6]:

[5] Note that this is a major change from the approach taken in our previous work. In that work we related cloning to the stimulation level and cloned when a node's stimulation level was above the clonal selection threshold. However, a node might have a lot of very similar neighbours that cause it to be cloned, even though it was not a good match for the current data. This had negative effects on the performance of the system as a whole. However, the stimulation level was important, and effective, as a reinforcement mechanism to ensure survival of nodes in the network. We thus made the match value directly influence the stimulation level.

[6] This is yet another departure from previous work. In our previous work we only considered doing nothing or matching. This approach was most similar to the natural immune system. However, for applications such as mortgage fraud we are looking for common patterns. Mutation may hit upon these patterns but equally it may miss them all together. By introducing generalization we have a better chance of generating nodes which represent a common set of patterns. Of

**Nothing.** The clone is left as an exact copy of the original.

**Generalization.** The clones, and the data that lead to the clone being created, are compared. All common elements (i.e. the fields which matched) remain in the clone, all other fields are replaced with wild cards (indicated by a * in Figure 11).

**Mutation.** The clone is mutated so that it can exactly match a slightly different new node (see Figure 11). Note that the mutation performed during this phase does not necessarily match that of the genetic algorithm community [Goldberg 1989]. This is discussed in more detail below.

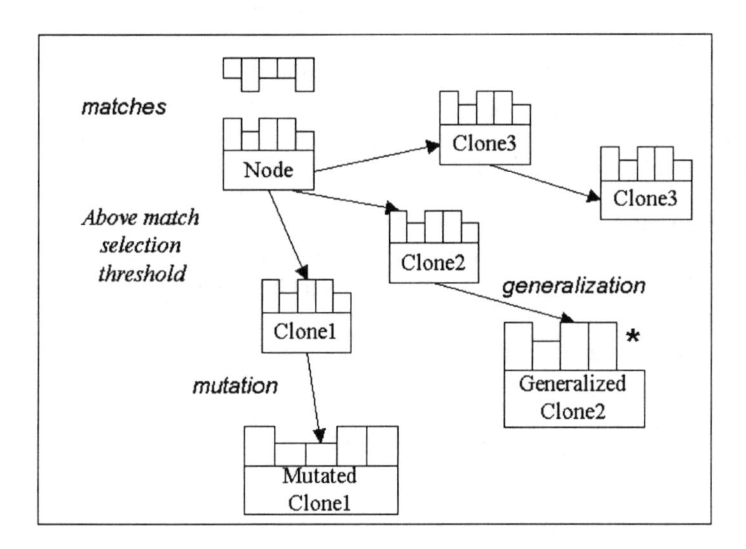


**Fig. 11.** Clonal selection and hypermutation

The current data item is then presented to each clone in turn to determine the clone's match value. The clone is then added to the node memory that is still ordered linearly (as well as being structured as a network). It will be integrated into the network structure and have its stimulation level set appropriately during the refinement step.

In this way nodes, which provide better matches for the new data item, clone themselves producing a greater number of matches for the new node. Note that if a generalization or mutation results in a node which is not consistent with the data (or which is a poor match for the data), its stimulation level will eventually fall way behind the stimulation levels of other nodes. This is important in the next stage of the learning process.

course, they may become too generalized in which case they are likely to die off as a wild card match will generate a lower value then an exact match.

### 3.7 Mutation within *Jisys*

When a node is cloned it may be mutated. This is determined by randomly generating a mutation indicator. If this mutation indicator is above the mutation threshold, then the clone will be mutated. Each type of field uses a different type of mutation, these are discussed below:

**Boolean fields.** To mutate this field, a new value is chosen at random from true and false.

**Numeric fields.** To mutate a numeric field we perform a type of real number creep. This is achieved by randomly generating a number between 0 and the field value. This number is then added or subtracted from the field value randomly.

**Enumerated fields.** To mutate an enumerated field, such as the days of the week, we randomly select a new value from the available set. This of course means that we may select the same value as the field already possesses.

**String fields.** These fields are mutated in one of two ways:

- Random mutation of the characters that comprise the string field.
- New value selection from an existing node. This is achieved by using a roulette wheel algorithm to select another node and then randomly selecting whether to take the value from the existing node or the selected node. Note that node selection is performed only once for a given clone.

The results of mutating the clone, of the node illustrated in Figure 6, are presented in Figure 12. The mutated fields are indicated in Italics.

### 3.8 The network memory: Refinement

During this step *Jisys* searches through all the nodes in the network to find all those nodes whose stimulation level is below the *stimulation threshold*. These nodes are deleted from the node memory. The stimulation threshold is set as a percentage of the average stimulation threshold and is application dependent.

The result of this node deletion process is that the node memory now contains the nodes that have been most use in categorizing the data presented to the system. That is, the more times a node successfully matched a new node, the higher its stimulation level. Next the node memory is re-transformed into the immune network (illustrated in Figure 7).

### 3.9 Classification

Once the immune network is constructed, this memory structure can be used to classify unseen data. To do this, the matching algorithm attempts to match any input data against all the fields in a node for all nodes. In this situation, the node memory is treated as a flat memory organization. Any nodes that

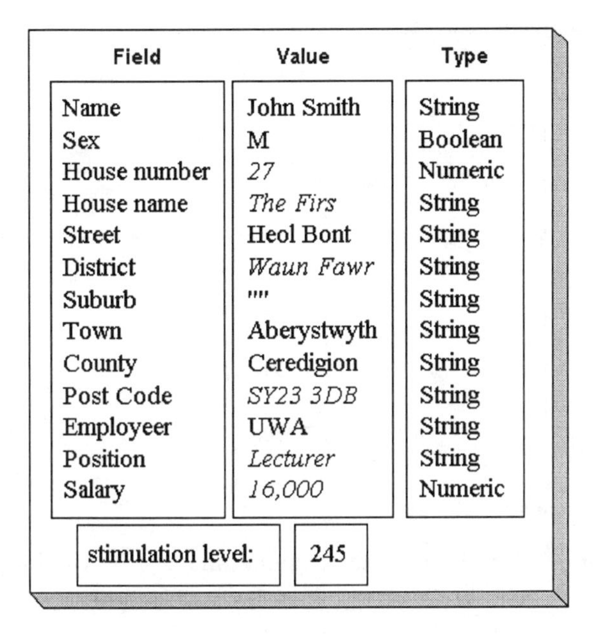


**Fig. 12.** A mutated clone

match the input node above the *clonal selection* threshold can then be said to classify the input data. These nodes are then presented to the user, indicating that they represent data that is in some way similar to that represented by the nodes (e.g. for mortgage fraud that the new application possesses some commonality with previous fraudulent applications). The number of nodes presented is user definable and can be 1 or more. The nodes are presented to the user with the closest match presented first. The analysis of the node network into a form that is more appropriate for tasks such as classification is the primary area of further work

## 4 Jisys System Structure

The Jisys system is comprised of a number of functional units, which together provide the functionality outlined in Figure 5. The physical structure of Jisys is illustrated in Figure 13.

There are 5 primary components to the Jisys system. Each of these performs a specific role that is summarised below:

- *Jidea.* This stands for **J**isys **I**sys **D**atabase for **E**xperimental **A**nalysis. It is the component that acts as the primary user interface. It allows a user

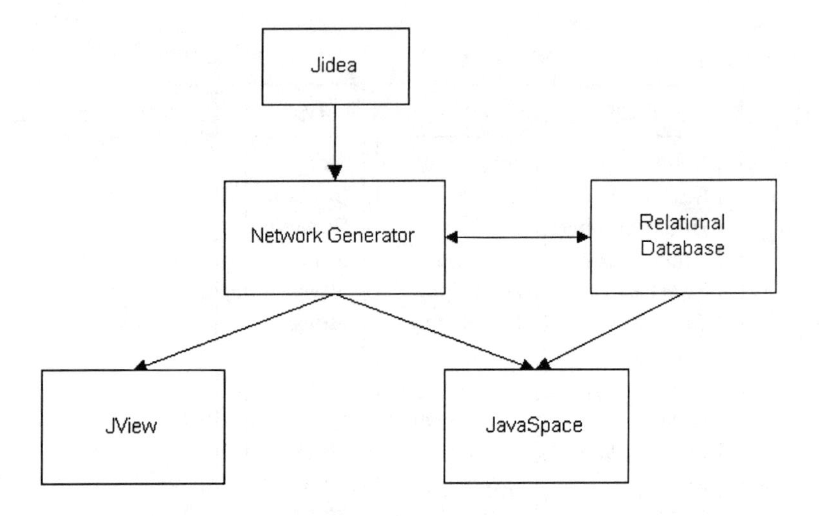


**Fig. 13.** The physical structure of *Jisys*

to select the data files to be used for training and testing the immune network, as well as providing a data file browser and editor. The *Jidea* interface is illustrated in Figure 14.

- *Network Generator.* This is the key component in the Jisys system. It initializes the node memory, generates the initial network, generalizes this network and refines it. It stores the nodes and links between the nodes in tables in the relational database. This also enables a previously generated network to be loaded from a database.
- *Relational database.* This is a relational DBMS that is used to provide not only efficient network generation and access but also persistence for the network. The original system used a purely object oriented approach, constructing a network of links between objects. Although the use of a relational database necessitates some transformation between objects and table entries, a major improvement in performance has been achieved. The database is accessed via the JDBC mechanism in Java 1.1, which insulates *Jisys* from any particular database system.
- *JavaSpace.* This is the network visualization tool described earlier in this chapter. It can display the node network as it evolves during the learning process or it can load a previously learnt network from a database for analysis.
- *JView.* This tool provides the classification operation of *Jisys.* At present this is the least developed part of the whole system (see further work).

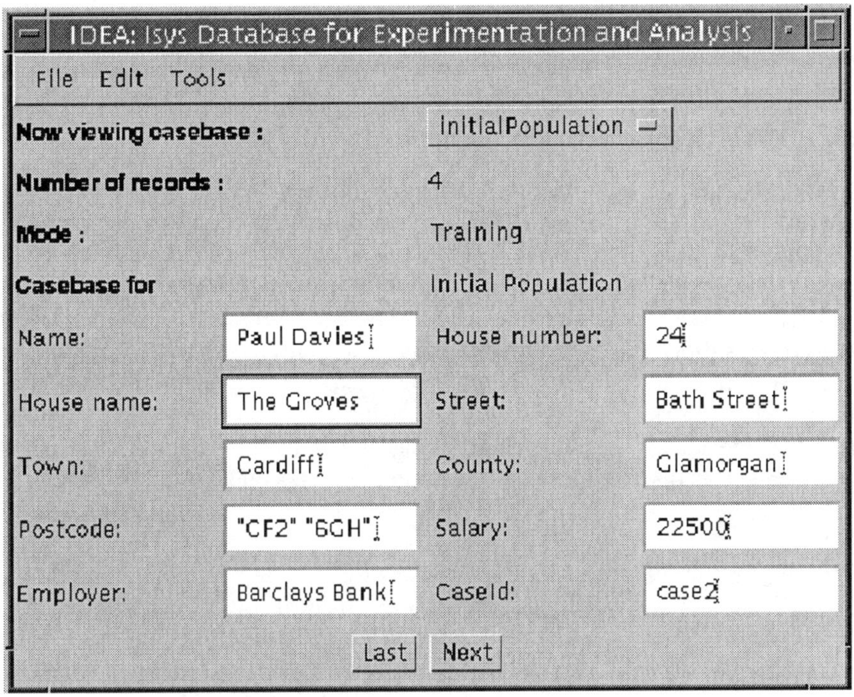

**Fig. 14.** The *Jidea* interface

## 5 The Mortgage Fraud Application

One estimate puts mortgage fraud in the UK at about £100 million per annum. Immunizing financial organizations against loan and mortgage fraud is therefore an important issue as well as a non-trivial computing problem. It involves the identification of valid, novel, potentially useful, and ultimately understandable patterns in very large amounts of data. The critical issue is that we are trying to extract knowledge from data. Depending on the techniques used, the identified knowledge can then be used to:

- Identify fraud in new applications.
- Explain existing fraud.
- Enable logical (as opposed to "graphical") data visualization to aid humans in discovering deeper fraud patterns.

An important issue relating to fraud is that as databases grow, fraud identification directly from their contents by humans becomes more and more difficult. A number of approaches have been developed to aid the human in their task. One such approach involves the use of A.I. techniques such as neural networks and machine induction. In this section we describe how the

*Jisys* system can be used to learn the patterns in a database relating to mortgage fraud.

### 5.1 Detecting patterns in mortgage fraud data

In this section we apply the AIS to the identification of fraud in mortgage applications. This is an extension of previous work done on data mining [Hunt and Fellows 1996] and is done by teaching the system on a database of known fraudulent, as well as non-fraudulent, mortgage applications. It then constructs a network of nodes which represent patterns in the network (note these nodes differ greatly from those found in neural networks as the nodes actually represent the patterns and the links represent similarity between nodes). This network can be examined, using a graphical network visualization tool, to identify significant groupings/areas in the network. The nodes can also act as discriminators for assessing new mortgage applications.

### 5.2 The data used

Mortgage fraud data can be categorized into two different types:

- mis-representation of the facts in order to obtain a mortgage that the applicant may otherwise have been ineligible for. In such circumstances, the applicant intends to repay the mortgage.
- fraudulent applications (for example, making up persons who do not exist in order to obtain money with no intention to repay that loan).

Both situations can result in bad debts that the vendor will wish to minimise. For example, one large loan vendor estimates that they have 3000 applications per day. Of these 10% are fraudulent. Each loan is on average worth about £5,000 that means that per day they are dealing with £1,500,000 worth of fraud. In such cases prosecution can be difficult, as it is necessary for the vendors to prove the intent to de-fraud. This is made more difficult as the law views those who default on payment as "intending to repay but being unable to do so" rather than being fraudsters - even if the information they provided was inaccurate. Thus prevention is much better than cure (although there is a tension between those marketing such loans and mortgages and those involved in fraud detection).

However, identifying fraudulent applications for a mortgage is made very difficult as the ways in which the fraudsters work continually changes. In these situations the greatest resource available to the vendors in their fight against fraud are the databases of past fraudulent applications. Encoded within these databases are the patterns of behaviour used by the fraudsters. However, these databases are very big. For example, a large loan vendor might well deal with many hundreds of applications every day of which 10%

may be fraudulent. Support from techniques that can analyse the resulting databases to identify such patterns is therefore desirable.

In this research, a data file of typical fraudulent patterns was prepared with the co-operation of a large mortgage vendor. This data file did not represent actual fraudulent applications; rather it was typical of the patterns of fraud, which are present in such data.

### 5.3 Domain knowledge

A key feature of the system is that existing domain knowledge should be easily integrated into Jisys. This knowledge will be used within the node matcher, within the mutation operators and (once these have been added) within the "histo-compatibility and self recognition" operators. The "histo-compatibility and self recognition operators" consider relationships within the pattern held by a node, as well as between this pattern and other patterns.

### 5.4 Analysis of mortgage fraud

The Jisys system has proved to provide an innovative solution to the identification and visualization of patterns of mortgage fraud. It can identify similar applications as groups of related nodes, as well as help to classify new applications. Current results suggest an accuracy of more than 90% on pattern identification and more than 80classification.

## 6 Analysis of *JISYS*

This section considers the success of Jisys as both a learning system for mortgage fraud data and as an artificial immune system.

### 6.1 Visualizing the immune network

Using the JavaSpace network visualization tool it is possible to explore the clusters present in the immune network. These clusters may indicate either fraudulent or non-fraudulent behavior. In the node of fraudulent behavior they may encapsulate some common fraud pattern. These patterns can be examined by human experts enabling a better understanding of the methods used by the fraudsters. This may allow human experts to redesign a mortgage application form or procedure to ensure that such fraud is easier to detect.

### 6.2 Identifying fraudulent applications

The information contained within the immune network can also be used as the basis of a fraud detection system. Just as in the natural immune system, once a particular fraud pattern has been encountered, it can be recognized in future applications. This means that if others try the same (or similar) fraud it can be caught.

### 6.3 Development of an artificial immune system

We have moved further away from the natural immune system with the development of *Jisys*. This is reflected not only in our adoption of the term node rather than B cell, but also by our use of techniques developed by the CBR community (such as nearest neighbour matching). However we believe that in adopting the strategy we have chosen we have addressed a number of the weaknesses with our original approach. For example, by allow the cloning of a node to be performed in a number of ways, rather than just using mutation the resulting cloned node has often proved to be far more useful. One additional method being considered is the use of crossover as another cloning operator as it can help combine useful features.

We believe that the pragmatic approach we have adopted to the application of various techniques is already returning dividends as our ability to apply *Jisys* to a real world problem, such as mortgage fraud analysis, illustrates.

## 7 Comparison with Related Work

The field of immunity based systems is growing rapidly (as evidenced by this book). However, no other system takes as literal an approach to the development of an artificial immune system as that presented in this chapter. For example, the work by [Kephart et al, 1997] on virus detection tends to focus on the analogy between their system and the immune system, rather than borrowing concepts directly from the immune system. In a similar vein [Dilger 1997] has employed immune system analogies for controlling an intelligent house.

Another trend amongst researchers in this area is to attempt to exploit immunity based concepts within other learning approaches. For example [Hoffmann, 1986] has compared the immune system, immune network and immune response to neural networks, while [Farmer et al 1986; Bersini and Varela, 1990] have compared them with learning classifier systems. This is a very different approach to that taken by the research presented in this chapter.

Another direction is that taken by researchers who attempt to elucidate the operation of the immune system by producing computer-based models, for example [Smith et al 1997]. Similarly, [Forrest et al 1993] use a genetic algorithm (GA) to model the evolution and the operation of the immune system. That is, they are using a GA to model the immune system to explore its behaviour.

From a machine learning perspective the two research groups closest to our own work are [Bersini, 1991; Bersini and Varela, 1990; Bersini and Varela, 1994] and [Gilbert and Routen, 1994]. Bersini and Varela have explored further the use of the immune network as an evolutionary learning mechanism. Their work concentrates almost solely on the immune network and ignores the genetic operation of the immune system. They have developed an approach which can be used for optimization of functions or controllers (e.g., they have applied their work to solving test functions, the travelling salesman problem, and optimizing a control function for the cart-pole balancing problem). In contrast, our approach learns about the data being presented to it in order to solve machine learning problems (e.g., classification, information extraction). This means that although the two approaches are both inspired by the immune system, the philosophy, architecture and abilities of the two approaches are vastly different.

Finally, [Gilbert and Routen, 1994] have used the concept of an immune network to create a content-addressable auto-associative memory. They have applied this system to the recording and recognition of 64 * 64 black and white pictures. Their system views the immune system as essentially a connectionist device in which localized nodes (B Cells) interact to learn new concepts or to recognize past situations. This differs greatly from our approach as is highlighted by Gilbert and Routen themselves when they state that they are only interested in "representing those aspects relevant from the point of view of their interactions .... only their combining regions". In contrast, in Jisys, we are not only interested in representing cells (as nodes in the network) but also in the genetic mechanisms by which new nodes are created and the network is evolved. It is also interesting to note that they failed to obtain a stable model that could remember patterns. This is in stark contrast to our approach in which we have successfully achieved memory in the Jisys system. This is due to the different manner in which we have used the network to support cells that represent patterns that have been learnt.

## 8 Future Work

Future work can be broken down into three distinct areas.

### 8.1 Further exploration of immunity concepts

We intend to extend the immune system metaphor further by exploring concepts such as killer nodes and hero nodes, T cells etc. The aim of such additions to Jisys would be to enhance its learning capabilities. Current work is considering the use of histo-compatibility and self-recognition operators. These are discussed further below.

**Histo-compatibility and self recognition operators.** Once the generalization stage (illustrated in Figure 5) is completed, the node memory can be scanned to find any nodes within which "histo-compatibility and self recognition" operators can be applied[7]. These operators are domain dependent and affect the stimulation level of the node. For example, a "histo-compatibility" operator may determine that the information within the node is not *consistent*, depending on the application this may have a negative or a positive effect on the node's stimulation level.

In turn the self-recognition operators may determine that a nodes' neighbours are all very similar to it. This may have a negative or positive influence on the node's stimulation level. This can be seen as a generalization of the influence of network neighbours in the *Pisys* system.

Figure 15 illustrates the resulting influences on the stimulation level of a node. For the mortgage fraud application histo-compatibility operators might consider whether the postcode is consistent with the address or whether the sex of the applicant is consistent with the name of the applicant, etc. In turn the self-recognition operators might consider whether there are a large number of applications from a similar geographic area all with common characteristics, etc.

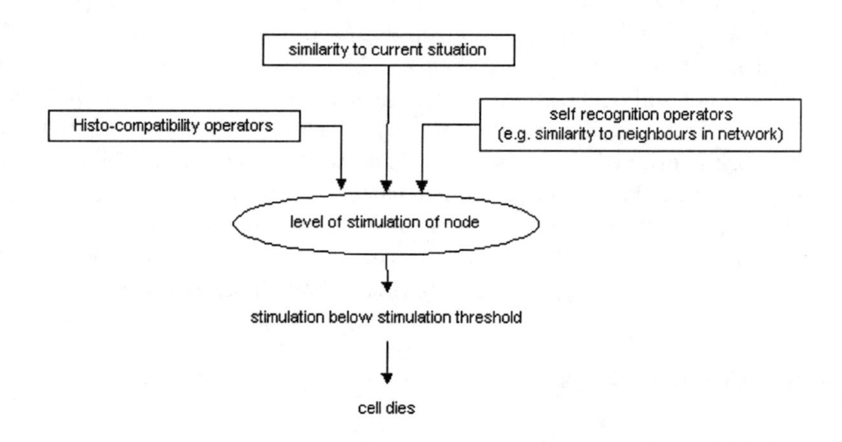


**Fig. 15.** Jisys influences on node stimulation level

[7] These concepts have been discussed numerous times by the members of the ISYS project and their use has been considered. However, they have not yet been implemented and this section represents a proposal for their implementation. The methodology presents has however been worked out using "thought experiments".

## 8.2 Generalization within *Jisys*

One of the cloning operators being consider performs a type of generalization on the node being created. Merging the new node with the original data item could do this. Any fields that did not match the original data item could then be replaced by a wild card. The result is a node that represents the common features between the matched data item and the matching node (an example of doing this is illustrated in Figure 16).

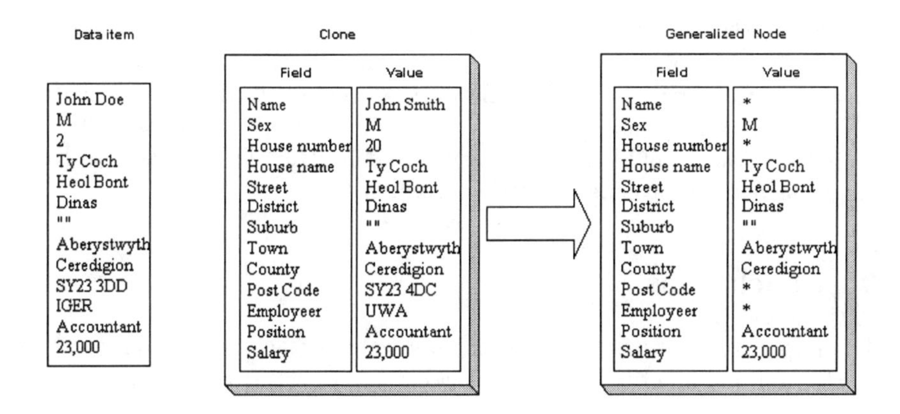


**Fig. 16.** Generalizing a clone

## 8.3 Immune network

A much larger and more significant area of research is the analysis of the immune network once the learning process has been completed. At present having completed the learning the whole network is used during classification (in a manner akin to a case based reasoning system) using the *JView* tool. Ideally this network should be compiled or compressed in some way. This is because in many cases it contains sets of related and very similar nodes. As a result the network is harder to understand for a user and less efficient for classification. There are a number of possible ways to compress the network. We outline some of them below.

**Option 1: Further analysis of the network.** Construction of the artificial immune system from a set of data results in a structure that classifies and relates that data in a useful way. It also however provides an effective set of summary cases that can be considered to be a data set in themselves. Large networks that are generated may not have any obvious overall structure, and by subsequently converting such networks into their corresponding data sets they can thus be analyzed in the same way as the original set of data. This process of treating an immune network as a set of data can thus be used repeatedly to generate hierarchical sets of immune networks that represent more and more general classes.

**Option 2: Exploiting inherent ordering of the network.** It seems clear that the construction of the immune network in the way presented produces a "topologically-ordered" network. That is to say that points that are closer in the network are also necessarily closer in the problem space under investigation. The fact that the network obeys this property will allow the development of more efficient insertion and deletion algorithms. Showing this result to be true for immune networks developed in this way no matter what the data set, and developing a coherent theoretical understanding of their behaviour, should then be possible and fruitful. This is likely to be a particularly useful avenue for further research.

## 9 Conclusions

The important features of the *Jisys* approach to machine learning (and to mortgage fraud identification in particular) are that it can:

1. Explicitly learn the patterns in the data. In our application this means that it learn patterns of fraudulent behaviour. A user can then examine these patterns. This can help them to determine whether it is necessary to change their mortgage policy.
2. Incorporate existing domain knowledge explicitly within the pattern recognition and learning processes. This can greatly improve the learning process.
3. Be capable of generalizing so that similar patterns are not missed, without the potential to become over generalized.
4. Generate pattern detectors. Thus allowing new mortgage applications to be automatically processed to determine if they are fraudulent or not.

No other immunity-based approach possesses all these features. This makes the *Jisys* system unique and enables it to address problems in a wide range of real world applications.

## References

1. [Bersini and Varela, 1990] H. Bersini and F. Varela. Hints for adaptive problem solving gleaned from immune networks. Proceedings of the First Conference on Parallel Problem Solving from Nature, 1990, pp. 343-354.

2. [Bersini, 1991] H. Bersini. Immune network and adaptive control. Proceedings of the First European Conference on Artificial Life. (Ed. F. J. Varela and P. Bourgine), 1991, pp. 465-465, MIT Press.
3. [Bersini and Varela 1994] H. Bersini, and F. Varela. The Immune Learning Mechanisms: Reinforcement, Recruitment and their Application, Computing with Biological Metaphors, ed. R. Paton, Pub. Chapman and Hall, London, 1994, pp. 166-192.
4. [Cooke and Hunt, 1995] D. E. Cooke and J. E. Hunt, Recognising Promoter Sequences Using an Artificial Immune System, in Proc. Intelligent Systems in Molecular Biology (ISMB'95), Pub AAAI Press, 1995, pp. 89-97.
5. [Dilger, 1997] W. Dilger. Decentralized Autonomous Organization of the Intelligent Home According to the Principle of the Immune System, 1997, pp. 351-356, IEEE SMC.
6. [Forrest et al 1993] S. Forrest, B. Javornik, R.E. Smith and A.S. Perelson. Using genetic algorithms to explore pattern recognition in the immune system. Evolutionary Computation, 1, 1993, pp. 191-211.
7. [Gilbert and Routen, 1994] C.J. Gilbert and T.W. Routen. Associative memory in an immune-based system. Proceedings of AAAI, 2, 1994, pp. 852-857.
8. [Goldberg 1989] D. Goldberg, Genetic Algorithms in Search, Optimization and Machine Learning, Pub. Addison Wesley, 1989.
9. [Hoffmann, 1986] G.W. Hoffmann. A neural network model based on the analogy with the immune system. Journal of Theoretical Biology, 122, 1986, pp. 33-67.
10. [Hunt et al. 1995] J. E. Hunt, D. E. Cooke and H. Holstein, Case memory and retrieval Based on the Immune System, in the First International Conference on Case Based Reasoning, Published as Case-Based Reasoning Research and Development, Ed. Manuela Weloso and Agnar Aamodt, Lecture Notes in Artificial Intelligence 1010, 1995, pp. 205 -216.
11. [Hunt and Cooke 1995] J. E. Hunt and D. E. Cooke, An Adaptive, Distributed Learning System, based on the Immune System, in Proc. of the IEEE International Conference on Systems Man and Cybernetics, 1995, pp. 2494 - 2499.
12. [Hunt and Cooke, 1996] J. E. Hunt and D. E. Cooke, Learning Using An Artificial Immune System, in Journal of Network and Computer Applications: Special Issue on Intelligent Systems: Design and Application, Vol. 19, 1996, pp. 189-212.
13. [Hunt and Fellows 1996] J. E. Hunt and A. Fellows, Introducing an Immune Response into a CBR system for Data Mining, in BCS ESG'96 Conference and published as Research and Development in Expert Systems XIII, 1996.
14. [Kephart et al, 1997] J. O. Kephart, G. B. Sorkin, D. M. Chess and S. R. White. Fighting Computer Viruses, Scientific American, November 1997, pp. 56-61.

15. [Kolodner 1993] J. L. Kolodner, Case-Based Reasoning, Morgan Kaufmann, 1993.
16. [Perelson, 1989] A. S. Perelson. Immune Network Theory, Immunological Review, 110, 1989, pp. 5-36.

**Dr. John Hunt** is the head of the Software Engineering Research Group in the Computer Science Department of the University of Wales, Aberystwyth, UK. His research interests are in immune network based software visualization for component reuse, model-based software diagnosis and the application of artificial immune systems to classification tasks. His current work involving the ISYS project is applying network concepts developed in the field of immunity-based systems to the visualization of reusable components. He is the director of a European Network of Excellence called MONET.

**Dr. Mark Neal** is currently a lecturer at the University of Wales Aberystwyth, the institution at which he obtained his PhD on "combined conventional and neural processing". Prior to working as a lecturer he was involved with various research projects involving the use of artificial intelligence techniques. Much of his work involved the development of the techniques so that they could be applied to a variety of real-world problems including multi-dimensional data-analysis and robotic control.

**Jonathan Timmis** is a full time researcher at the University of Wales, Aberytwyth. After graduating with a first class honours degree in Computer Science he began work on the ISYS project. His work is concerned with using metaphores taken from the human immune system, applying them the domain of machine learning and extending the application of Artificial Immune Networks to other complex real world problems.

# Decentralized Behavior Arbitration Mechanism for Autonomous Mobile Robot Using Immune Network

Yuji Watanabe, Akio Ishiguro, and Yoshiki Uchikawa

Department of Information Electronics
Graduate School of Engineering
Nagoya University
Furo-cho, Chikusa-ku Nagoya 464-01, Japan

**Abstract.** In recent years much attention has been focused on behavior-based artificial intelligence, (AI) which has already demonstrated its robustness and flexibility against dynamically changing world. However, in this approach, the followings problems have not yet been resolved: 1) how do we construct an appropriate arbitration mechanism, and 2) how do we prepare appropriate competence modules (behavior primitives). One of the promising approaches to tackle the problems is a biologically inspired approach. Among them, we particularly focus on the immune system, since it is dedicated to self-preservation under hostile environment (needless to say autonomous mobile robots must cope with dynamically changing environment). Therefore, we construct a new decentralized behavior arbitration mechanism inspired by the biological immune system. And we apply it to the garbage-collecting problem of autonomous mobile robot that takes into account of the concept of self-sufficiency. To verify the feasibility of our method, we carry out some experiments using a real robot. In addition, we investigate two types of adaptation mechanisms to construct an appropriate artificial immune network without human intervention.

## 1 Introduction

In recent years much attention has been focused on *behavior-based AI*, which has already demonstrated its robustness and flexibility against dynamically changing world. In this approach, intelligence is expected to result from both mutual interactions among competence modules (behavior primitives) and interaction between the robot and environment. However, there are still open questions: (1) how do we construct a mechanism that realizes appropriate arbitration among multiple competence modules? (2)How do we prepare appropriate competence modules?

*Brooks* recently showed a solution to the former problem with the use of the *subsumption architecture*[1,2]. Although this method demonstrates highly robustness, it should be noted that this architecture arbitrates the prepared competence modules on a *fixed priority* basis. It would be quite natural to vary the priorities of the prepared competence modules according to the situation.

*Maes* proposed an another flexible mechanism called the *behavior network system*[3,4]. In this method, agents (i.e. competence modules) form a network based on their cause-effect relationship, and an agent suitable for the current situation and the given goals emerges as the result of activation propagation among agents. This method, however, is difficult to apply to a problem where it is hard to find the cause-effect relationship among agents.

One of the promising alternative approaches to tackle the above-mentioned problems is a biologically inspired approach. Among the biological systems, we particularly focus on the immune system, since this system is dedicated to self-preservation under hostile environment (needless to say autonomous mobile robots must cope with dynamically changing environment). This system additionally has various interesting features such as *immunological memory, immunological tolerance, pattern recognition*, and so on viewed from the engineering standpoint.

Recent studies on immunology have clarified that the immune system does not just detect and eliminate non-self substances called *antigen* such as virus, cancer cells and so on, rather plays important roles to maintain its own system against dynamically changing environments through the interaction among *lymphocytes* and/or *antibodies.* Therefore, the immune system would be expected to provide a new methodology suitable for dynamic problems dealing with unknown/hostile environments rather than static problems.

Based on the above facts, we have been trying to engineer methods inspired by the biological immune system and the application to robotics [5–8]. We expect that there would be an interesting AI technique suitable for dynamically changing environments by imitating the immune system in living organisms.

In this chapter, we particularly pay close attention to the regulation mechanisms in the immune system, and propose a new decentralized behavior arbitration mechanism for an autonomous mobile robot based on the immune network architecture. We then apply our proposed method to the *garbage-collecting problem* that takes into account of the concept of *self-sufficiency.* In order to verify our method, we perform some experiments using a real robot (*Khepera*). In addition, to autonomously construct appropriate immune networks, we try to incorporate adaptation mechanisms into our proposed artificial immune network based on *adjustment* and *innovation* mechanisms.

## 2 Biological Immune System

### 2.1 Overview

The basic components of the biological immune system are *macrophages, antibodies* and *lymphocytes* that are mainly classified into two types, that is, *B-lymphocytes* and *T-lymphocytes.*

B-lymphocytes are the cells stemming from the *bone marrow*. Roughly $10^7$ distinct types of B-lymphocytes are contained in a human body, each of which has distinct molecular structure and produces "Y" shaped antibodies from its surfaces. The antibody recognizes specific antigens, which are the foreign substances that invade living creature, such as virus, cancer cells and so on. The antigen-antibody reaction is often likened to a *key and keyhole relationship*. For the sake of convenience in the following explanation, we introduce several terms from immunology. The key portion on the antigen recognized by the antibody is called an *epitope* (antigen determinant), and the keyhole portion on the corresponding antibody that recognizes the antigen determinant is called a *paratope* (see Figure 1).

On the other hand, T-lymphocytes are the cells maturing in thymus, and they generally perform to kill infected cells and regulate the production of antibodies from B-lymphocytes as outside circuits of B-lymphocyte network (*idiotypic network*) discussed later.

### 2.2 Jerne's idiotypic network hypothesis

Recent studies in immunology have clarified that each type of antibody also has its specific antigen determinant called an *idiotope*. Based on this fact, Jerne proposed a remarkable hypothesis called the *idiotypic network (immune network) hypothesis* [9–13]. This network hypothesis is the concept that antibodies/lymphocytes are not just isolated, namely they are communicating to each other among different species of antibodies/lymphocytes. This idea of Jerne's is schematically shown in Figure 1.

In the figure, the idiotope of antibody 1 (**Id1**) stimulates the B-lymphocyte 2, which attaches the antibody 2 to its surface, through the paratope of antibody 2 (**P2**). Viewed from the standpoint of antibody 2, **Id1** works as an antigen. As a result, antibody 2 suppresses the B-lymphocytes 1 with antibody 1.

On the other hand, the idiotope of antibody 3 (**Id3**) stimulates antibody 1 since it works as an antigen in view of antibody 1. In this way, the stimulation and suppression chains among antibodies form a large-scaled network and work as a self and non-self recognizer. We expect that this regulation mechanism provides a new parallel decentralized processing mechanism.

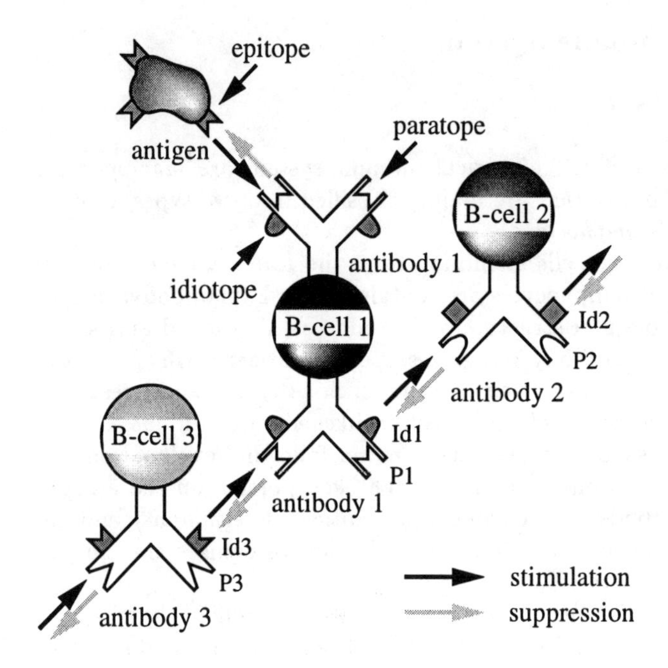


**Fig. 1.** Jerne's idiotypic network hypothesis

## 2.3 Metadynamics

In the biological immune system, the structure of the network is not fixed, rather variable continuously. It flexibly self-organizes according to dynamic changes of environment. This remarkable function, called the *metadynamics function* [14–16], is mainly realized by incorporating newly generated cells and removing useless ones. Figure 2 schematically illustrates the metadynamics function.

The new cells are generated by both gene recombination in bone marrow and mutation in the proliferation process of activated cells (the mutant is called *quasi-species*). Although many cells are newly generated every day, most of them have no effect on the existing network and soon die away without any stimulation. Due to such enormous loss, the metadynamics function works to maintain appropriate repertoire of cells so that the system could cope with environmental changes. The metadynamics function would be expected to provide feasible ideas to engineering field as an emergent mechanism.

Furthermore, new types of T-lymphocyte, which are also generated by gene recombination, undergo the selection in the thymus before they are incorporated into the body. In the selection mechanism, over 95% of them would be eliminated (*apoptosis*). The eliminated T-lymphocytes would strongly re-

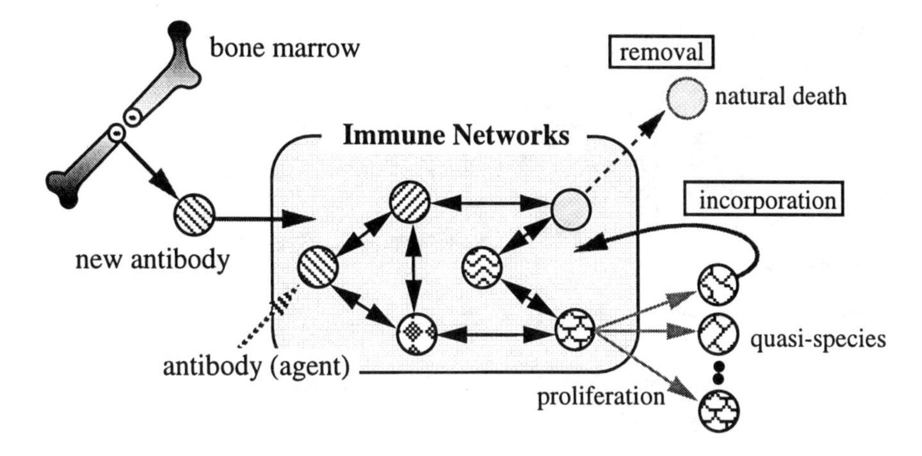


**Fig. 2.** Metadynamics function

spond to self or not respond to self at all. In other word, the selection mechanism accelerates the system to incorporate new types effectively.

# 3 Proposed Behavior Arbitration Mechanism Based on the Immune System

## 3.1 Behavior selection mechanism and the immune network

As described earlier, in the behavior-based AI, how to construct an appropriate arbitration mechanism among prepared competence modules must be solved. We approach to this problem from the immunological standpoint, more concretely with the use of immune network architecture. Figure 3 schematically shows the behavior selection system for an autonomous mobile robot and the immune network architecture.

From the figure, we should notice that there are some similarities between these systems. That is, current situations, (e.g. distance and direction to the obstacle, etc.) detected by installed sensors, work as multiple antigens, and a prepared competence module (i.e. simple behavior) is regarded as an antibody (or B-lymphocyte), while the interaction between modules is replaced by the stimulation and suppression between antibodies. The basic concept of our method is that the immune system equipped with the autonomous mobile robot selects a competence module (antibody) suitable for the detected current situation (antigens) in a bottom-up manner.

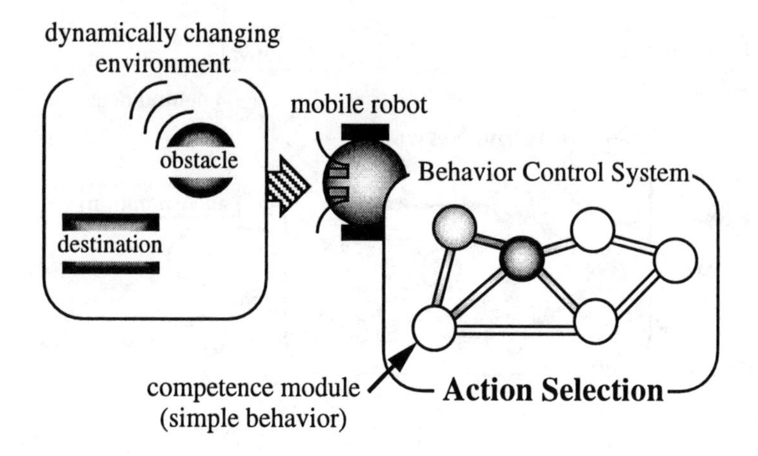


(a) An autonomous mobile robot with a behavior selection mechanism

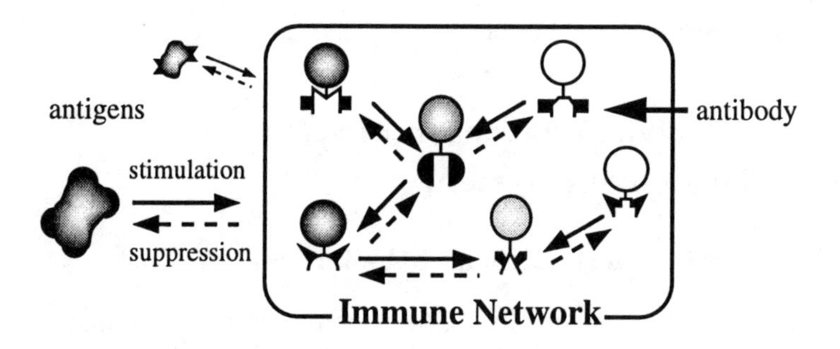


(b) Immune network architecture.

**Fig. 3.** Basic concept of our proposed method

### 3.2 The problem

For the ease of the following explanation, we firstly describe the problem used to confirm the ability of an autonomous mobile robot with our proposed immune network-based behavior arbitration mechanism (for convenience, we dub the robot *immunoid*).

To be really autonomous, robot must not only accomplish the given task, but also be self-sufficient [17,18]. Inspired by their works, we adopt the following garbage collecting problem that takes into account of the concept of self-sufficiency. Figure 4 shows the environment. As can be seen in the figure, this environment, surrounded by walls, has a lot of garbage to be collected. And there exist garbage cans and a battery charger in the home base. The task of immunoid is to collect the garbage into the garbage can without running out of its internal energy (i.e. battery level). Note that immunoid consumes some energy as it moves around the environment. This is similar to the *metabolism* in the biological system.

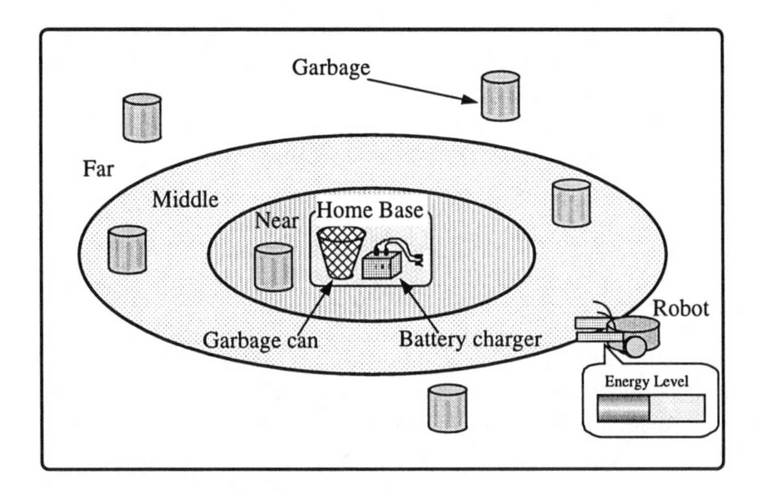


**Fig. 4.** The Problem Environment

In this study, we assume that prespecified quantity of initial energy is given to immunoid, and the simulated internal sensor installed in immunoid can detect the current energy level. For quantitative evaluation, we also use the following assumptions:

- Immunoid consumes energy $E_m$ with every step.
- Immunoid loses additional energy $E'_m$ when it carries garbage.
- If immunoid collides with garbage or a wall, it loses some energy $E_c$.
- If immunoid reaches the home base, it instantaneously gains full energy.
- If the energy level of immunoid is high, *go to home base* behavior might not emerge to avoid over-charging.

Based on the above assumptions, we calculate current energy level as:

$$E(t) = E(t-1) - E_m - k_1 E'_m - k_2 E_c, \tag{1}$$

$$k_1 = \begin{cases} 1 : \text{garbage is in the hand} \\ 0 : \text{otherwise} \end{cases}$$

$$k_2 = \begin{cases} 1 : \text{collision with wall/garbage} \\ 0 : \text{otherwise} \end{cases}$$

where $E(t)$ denotes the energy level at time $t$. For ease of understanding, we explain why this problem is suitable for the behavior arbitration problem in detail using the following situations. Assume that immunoid is in the far distance from the home base, and its energy level is low. In this situation, if immunoid carries the garbage, it will run out of its energy due to the term $E'_m$ in equation (1). Therefore, immunoid should select the *go to home base* behavior to fulfill its energy. In other word, the priority of the *go to home base* behavior should be higher than that of the *garbage-collecting* behavior.

On the other hand, if immunoid is in the near distance from the home base. In this situation, unlike the above situation, it would be preferable to select the *garbage-collecting* behavior. From these examples, it is understood that immunoid should select an appropriate competence module by flexibly varying the priorities of the prepared competence modules according to the internal/external situations.

### 3.3 Description of the antigens and antibodies

As described earlier, the detected current internal/external situation and the prepared simple behavior work as an antigen and an antibody, respectively. In this study, each antigen informs the existence of garbage (direction), wall (direction) and home base (direction and distance), and also current internal energy level. For simplicity, we categorize direction and/or distance of the detected objects and the detected internal energy level as:

- direction → front, right, left, back
- distance → far, middle, near
- energy level → high, low.

Next, we explain how we describe an antibody in detail. To make immunoid select a suitable antibody against the current antigen, we must look carefully into the definition of the antibodies. Moreover, we should recall that our immunological arbitration mechanism selects an antibody in a bottom-up manner through the interaction among antibodies.

To realize the above requirements, we define the description of antibodies as follows. As mentioned in the previous section, the identity of each antibody is generally determined by the structure (e.g. molecular shape) of its paratope and idiotope. Figure 5 depicts our proposed definition of antibodies. As depict in the figure, we assign a pair of precondition and behavior to the paratope, and the ID-number of the stimulating antibody and the degree of stimuli to the idiotope, respectively. The structure of the precondition is the same as the antigen described above. We prepare the following behaviors for immunoid in the garbage-collecting problem: *move forward, turn right, turn left, explore, catch garbage, and search for home base.*

For an antibody selection, an index that quantitatively represents suitableness under the current situation is necessary. We assign one state variable called *concentration of antibody* to each antibody (discussed later in section 3.5).

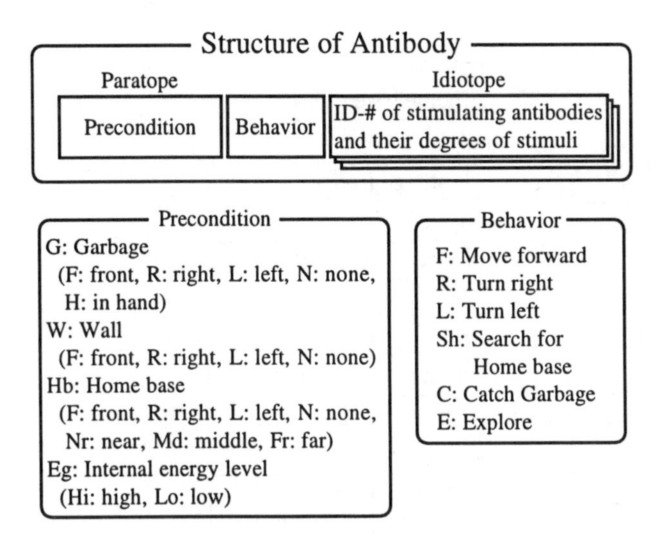


**Fig. 5.** Description of the antibodies

### 3.4 Interaction among antibodies

Next, we explain the interaction among antibodies, that is, the basic principle of our immunological consensus-making networks in detail. For the ease of understanding, we assume that immunoid is placed in the situation shown in Figure 6 as an example. In this situation, three antigens possibly invade immunoid's interior.

Suppose that the listed four antibodies are prepared in advance that respond to these antigens. For example, **antibody 1** means that if immunoid detects the home base in the right direction, this antibody is activated and then would cause *turn right* behavior. However, if the current energy level is high, this antibody would give way to other antibodies represented by its idiotope (in this case, **antibody 4**) to prevent over-charging.

Now assume that immunoid has enough energy, in this case **antibodies 1, 2** and **4** are simultaneously stimulated by the antigens. As a result, the concentration of these antibodies increases. However, due to the interactions indicated by the arrows among the antibodies through their paratopes and idiotopes, the concentration of each antibody varies. Finally, **antibody 2** will have the highest concentration, and then is allowed to be selected. This means that immunoid catches the garbage.

In the case where immunoid has not enough energy, **antibody 1** tends to be selected in the same way. This means that immunoid ignores the garbage and tries to recharge its energy. As observed in this example, the interactions among the antibodies work as a priority adjustment mechanism.

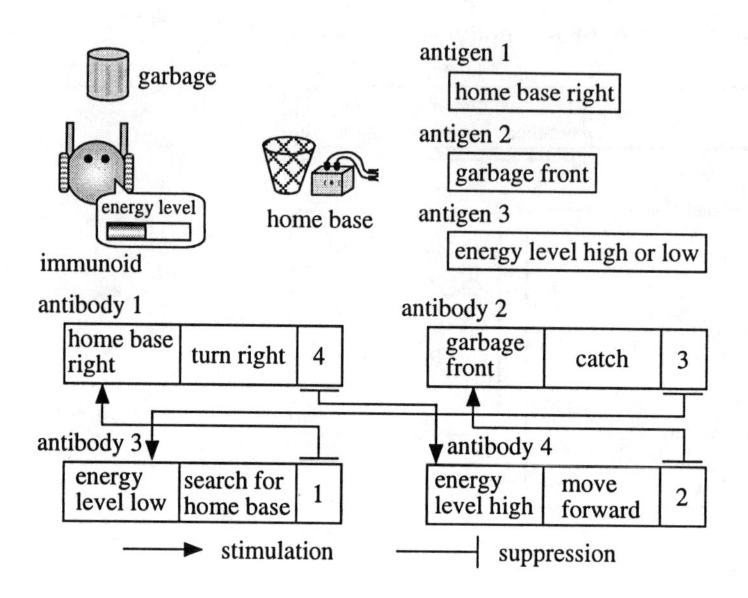


**Fig. 6.** An example of consensus-making network by interacting among antibodies

### 3.5 Dynamics

The concentration of $i$-th antibody, which is denoted by $a_i$, is calculated as follows:

$$\frac{dA_i(t)}{dt} = \left\{ \alpha \sum_{j=1}^{N} m_{ji} a_j(t) - \alpha \sum_{k=1}^{N} m_{ik} a_k(t) + \beta m_i - k_i \right\} a_i(t) \, , \tag{2}$$

$$a_i(t+1) = \frac{1}{1 + \exp(0.5 - A_i(t))} \, , \tag{3}$$

where, in equation (2), $N$ is the number of antibodies. $m_{ji}$ and $m_i$ denote affinities between antibody $j$ and antibody $i$ (i.e. the degree of disallowance), and between antibody $i$ and the detected antigen, respectively. The first and second terms of the right hand side denote the stimulation and suppression from other antibodies, respectively. The third term represents the stimulation from the antigen, and the forth term the dissipation factor (i.e. natural death). Equation (3) is a squashing function used to ensure the stability of the concentration. In this study, selection of antibodies is simply carried out on a *roulette-wheel manner* basis according to the magnitude of concentrations of the antibodies. Note that only one antibody is allowed to activate and act its corresponding behavior to the world.

### 3.6 Experimental results

To verify the feasibility of our proposed method, we carry out some experiments. In the experiments, we use the *Khepera* robot, which is widely used for experiments, as immunoid. The robot has a gripper to catch the garbage and it is equipped with 8 infrared proximity sensors, eight photo sensors, and one color CCD camera. Each infrared sensor detects garbage or a wall of its corresponding direction. The photo sensors recognize the direction of the electric-light bulb (i.e. the home base). The CCD camera detects the color (red (far), green (middle), and blue (near)) at the current position and this in turn tells immunoid the current distance to the home base (see Figure 7).

As a rudimentary stage of investigation, we prepare 24 antibodies of which the paratope and the idiotope are described a priori. Figure 8 shows the structure of the immune networks by the prepared antibodies. In the figure, the degrees of stimuli (affinities) in each idiotope are omitted for lack of space.

At the beginning, we equip immunoid with the maximum energy level (i.e. 1000). We set $E_m = 1$, $E'_m = 3$, and $E_c = 5$. Typical results obtained in the experiments are as follows: while the energy level is enough, immunoid tries to collect garbage into the home base. As the remaining energy runs out, immunoid tends to select an antibody concerned with *go to home base* and/or *search for home base* behaviors. After successful reaching the home base, immunoid starts to explore again. Such a regular behavior could be frequently observed in the experiments.

In order to evaluate the ability of our proposed arbitration mechanism, we furthermore carry out simple experiments by varying the initial energy level. Figure 9(a) and (b) are the resultant trajectories of immunoid in the case where the initial energy level is set to 1000 (maximum) and 300, respectively. In case 1, due to the enough energy level, immunoid collects the garbage $B$ and successfully reach the home base. On the other hand, in case 2, due to the critical energy level, immunoid ignores the garbage $B$ and then collects the garbage $A$.

In spite of simple experiments, we can see from the figure that immunoid selects an appropriate antibodies according to both the internal and external situations by flexibly changing the priorities among the antibodies.

## 4 Adaptation Mechanisms

### 4.1 Classification of adaptation mechanisms

In the previous section, we manually prepared antibodies and designed the immune network architecture. However, such a design approach would collapse as the number of the antibodies increased. Therefore, for more usefulness, the introduction of some adaptation mechanisms is highly indispensable. The adaptation mechanism is usually classified into two types: *adjustment*

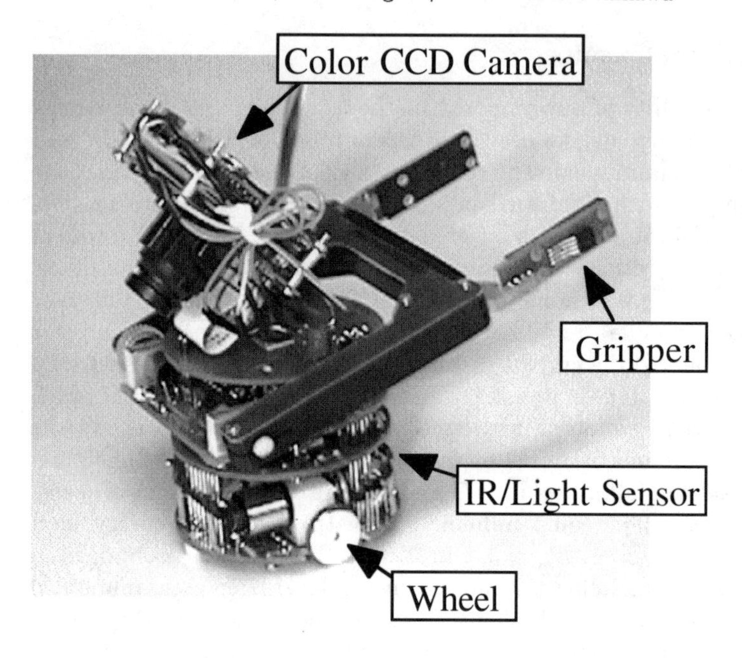


(a) Immunoid

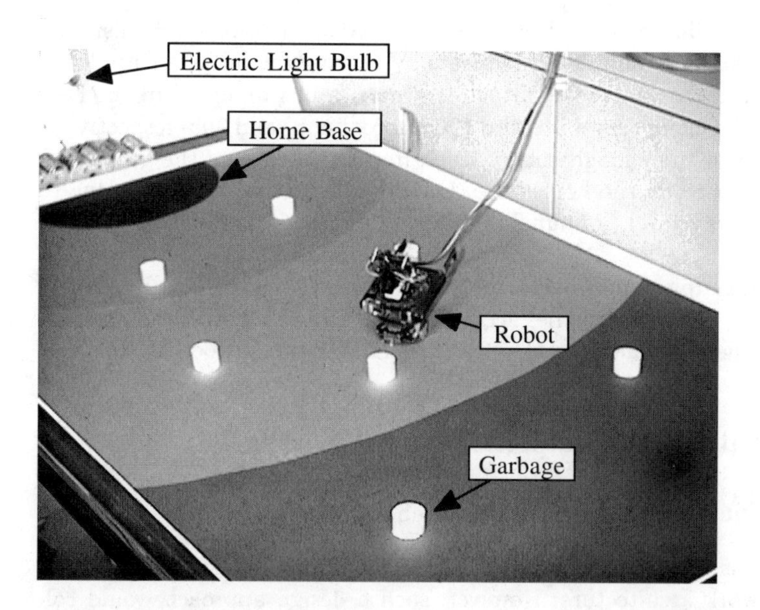


(b) Experimental environment

**Fig. 7.** Experimental system

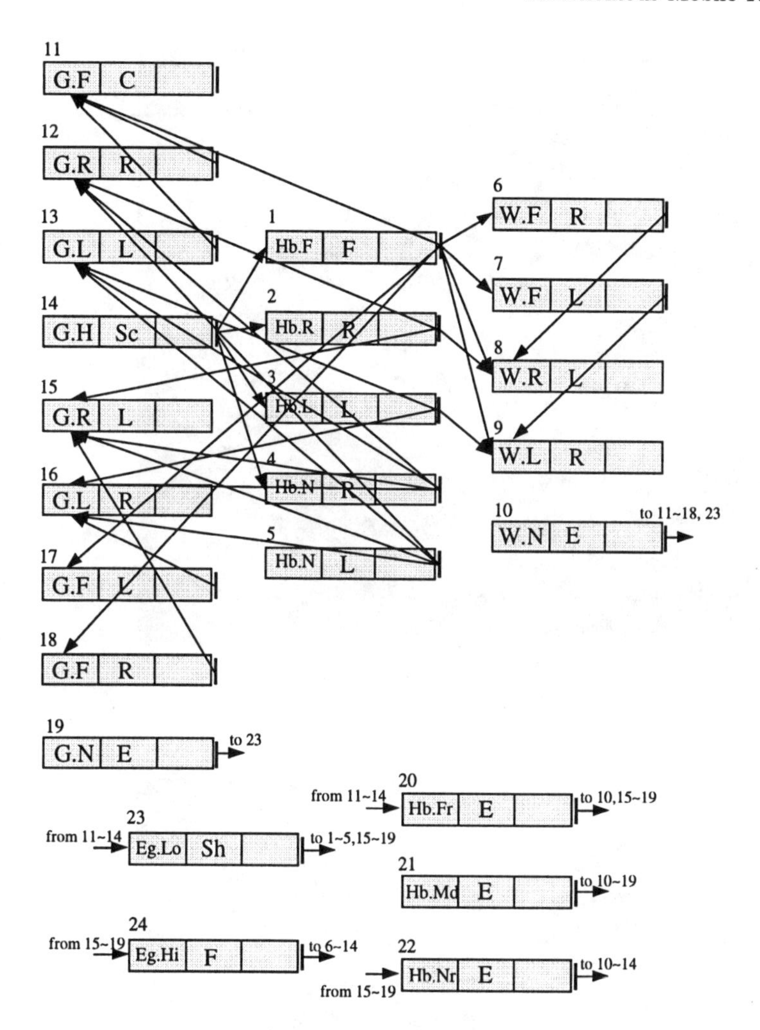


**Fig. 8.** Structure of the immune network

and *innovation* [19,20]. The adjustment can be considered as the adaptation by changing parameters in systems, e.g. modification of synaptic weights in neural networks, while the innovation as the adaptation by selection mechanisms. In the followings, we propose two types of adaptation mechanisms based on the adjustment and the innovation mechanisms to construct an appropriate artificial immune network without human intervention.

### 4.2 Adjustment mechanism

For an appropriate arbitration, it is necessary to appropriately determine the ID-number of the stimulating antibody and its degree of stimuli $m_{ij}$, which are described in each idiotope. To realize this aim, we propose the

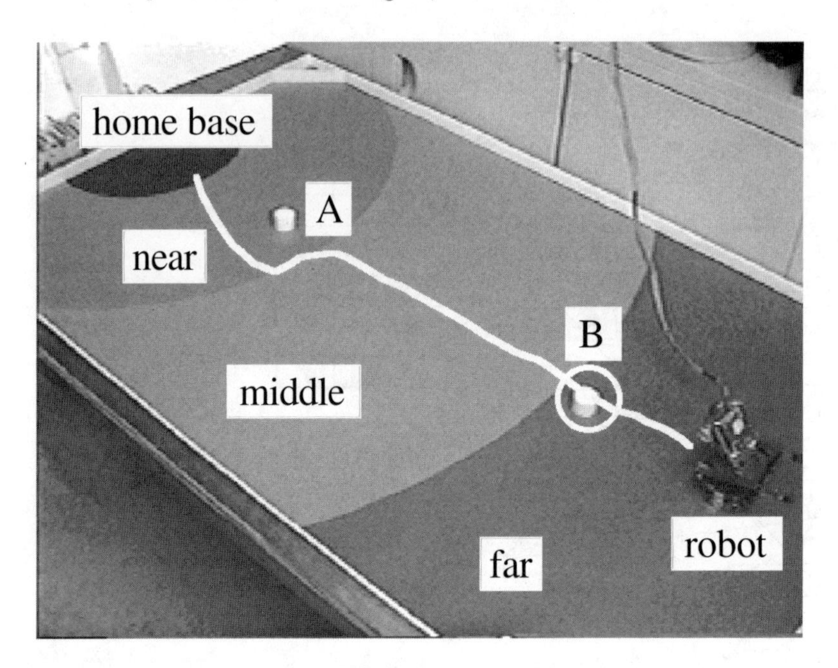


(a) Case 1 (initial energy level = 1000).

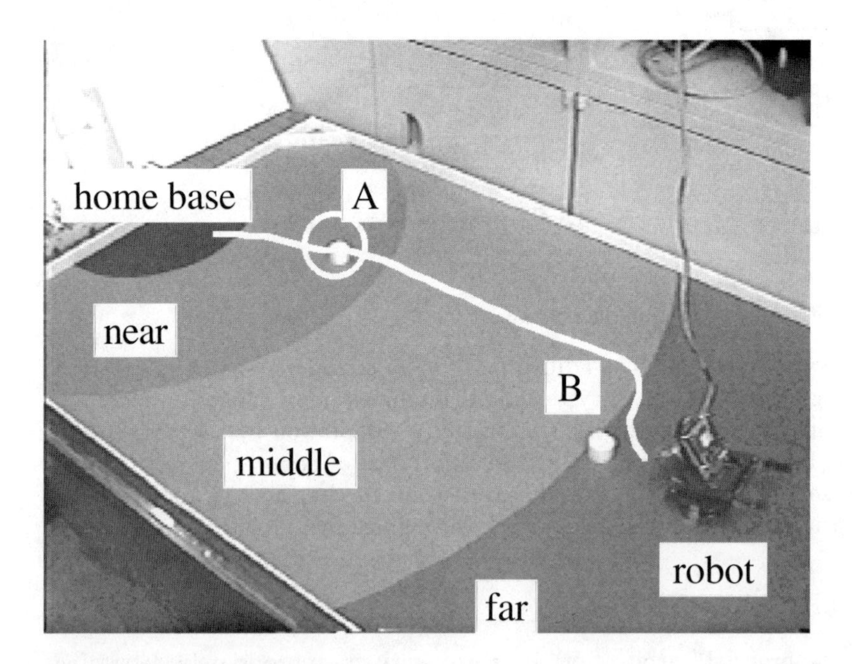


(b) Case 2 (initial energy level = 300).

**Fig. 9.** Resultant trajectories

on-line adjustment mechanism that initially starts from the situation where the idiotopes of the prepared antibodies are undefined, and then obtains the idiotopes using reinforcement signals.

For the following explanation, we assume that antigen 1 and 2 invade immunoid's interior (see Figure 10). In this example, each antigen simultaneously stimulates antibody 1 (**Ab1**) and 2 (**Ab2**). Consequently, the concentration of each antibody increases. However, since the priority between **Ab1** and **Ab2** is unknown (because idiotopes are initially undefined, there are no stimulation/suppression chain), in this case either of them can be selected randomly.

Now, assuming that immunoid randomly selects **Ab1** and then receives a positive reinforcement signal as a reward. To make immunoid tend to select **Ab1** under the same or similar antigens (situation), we record the ID-number of **Ab1** (i.e. 1) in the idiotope of **Ab2** and increase a degree of stimuli $m_{21}$. In this study, we simply modify the degree of stimuli as:

$$m_{12} = \frac{T_p^{Ab_1} + T_r^{Ab_2}}{T_{Ab_2}^{Ab_1}} \tag{4}$$

$$m_{21} = \frac{T_r^{Ab_1} + T_p^{Ab_2}}{T_{Ab_2}^{Ab_1}} \quad , \tag{5}$$

where $T_p^{Ab1}$ and $T_r^{Ab1}$ represent the number of times of receiving penalty and reward signals when **Ab1** is selected. $T_{Ab2}^{Ab1}$ denotes the number of times when both **Ab1** and **Ab2** are activated by their specific antigens. We should notice that this procedure works to raise the relative priority of **Ab1** over **Ab2**. In the case where immunoid receives a penalty signal, we record the ID-number of **Ab2** (i.e. 2) in the idiotope of **Ab1** and modify $m_{12}$ in the same way. This works to decrease the relative priority of **Ab1** over **Ab2**.

To confirm the validity of this adjustment mechanism, we carry out some simulations. In the simulations, the following reward and penalty signals are used:

**Reward**

- Immunoid recharges with low energy level.
- Immunoid catches garbage with high energy level.

**Penalty**

- Immunoid catches garbage with low energy level.
- Immunoid collides with garbage or a wall.

Figure 11 denotes the transitions of the resultant life time and collection ratio.

From these results, it is understood that both are improved gradually as iterated.

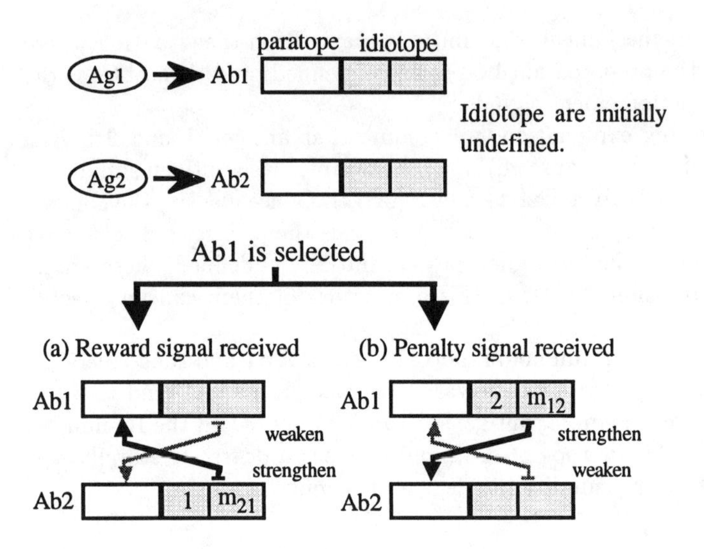


**Fig. 10.** Proposed adjustment mechanism

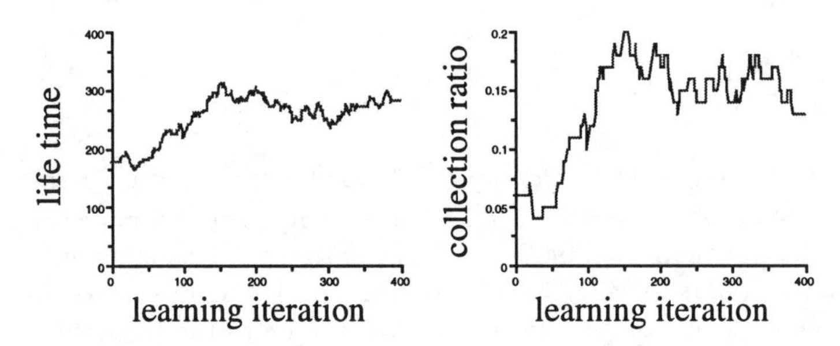


**Fig. 11.** Transitions of life time and collection ratio

Figure 12 illustrates an example of the obtained immune networks through our proposed learning process. In this figure, for easy understanding, only the connections with high affinities ($m_{ij} > 0.6$) are shown. ¿From this figure, this network makes immunoid to search for the charging station when the current energy level is low. And it is also comprehended from this network that if the energy level is high, immunoid tends to select a garbage-collecting behavior. In spite of no explicit reinforcement signals concerned with distance to the home base, immunoid tends to search charging station if the distance to the charging station is far. While distance is near, it tends to collect garbage. We are currently implementing this mechanism into the real experimental system.

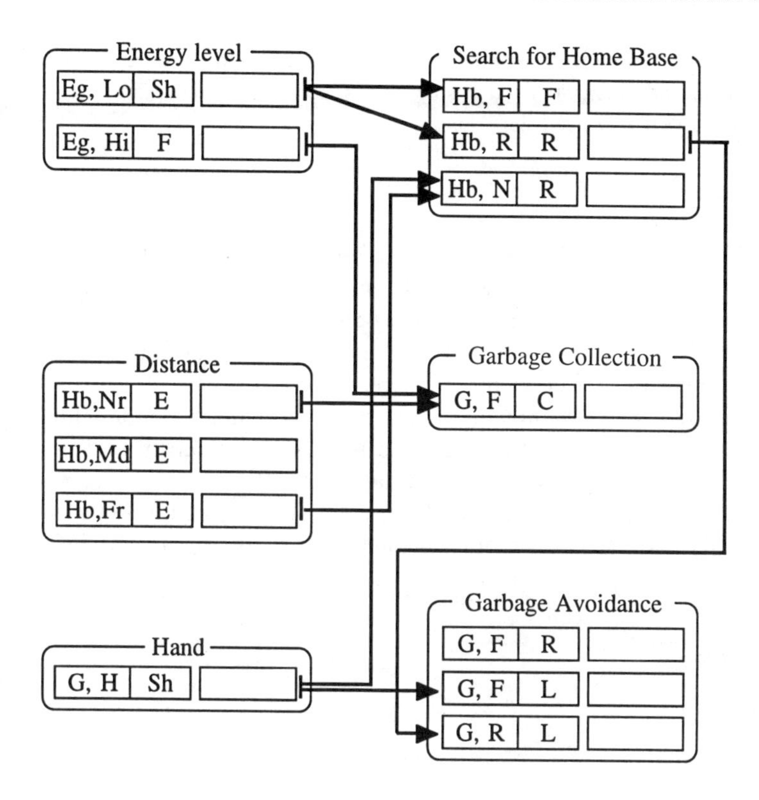


**Fig. 12.** An example of the obtained immune network

### 4.3 Innovation mechanism

In the above adjustment mechanism, we should notice that we must still describe the paratope of each antibody in a top-down manner. One obvious candidate to avoid such difficulties is to incorporate an innovation mechanism. As described in section 2.3, in the biological immune system, the metadynamics function can be instantiated as an innovation mechanism. Therefore, we propose the following innovation mechanism inspired by the biological immune system.

Figure 13 schematically depicts the proposed innovation mechanism. Initially, the immune network consists of $N$ antibodies, each of them is generated by gene recombination and given one state variable named *concentration of B-cell*. In order to relate this variable to the action selection process, we modify the equation (2) as follows:

$$\frac{dA_i(t)}{dt} = \left\{ \alpha \sum_{j=1}^{N} m_{ji} a_j(t) - \alpha \sum_{k=1}^{N} m_{ik} a_k(t) + \beta m_i - k_i \right\} a_i(t) b_i(T) \quad (6)$$

$b_i(T)$ is the concentration of B-cell $i$ in the $T$-th time step. If an antibody receives a reinforcement signal as a result of its action, the corresponding concentration of B-cell is varied as:

$$\frac{db_i(T)}{dT} = r_i \Delta b - K b_i(T) \tag{7}$$

where $r_i = 1$ if the antibody $i$ is selected and receives a reward signal, $r_i = -1$ if the antibody $i$ receives a penalty signal, and $r_i = 0$ if the antibody $i$ is not selected. $K$ is the dissipation factor of the B-cell. If $b_i(T)$ becomes below 0, then the corresponding antibody is removed, and a new antibody is incorporated through the selection mechanism.

For quick improvement, we introduce a selection mechanism by modeling the function in *thymus*. Next, we explain this selection mechanism in more detail. First, we randomly generate $m$ candidates for antibodies by gene recombination process. Then we calculate their sensitivities $\sigma_i$ and $\delta_i$ between each new antibody and the existing immune network. $\sigma_i$ and $\delta_i$ are obtained as:

$$\sigma_i = \sum_{j=1}^{N} m_{ji} a_j, \tag{8}$$

$$\delta_i = \sum_{j=1}^{N} m_{ij} a_j \tag{9}$$

As described earlier, each antibody has the interactions, i.e. stimulation and suppression. Sensitivity $\sigma_i$ represents the sum of stimulation from the existing network, while sensitivity $\delta_i$ is the sum of suppression. Finally, only one antibody is allowed to be incorporated based on the predetermined criterion. In this study, we used $\max \sigma_i$ and $\max |\sigma_i - \delta_i|$ as criteria.

To confirm the ability of the proposed innovation mechanism, we apply to a simple example, i.e. obstacle avoiding problem. The simulated environment contains immunoid, multiple obstacles and one charging station. The aim of immunoid is to reach the charging station regularly in order to fulfill its energy level while at the same time avoiding collisions. In the simulations, the following reward and penalty signals are used:

**Reward**

- Immunoid approaches near the charging station with low energy level.
- Immunoid moves forward without collisions.

**Penalty**

- Immunoid collides with an obstacle or a wall.
- Immunoid does not move forward when there is no obstacle around it.

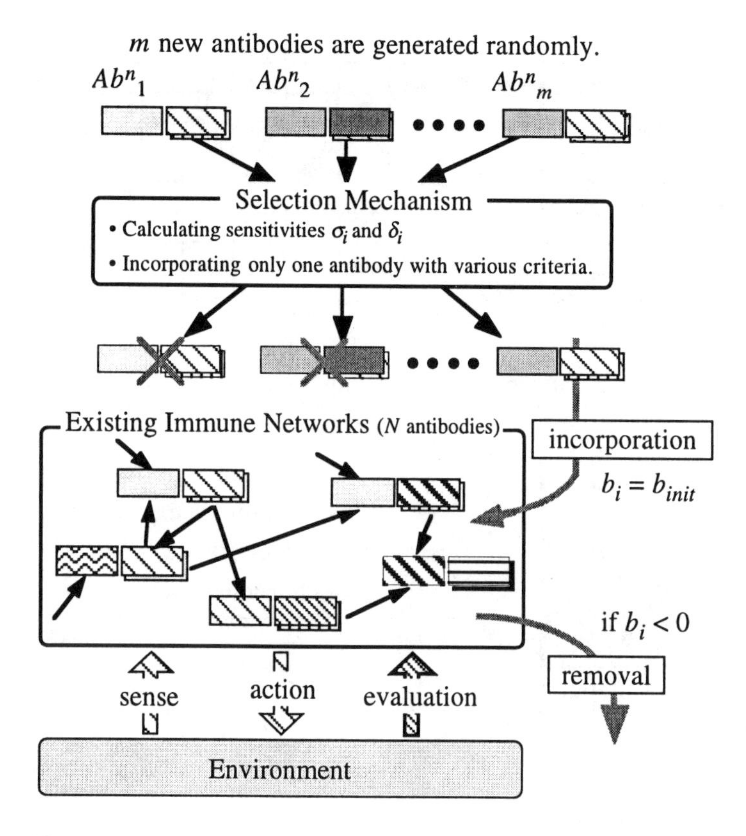


**Fig. 13.** Proposed innovation mechanism

Additionally, we assume that the number of antibody $N$ is set to 50, and the number of new antibody $m$ to 20. Figure 14 denotes the transitions of the resultant lifetime, the number of move-forward actions and the number of collisions in three cases.

In case (a), the selection mechanism is not used, namely one randomly generated antibody is incorporated, while in case (b) and (c), the selection mechanism is used with the criterion $\max \sigma_i$ and $\max |\sigma_i - \delta_i|$, respectively. From these results, the selection mechanisms (particularly the criterion $\max \sigma_i$) improve the adaptation performance more rapidly than that without the selection mechanism. We are currently analyzing these results in detail.

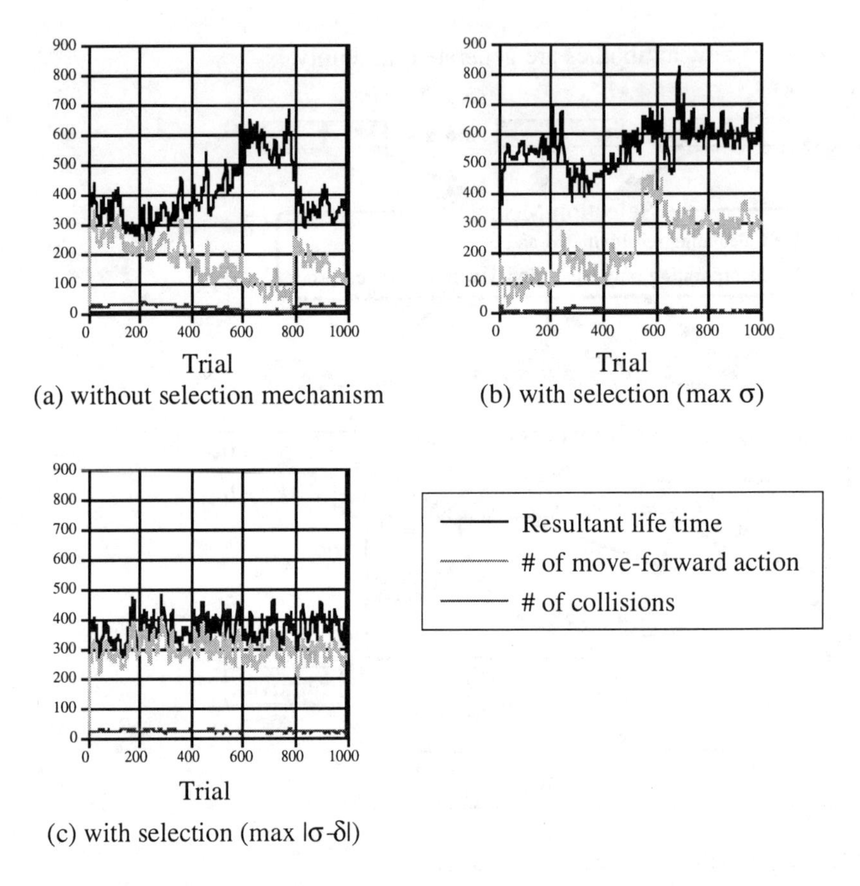


**Fig. 14.** Simulation results under three different selection criteria

## 5 Conclusions and Further Work

In this paper, we proposed a new decentralized behavior arbitration mechanism based on the biological immune system and confirmed the validity of our proposed system in some experiments. And we proposed two types of adaptation mechanism for an appropriate arbitration using reinforcement signals.

As artificial systems increase their complexities, the concept of self-maintenance and self-preservation become highly indispensable. For this, we believe that the immune system would provide fruitful ideas such as on-line maintenance mechanisms and robustness against hostile environments. This research is a first step toward the realization of artificial immune systems.

## Acknowledgements

This research was supported in part by a Grant-in Aid for Scientific Research on Priority Areas from the Ministry of Education, Science, Sports and Culture, Japan (No.07243208, 08233208), and Mechatronics Technology Foundation.

## References

1. R.Brooks: A Robust Layered Control System for a Mobile Robot, *IEEE Journal R&A*, Vol.2, No.1, pp.14-23, 1986.
2. R.Brooks: Intelligence Without Reason, *Proc. of the IJCAI-91*, pp.569-595, 1991.
3. P.Maes: The dynamic action selection, Proc. of IJCAI-89, pp.991-997, 1989.
4. P.Maes: Situated agent can have goals, *Designing Autonomous Agents*, pp.49-70, MIT Press, 1991.
5. A. Ishiguro, S. Ichikawa and Y. Uchikawa: A Gait Acquisition of 6-Legged Walking Robot Using Immune Networks, Journal of Robotics Society of Japan, Vol.13, No.3, pp.125-128, 1995 (in Japanese), also in Proc. of IROS'94, Vol.2, pp.1034-1041, 1994.
6. A.Ishiguro, Y.Watanabe and Y.Uchikawa: An Immunological Approach to Dynamic Behavior Control for Autonomous Mobile Robots, *in Proc. of IROS '95*, Vol.1, pp.495-500, 1995.
7. A.Ishiguro, T.Kondo, Y.Watanabe and Y.Uchikawa: Dynamic Behavior Arbitration of Autonomous Mobile Robots Using Immune Networks, *in Proc. of ICEC'95*, Vol.2, pp.722-727, 1995.
8. A. Ishiguro, T. Kondo, Y. Watanabe and Y. Uchikawa: Immunoid: An Immunological Approach to Decentralized Behavior Arbitration of Autonomous Mobile Robots, *Lecture Notes in Computer Science 1141*, Springer, pp.666-675, 1994.
9. N.K.Jerne: The immune system, *Scientific American*, Vol.229, No.1, pp.52-60, 1973.
10. N.K.Jerne: The generative grammar of the immune system, *EMBO Journal*, Vol.4, No.4, 1985.
11. N.K.Jerne: Idiotypic networks and other preconceived ideas, *Immunological Rev.*, Vol.79, pp.5-24, 1984.
12. H.Fujita and K.Aihara: A distributed surveillance and protection system in living organisms, *Trans. on IEE Japan*, Vol. 107-C, No.11, pp.1042-1048, 1987. (in Japanese)
13. J.D.Farmer, N.H.Packard and A.S.Perelson: The immune system, adaptation, and machine learning, *Physica 22D*, pp.187-204, 1986.

14. F.J.Valera, A.Coutinho, B.Dupire and N.N.Vaz.: Cognitive Networks: Immune, Neural, and Otherwise, *Theoretical Immunology*, Vol.2, pp.359-375, 1988.
15. J.Stewart: The Immune System: Emergent Self-Assertion in an Autonomous Network, *in Proceedings of ECAL-93*, pp.1012-1018, 1993.
16. H.Bersini and F.J.Valera: The Immune Learning Mechanisms: Reinforcement, Recruitment and their Applications, *Computing with Biological Metaphors*, Ed. R.Paton, Chapman & Hall, pp.166-192, 1994.
17. R.Pfeifer: The Fungus Eater Approach to Emotion -A View from Artificial Intelligence, *Technical Report, AI Lab, No. IFIAI95.04*, Computer Science Department, University of Zurich, 1995.
18. D.Lambrinos and C.Scheier: Extended Braitenberg Architecture, *Technical Report, AI Lab, No. IFIAI95.10*, Computer Science Department, University of Zurich, 1995.
19. B.Manderick: The importance of selectionist systems for cognition, *Computing with Biological Metaphors*, Ed. R.Paton, Chapman & Hall, 1994.
20. J.D.Farmer, S.A.Kauffman, N.H.Packard and A.S.Perelson: Adaptive Dynamic Networks as Models for the Immune System and Autocatalytic Sets, *Technical Report LA-UR-86-3287*, Los Alamos National Laboratory, Los Alamos, NM, 1986.

**Mr. Yuji Watanabe** was born in Gifu, Japan, on 1972. He received the BS degree and the MS degree in Electronic-Mechanical Engineering from Nagoya University, Japan, in 1994 and 1996,respectively. Since 1996, he has been a Ph.D. candidate of the Department of Information-Electronics of Nagoya University. His current research interests are engineering biological immune systems and its application to robotics. He is a member of the Robotics Society of Japan, and the Society of Instrument and Control Engineers of Japan.

**Dr. Akio Ishiguro** born in Kochi, Japan, on 1964. He received the BS, MS and Ph.D. degrees in Electronic-Mechanical Engineering from Nagoya University, Japan, in 1987, 1989, 1991, respectively. From 1991 to 1993, he was with the Department of Electronic-Mechanical Engineering of Nagoya University, from 1993 to 1997, he was with the Department of Information-Electronics of Nagoya University as an Assistant Professor, respectively. Since 1997, he has been as an Associate Professor of the Department of Computational Science and Engineering of Nagoya University. His research interests are in emergent computations, robotics, biological information processing systems and artificial life. He is a member of the Robotics Society of Japan, the Society of Instrument and Control Engineers of Japan, the Institute of Electrical Engineers of Japan, and the Institute of Electrical and Electronics Engineers.

**Dr. Yoshiki Uchikawa** born in Aichi, Japan, in 1941. He received the BE, ME and Ph.D. degree in Electrical Engineering from Nagoya University, Japan, in 1964, 1966 and 1971, respectively. From 1969 to 1984, he was with the Department of Electrical Engineering of Nagoya University as an Assistant Professor. From 1985 to 1993, he was with the Department of Electronic-Mechanical Engineering of Nagoya University. From 1994 to 1996, he was with the Department of Information-Electronics of Nagoya University as a Professor. Since 1997, he has been with the Department of Computational Science and Engineering of Nagoya University as a Professor. His research interests are in the areas of electronic mechanics, electron microscopy, fuzzy modeling and neural networks. He is a member of the Institute of Electrical Engineers of Japan, the Society of Instrument and Control Engineers of Japan, the Robotics Society of Japan, the Japan Society of Electron Microscopy, the Japan Society of Applied Physics, the Japan Society of Applied Electromagnetics, the Japan Society of Precision Engineering, and the Institute of Institute of Electrical and Electronics Engineers.

# Parallel Search for Multi-Modal Function Optimization with Diversity and Learning of Immune Algorithm

Toyoo Fukuda[1], Kazuyuki Mori[2] and Makoto Tsukiyama[2]

[1] School of Policy Studies
Kwansei Gakuin University
2-1 Gakuen, Sanda, Hyogo 669-13
JAPAN

[2] Industrial Electronics & Systems Laboratory
Mitsubishi Electric Corporation
Amagasaki, Hyogo 661
JAPAN

**Abstract.** Immune System in the higher mammal has interesting characteristics and powerful abilities from the information view points, such as recognition of antigen, production of antibody and learning with memory cell. This paper proposes an optimization algorithm imitating the immune system to solve the multi-modal function optimization problem partly using a genetic algorithm. The proposed algorithm is shown to be effective for searching for a set of solutions as well as local solutions. The illustrative examples are shown for multi-modal functions such as multi-peaks function and Shubert function.

## 1 Introduction

The artificial immune algorithm for parallel search is shown with illustrative examples. Immune system has fundamental ability to produce new types of antibody or to find the best fitted antibody which is able to attack the antigen invading into the body. Against the unnumerable types of unknown antigen, the immune system produces a great many types of antibody by trial and error. To realize the diversity of antibody types is essential adaptability against the foreign virus and bacteria in the environment. The diversity of the immune system can be mathematically formulated as a multi-modal function optimization problem, which has multiple solutions not single solution. The proposed algorithm is aimed on how to keep the parallel search vectors for multiple solutions. The index of diversity is introduced and multiple solution vector is kept as memory cell mechanism in the immune system. The antigen can be considered as a problem to be solved and antibody as solution vector best fitted to solve the problem.

Many engineering problems can be formulated as optimization problems which optimize some objective function. Meanwhile most cases show the multi-modal function as objective function. It is not easy to solve such multi-modal function problem by the conventional optimization methods. Therefore, a method to get a set of solution is needed in the real world. Meanwhile, the immune system in a higher mammal eliminates antigens by the genetic evolution of a lymphocyte population which has capability to produce antibodies (see Figure 1). Many types of antibody are produced by combinations of gene by way of trial because the type of antigen is not known a priori. From among the varieties of antibody candidates a unique antibody is selected to destroy the antigen successfully by bio-chemically pattern matching between antigen and antibody. So the process of immune system can be considered as an optimization process. The process is to select a type of antibody from among a great many solution candidates that is the best fitted with the unknown antigen. Then the immune process is considered to be a kind of combinatorial optimization process[2].

This paper proposes an immune algorithm(IA) imitating the physiological immune system, that is based on somatic theory [1] and the network hypothesis [3]. The somatic theory describes that somatic recombination and mutation contribute to increasing the diversity of the antibodies. The network hypothesis describes that a mutual recognition network among the antibodies contributes to control of the proliferation of clones[1],[4],[6],[7]. A few numerical examples of test functions such as five-peaks function and Shubert functions are illustrated to show the abilities of immune algorithm for multi-modal function.

## 2 Immune Algorithm

### 2.1 Diversity and Affinity of Antibodies

In order to observe the diversity of antibodies produced from a lymphocyte population, it is necessary to define a measure of that diversity. A model of a lymphocyte population consisting of antibodies is shown in Figure 2.

The informative entropy of locus $j$ in the lymphocyte population is represented by

$$H_j(N) = \sum_{i=1}^{S} -p_{i,j} \log p_{i,j} \tag{1}$$

where $N$ is the size of the antibodies in a lymphocyte population, $S$ is the variety of allele and $p_{i,j}$ means the probability that locus $j$ is allele $i$.

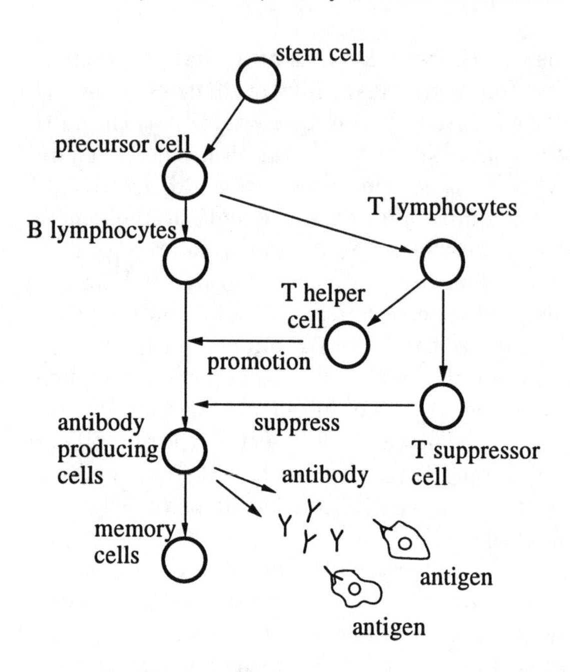


**Fig. 1.** The production mechanism of antibodies in an immune system

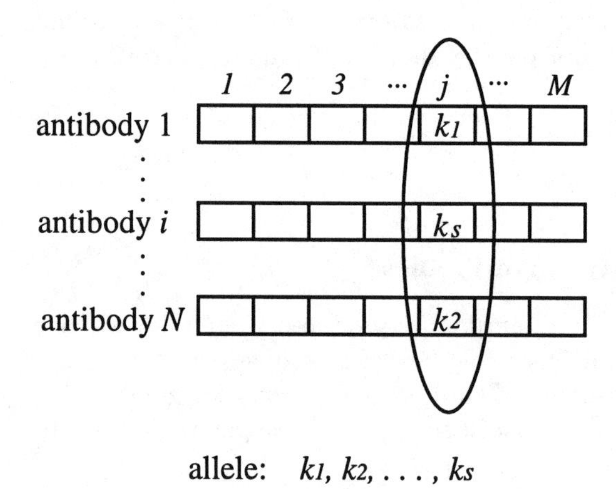


**Fig. 2.** The informative entropy of antigens

Therefore, the mean of the informative entropy in a lymphocyte population can be represented by

$$H(N) = \frac{1}{M} \sum_{j=1}^{M} H_j(N) \tag{2}$$

where $M$ is the size of the genes in an antibody. This entropy can show the diversity of the lymphocyte population. The affinity $ay_{v,w}$ between two antibodies $v$ and $w$ can also be represented by equation (3).

$$ay_{v,w} = \frac{1}{1 + H(2)} \tag{3}$$

The affinity between antigen and antibody is defined by equation (4)

$$ax_v = opt_v, \tag{4}$$

where $opt_v$ means the evaluated value to show the connectedness between antigen and antibody $v$.

## 2.2 Proposition of Immune Algorithm

This section proposes an immune algorithm based on somatic theory and the network hypothesis. According to the somatic theory, the genetic information is contained in multiple gene segments scattered along a chromosome. During the development of bone marrow-derived lymphocytes, those gene segments are brought together to form a complete immunoglobulin gene active in B lymphocytes by genetic recombination. In addition hyper mutations are introduced somatically into an immunoglobulin gene at a high rate. Both somatic recombination and mutation contribute greatly to an increase in the diversity of antibody [1]. This immune algorithm can produce the required diversity of antibodies and regulate the proliferation of clones as though in the real immune system. The natural immune system is illustrated in Figure 3 from the view points of information and control mechanism.

From this scheme of the natural immune system, the mathematical optimization framework can be modelled as an algorithm as shown in Figure 4 which we are proposing. The algorithm can be realized by the following six steps as shown in Figure 4.

*Immune system and Algorithm*

[step 1] Recognition of antigen: The natural immune system recognizes the invasion of antigen and whether it is foreign cells or not for the body. This process corresponds to the identification of the optimization problem.

[step 2] Production of antibody from memory cell: The memory cells are activated to produce the antibodies which were effective to kill the antigen in the past. This corresponds to recalling a past successful solution of a similar problem.

[step 3] Calculation of affinity: Against the new antigen the better fitted antibody cells are selected which can be done by bio-chemical pattern affinity. The affinities $ay_{v,w}$ and $ax_v$ are calculated by equations (3) and (4), which correspond to searching for the optimal solution.

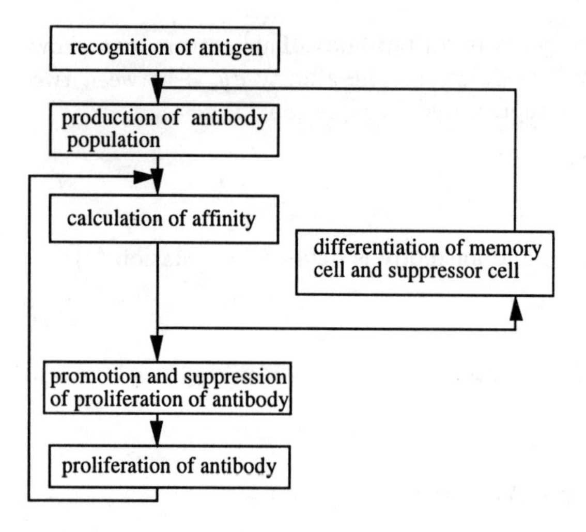


**Fig. 3.** Immune system

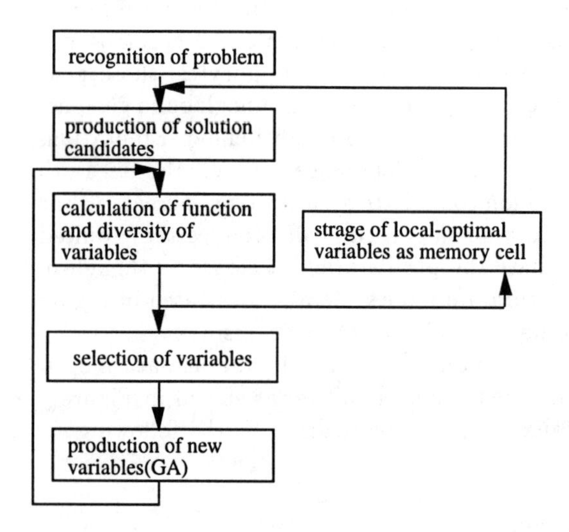


**Fig. 4.** Immune algorithm(optimization)

[step 4] Differentiation of lymphocyte: The B-lymphocyte cell, the antibody of which matched the antigen, is dispersed to the memory cells and suppressor cells when the concentration $c_v$ of antibody exceeds over a threshold level $Tc$. This process can be seen as keeping good solution as memory for the next step search. The suppressor works to eliminate the surplus of solution candidates.

$$c_v = \frac{1}{N}\sum_{w=1}^{N} ac_{v,w} \tag{5}$$

$$ac_{v,w} = \begin{cases} 1 & ay_{v,w} \geq Tac1 \\ 0 & otherwise \end{cases} \tag{6}$$

[step 5] Proliferation and suppression of antibody: The expected value $e_v$ of the proliferation of the antibody is defined by equation (7),

$$e_v = \frac{ax_v \prod_{s=1}^{S}(1 - as_{v,s})}{c_v \sum_{i=1}^{N} ax_i} \tag{7}$$

$$as_{v,s} = \begin{cases} ay_{v,s} & ay_{v,s} \geq Tac2 \\ 0 & otherwise \end{cases} \tag{8}$$

Equation (7) regulates the concentration and the variety of antibodies in the lymphocyte population. As an antibody obtains a higher affinity against an antigen, the antibody proliferates, while proliferation of an antibody of excessive higher concentration is suppressed. This corresponds to maintaining the diversity of searching directions as well as to focusing on a local maximum.

[step 6] Proliferation of antibody: To respond to the unknown antigen, new lymphocytes are produced in the bone marrow in place of the antibody eliminated in step 5. This procedure can generate a diversity of antibodies by a genetic reproduction operator of the genetic algorithm (GA)[5] such as mutation or crossover. These genetic operators are expected to be more efficient than random generation of antibodies.

### 2.3 Characteristics of the Immune Algorithm

As defined above, the immune algorithm is based on somatic theory and a network hypothesis. The former theory shows that somatic recombination and mutation contribute to increasing the diversity of antibodies, and correspond to step 6. The other shows that a mutual recognition network among the antibodies contributes to control of the proliferation of clones, and corresponds to step 5. Therefore, this algorithm can be expected to have the following characteristics.

(i) Diversity of solution candidate
Generating the diversity of solution candidates based on the above theories can be expected to perform the parallel search and as a result to find a global solution as well as local optimal solutions.

(ii) Parallel efficient search
Parallel searching in a neighbourhood space by a number of antibodies can be expected to search more quickly and efficiently.

# 3 Experiments and Implementation Details

## 3.1 Test function 1(Decreasing peak function)

Equation (9) describes the decreasing peaks function with five peaks as shown Figure 5 and 6.

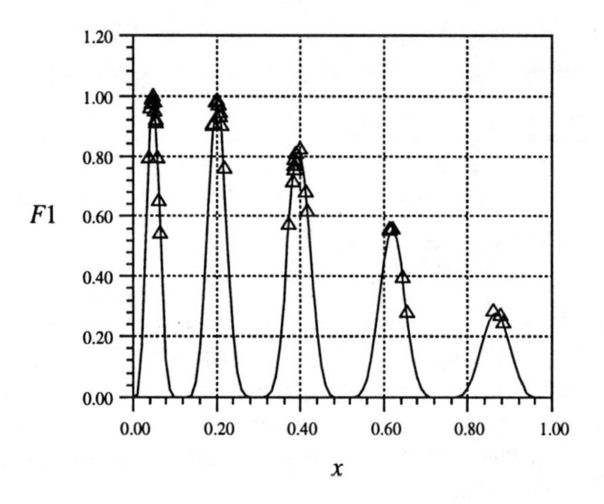


**Fig. 5.** State of the memory cells on function F1 after 200 generations

$$F1(x) = \exp(-2\log_2(\frac{x-0.1}{0.8})^2)\sin^6 5\pi x^{\frac{3}{4}} \tag{9}$$

## 3.2 Test function 2(Shubert function)

Equation (10) describes the Shubert function with 18 global maximum value in 2-dimensional space as shown in Figure 7.

$$F2(x,y) = -\sum_{i=1}^{5} i\cos((i+1)x+i) \times \sum_{i=1}^{5} i\cos((i+1)y+i) \tag{10}$$

## 3.3 Implementation Details

We have carried out the simulations for determining the maximum values of the functions $F1$ and $F2$ by the IA and simple GA. The codings to the genes of the problem are 16 bits as one antibody (individual) for $F1$ and 42 bits as ane antibody for $F2$. The values of various parameters as well as the genetic operation methods of the crossover and mutation used in the experiments are shown in the following.

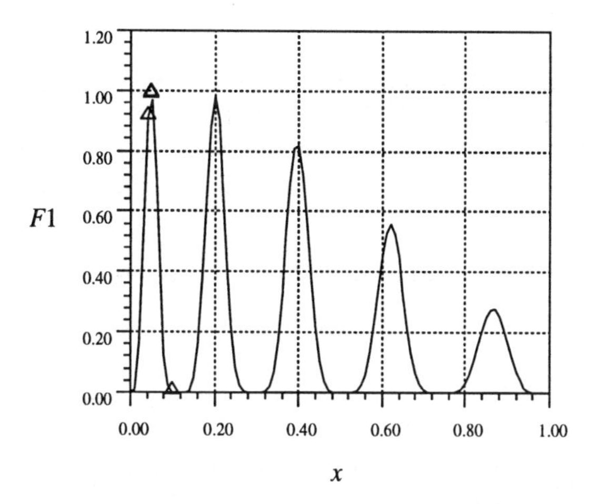


**Fig. 6.** State of the population of function F1 after 200 generations

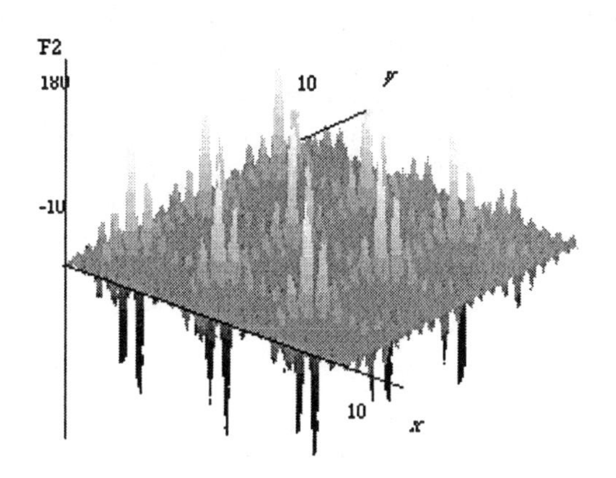


**Fig. 7.** The Shubert function

- $F1$(IA)
  Number of antibodies (individuals): $N = 100$, number of generations: $G = 200$, crossover probability: $P_c = 1.0$, mutation probability: $P_m = 0.01$, crossover operation: one–point crossover, mutation operation: reversion of arbitrary one bit, $Tc = 0.45$, $Tac1 = 0.5$ and $Tac2 = 0.5$
- $F1$(simpleGA)
  Number of antibodies (individuals): $N = 100$, number of generations: $G = 200$, crossover probability: $P_c = 1.0$, mutation probability: $P_m = 0.01$, crossover operation: one–point crossover, mutation operation: reversion of arbitrary one bit,

- $F2$(IA)
  Number of antibodies (individuals): $N = 100$, number of generations: $G = 2000$, crossover probability: $P_c = 1.0$, mutation probability: $P_m = 0.5$, crossover operation: one–point crossover, mutation operation: reversion of arbitrary one bit, $Tc = 0.7$, $Tac1 = 0.5$ and $Tac2 = 0.5$

### 3.4 Experimental Results and Considerations

In Figure 5, the symbol $\triangle$ indicates the degree of affinity of memory cells generated by IA up to 200 generations for function $F1$. $\triangle$ shown in Figure 6 plots the value of fitness of individuals in the 200-th generation by GA for function$F1$.

Figure 8 shows the distribution of 47 of the $x$–$y$ coordinates of phenotype of memory cells plotted by the character + and 18 of the $x$–$y$ coordinates of global maximum solution points plotted by the character $\times$, respectively.

**(i) Search results** It is seem from Figure 7 that the majority of individuals in GA gathers at one peak. On the other hand, it is seem from Figure 6 that the memory cells corresponding to the respective peaks are generated in IA. Moreover, it is seen from Figure 8 that the memory cells close to 18 peaks are also generated for $F4$. However, the memory cells of more than the number of peaks are generated in all functions. This may be caused by the fact that the IA has attempted to generate the memory cells up to the upper limit of the total number of the memory cells.

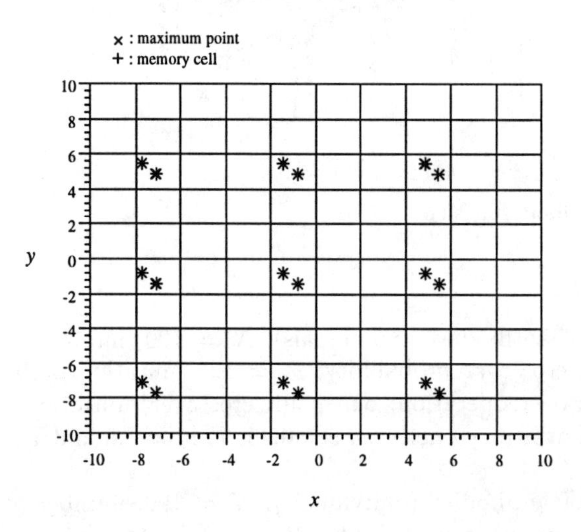


**Fig. 8.** State of the memory cells on function F2 after 2000 generations

**(ii) Diversity** Figure 9 shows the changing of the diversity of both antibodies and individuals while searching advances. It is seem from this figure that the diversity of the population in GA is lost as the generation advances. On the contrary, the diversity of population in IA is maintained by the production of the new antiboies. An important ability to find the global maxima comes from the fact that the diversity of antibodies is maintained in the IA.

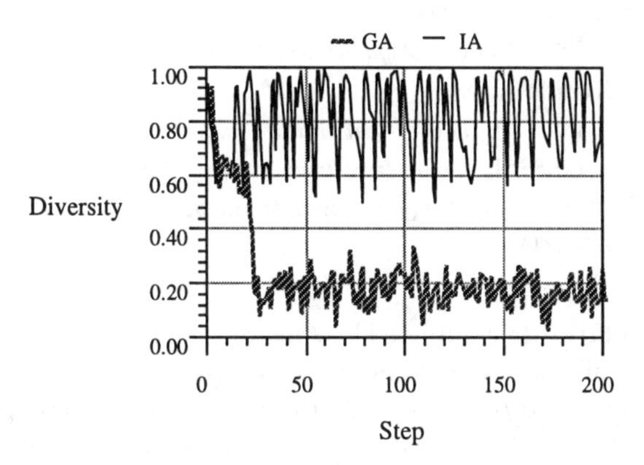


**Fig. 9.** The changing of the diversity in the GA and IA

## 4 Conclusion

It is shown that the proposed artificial immune algorithm is effective for parallel search the optimal solutions of multi-modal function optimization. In comparison with the Genetic Algorithm, the proposed artificial immune algorithm includes the genetic algorithm in its own algorithm. So, the artificial immune algorithm is considered as a meta-level algorithm including genetic algorithm. The characteristic properties of immune algorithm are keeping diversity of a set of solution vector and learning mechanism which the GA does not have.

As a conclusion, the proposed artificial immune algorithm shows the important properties such as the producability of solution candidates diversifying in the global space, the mass production of search directions around the efficient starting points in the sense of trial and error, and the parallel search efficiently from a set of memorized points kept by the learning function.

## References

1. Atlan, H. and I. R. Cohen (1989); *Theories of Immune Networks*; Springer-Verlag.

2. Bersini, H. and F. J. Varela (1991); The Immune Recruitment Mechanism: A Selective Evolutionary Strategy; *Proc. ICGA 91*(pp.520–526).
3. Farmer, J. D., N. H. Packard and A. A. Perelson (1986); The Immune System, Adaptation, and Machine Learning, *Physica*; 22D (pp. 187–204).
4. Forrest, S. and A. A. Perelson (1990); Genetic Algorithms and the Immune System; *Proc. of 1st Workshop of PPSN (G. Goos and J. Hartmanis, Ed.)*, Springer-Verlag (pp. 320–325).
5. Goldberg, D. (1989); *Genetic Algorithms in Search, Optimization, and Machine Learning*; Addison Wesley.
6. Perelson, A. A. (1988a); *Theoretical Immunology Part One*, Addison Wesley.
7. Perelson, A. A. (1988b); *Theoretical Immunology Part Two* Addison Wesley.
8. Tonegawa, S. (1983); Somatic generation of antibody diversity; *Nature*,Vol. 302, 14 April (pp.575-581).

**Dr. Toyoo Fukuda** completed his Master's course at the Engineering Research Division of the Graduate School of Kyoto University, 1970. He joined Mitsubishi Electric Corporation in April of that year. He completed in 1975 a Master's course in the Department of Applied Mathematics at Harvard University. In April 1995, He became a Professor in the School of Policies of Kwansei Gakuin University. He is engaged in research on systems science. He has a Doctor of Engineering degree. He is a member of the Society of Instrument and Control Engineers, the Institute of Electrical Engineers of Japan, and IEEE. He received a Paper Award of the Institute of Electrical Engineers of Japan in 1994.

**Mr. Kazuyuki Mori** completed his Master's course at the Science and Engineering Research Division of the Graduate School of the Science University of Tokyo, 1987. He Joined Mitsubishi Electric Corporation in April of that year. He is currently engaged in research on analysis and scheduling of discrete event systems at Industrial Electronics & Systems Laboratory. He is a member of the Society of Instrument and Control Engineers, and the Institute of Electrical Engineers of Japan. He received a Paper Award of the Institute of Electrical Engineers of Japan in 1994.

**Dr. Makoto Tsukiyama** completed his Master's course at the Engineering Research Division of the Graduate School of Kyushu Institute of Technology, 1978. He joined Mitsubishi Electric Corporation in April of that year. He is currently engaged in research on discrete event systems, scheduling and operation optimization of systems at Industrial Electronics & Systems Laboratory. He has a Doctor of Engineering degree. He is a member of the Society of Instrument and Control Engineers, and the Institute of Electrical Engineers of Japan. He received a Paper Award of the Institute of Electrical Engineers of Japan in 1994.

# Immunized Adaptive Critic for an Autonomous Aircraft Control Application

Kalmanje KrishnaKumar and James Neidhoefer

Department of Aerospace Engineering and Mechanics
The University of Alabama
Tuscaloosa, AL 35487-0280, USA

**Abstract.** Immunized Computational Systems combine *a priori* knowledge with the adapting capabilities of immune systems to provide a powerful alternative to currently available techniques for intelligent control. In this paper, we present a perspective on various levels of intelligent control and relate them to similar functioning in human immune systems. A technique for implementing immunized computational systems as adaptive critics is presented and the technique is then applied to a flight path generator for level 2, non-linear, full-envelope, intelligent aircraft control problem.

## 1 Introduction

Biological immune systems use a finite number of discrete "building blocks" derived from the DNA molecule to achieve both robustness and adaptiveness. These building blocks, that are evolved, can be thought of as pieces of a puzzle that must be put together in a specific way to neutralize, remove, or destroy each unique disturbance the system encounters. One can define and learn linear and non-linear building blocks (analogous to DNA building blocks) to design complex intelligent control architectures. The building blocks are processed on-line for system adaptation. Building blocks can be linear, neural, or fuzzy. Neural building blocks are utilized for non-linear mapping and for on-line learning. Linear building blocks are utilized in situations where linear control solutions are readily available and are necessary and sufficient (small perturbations about equilibrium). Linear building blocks also provide a sound theoretical foundation for arriving at stability proofs. Fuzzy building blocks could be used for handling human rules-of-thumb. In summary, the "learning" capabilities of artificial neural networks and theoretical foundations of linear controllers are combined with the "adapting" capabilities of immune systems to arrive at a new breed of immunized computational systems (ICS).

The capabilities of ICS were demonstrated on several problems: (a) on-line identification and adaptive control of an uncertain system [5,6]; (b) synthesis of complex controllers using man-in-the-loop simulation [7]; and (c) all envelope stabilizing controllers [8]. Experimental verification using an intelligent aircraft control test bed is in progress.

One of the necessary characteristics of any truly adaptive system is the system's ability to forecast performance into the future correctly. Critics, both adaptive [1,9] and non-adaptive, have been proposed in the literature as Neural Network systems that can model future performance. There are a number of ways to adapt critic networks. One way is to implement the heuristic dynamic programming (HDP) technique discussed by Werbos [9]. Essentially, the critic, in addition to predicting the cost to go (future error), adapts itself with the help of the recursive relationship derived from approximate dynamic programming. Typically, back-propagation of error is used to update the weights of the critic. In this study, we apply the capabilities of immunized computational systems in arriving at the adaptive critic system.

The outline of the paper is as follows: we first present our perspective on levels of intelligent control and relate it to similar functioning in the human immune systems. Next, we present the aircraft autonomous control problem and the levels of intelligent control associated with that problem. Then we present the details of immunized computational systems. Finally, we define immunized adaptive critics and apply it to a non-linear full-envelope level 2 intelligent aircraft control problem.

## 2 Levels of Intelligent Control

Intelligent Control is currently a hotly debated topic in the control community. It is so current that in spite of the fact that it is accepted as an established area within the field of control systems, no standardized definition of exactly what intelligent control is has been accepted. However, many researchers have expressed their views on intelligent control in various forums, and many different definitions with common themes have been offered. There are certain themes on which these definitions agree and we can say in a general sense, that the intelligence of a control system is characterized by its ability to manage and process uncertain and imprecise information with attributes such as adaptability, memory, and learning. Capabilities such as information gathering, making inferences, and applying it to understand and solve old and new problems efficiently are observed to be critical features of such systems. Intelligent control as practiced today encompasses many fields from conventional control such as optimal control, robust control, stochastic control, linear control, and nonlinear control, as well as the more recent fuzzy, genetic, and neuro-control technologies. Intelligent control can also be considered to be the juxtaposition of several already well-established disciplines including: artificial and computational intelligence, classical control theory, operations research, and computer science.

Intelligent Control focuses on control problems that otherwise cannot be solved, or cannot be solved in a satisfactory way by traditional control techniques. It has been well accepted that certain tasks are better done using linear control laws as compared to fuzzy or neuro-control (Ex: small perturbations about equilibrium). What fuzzy and neural methods provide us is the ease with which complex control architectures can be implemented. For example, it has been shown that Fuzzy Logic controllers provide good uncertainty management without having to design for it. Another example is the ease with which system sensitivities can be computed using Neural Networks. These sensitivities can then be used for real-time adaptive control that minimizes a measure of performance over time.

It cannot be denied that the need for improved control technologies is motivated by the need to improve efficiency and performance of current systems. Another aspect that is not so obvious is the need to speed-up the innovation cycle (theory to modeling to practice). Intelligent control (intelligent systems in general) is being sold as a way to realize the above needs. Unfortunately, the understanding of what exactly is intelligence and specifically what is intelligent control is incomplete to say the least.

A useful way to define intelligent control is to quantize the definition based upon the notion that different systems have various levels of capability for self-improvement (See Table 1).

**Table 1.** The Levels of Intelligent Control.

| Level | Self improvement of | Description |
|---|---|---|
| 0 | Tracking Error (TE) | Robust Feedback Control: Error tends to zero. |
| 1 | TE + Control Parameters (CP) | Adaptive Control: Robust feedback control with adaptive control parameters (error tends to zero for non-nominal operations; feedback control is self improving). |
| 2 | TE + CP + Performance Measure (PM) | Optimal Control: Robust, adaptive feedback control that minimizes or maximizes a utility function over time. |
| 3 | TE+CP+PM+ Planning Function | Planning Control: Level 2 + the ability to plan ahead of time for uncertain situations, simulate, and model uncertainties. |
| 4 | Yet to be defined | |

It is emphasized here that self-improvement is an important goal of human intelligence. Self- improvement is quantifiable and measurable in various ways. By defining Intelligent Control with various levels of intelligence, the definition is left 'open ended' such that it will not become obsolete, and it will accommodate easily the innovations that will inevitably come from the contributions of such fields as cognitive science, computer hardware, sensors and actuators, learning theory, and control architectures.

In keeping with the idea of immunized computational systems, Table 2 presents the levels of intelligence required in an intelligent controller, and compares this to the levels of intelligence exhibited in an immune system. These levels are motivated by research done by the authors in immunized artificial systems and the quest to implement autonomous controllers.

**Table 2.** Levels of Intelligence and the Immune System.

| Immune Response | Level | Intelligent Control |
|---|---|---|
| Antigen is present in the system. | | Disturbance is present in the system. |
| Innate Immunity is the first line of defense. Alerts next level. | 0 | Robust feedback control (non-adaptive; Error tends to zero) |
| T cells activate the B cell response (adaptation) to counteract the antigen. | 1 | An error critic modifies the controller parameters to counteract the disturbances. |
| Macrophages present the antigen to the T cells and the T cell response (adaptation) is activated. | 2 | Some utility function translates the disturbances into an error function and presents it to the critic. The critic starts the adaptation process. |
| For certain antigen, the Macrophages adapt with the end product: antibody that modifies the specificity of controller from broad but weak to narrow but strong. | 3 | For certain classes of disturbances (Ex: control hardware failure), the utility function is adapted directly based on a planning function. |

## 3 The Autonomous Aircraft Control Problem

Autonomous Systems are systems that are capable of responding, reacting, and developing independently. An intelligent control architecture (based upon levels of intelligent control) for the autonomous aircraft control problem is presented in Figure 1. The intelligent control architecture was implemented on a six-DOF numerical aircraft simulation with full-envelope nonlinear aerodynamics, as well as nonlinear kinematics, and a first order full-envelope thrust model. The aircraft modeled is a high-performance, supersonic vehicle representative of modern fighters [11]. Another novel idea in the implementation of the architecture was the use of neural approximators to emulate the non-linear nature of the problem. This approach is suited well when good linear approaches are available for system design.

In the next few sections, each of the levels represented in the architecture is elaborated.

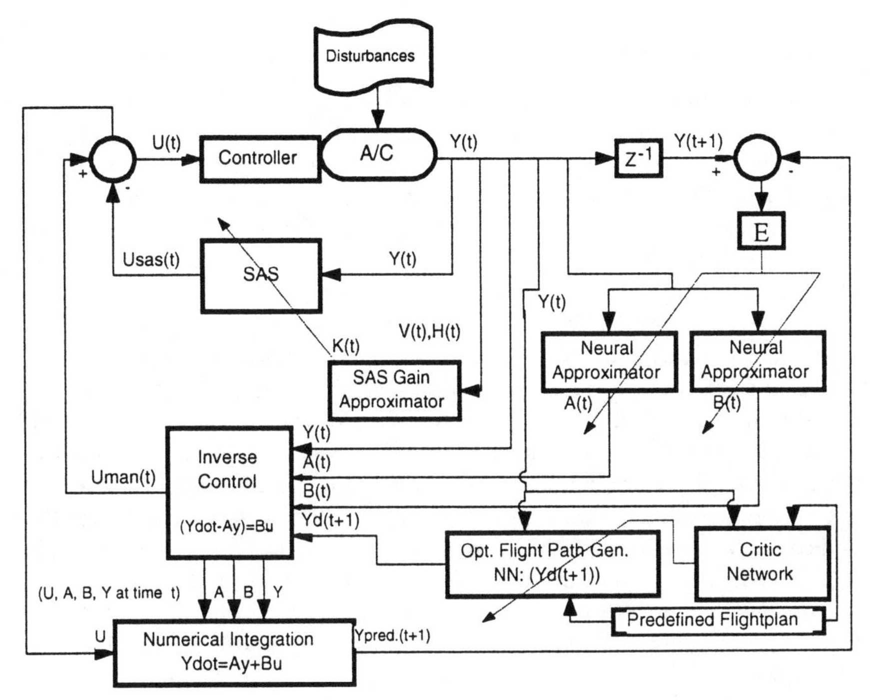


**Fig. 1.** Intelligent Control Architecture for the Autonomous Aircraft Control Problem

### 3.1 Level 0 Intelligent Control – A Robust Controller

Self-improvement of Tracking Error is an important goal of many control techniques. An example of one way to achieve this is to design robust feedback controllers with constant gains that improve the error as time goes to infinity. This has been defined as "Level 0 Intelligent Control".

In this application, the level 0 controller plays the role of a stability augmentation system (SAS). The controller is based on the idea of neural approximators for nonlinear control. Specifically, neural approximators are used to approximate inner loop feedback gains in a stability augmentation controller for the high performance aircraft model. The idea behind the architecture is best understood by thinking of the gain approximator block as a continuous gain scheduler. In fact, the gain approximator is a neural network whose inputs are the scheduling variables, altitude and airspeed, and the outputs were sensitive gains. It is desired that the level 0 SAS controller place the closed loop poles of the plant to provide stable, and desirable handling characteristics throughout the operational envelope [11].

### 3.2 Level 1 Intelligent Control – An Adaptive Controller

Self-improvement of control parameters towards the goal of achieving better tracking error or some error oriented goal, is the next level in intelligent control. This has been defined as "Level 1 Intelligent Control". An example of a level 1 intelligent controller is a robust feedback controller with adaptive parameters (such as model reference adaptive control, or neural adaptive control) that helps the error tend to zero for non-nominal operations. Thus, the feedback controller is self-improving.

The level 1 controller for the autonomous aircraft problem is shown in Figure 1. The idea behind this architecture is best understood by thinking of the gain approximator block as a continuous approximation of the nonlinear mapping between different linear representations of the aircraft model. In fact, the gain approximator is a neural network whose inputs are the scheduling variables, and whose outputs are an approximation of the aircraft plant-system Jacobians (state space A, and B matrices) that are valid for the specified flight condition. In this implementation, the inputs were altitude and airspeed, and the outputs were sensitive elements of A and B matrices. Also, in this implementation, desired trim values for certain states and the Neural Approximator output control variables. The performance objective for the level 1 tracking controller was to control the system state to follow a predefined path (assumed flight path).

### 3.3 Level 2 Intelligent Control – An Optimal Controller

Self-improvement of an estimate of the performance error (or some measure of performance over time) towards the goal of minimization or maximization of a utility function over time (error tends to zero and a measure of performance is optimized) is the next level in intelligent control. This is defined as "Level 2 Intelligent Control". This level is essentially a robust feedback controller with adaptive parameters that helps the error tend to zero for non-nominal operations, feedback controller is self improving, and a measure of performance that is self-improving is optimized over time. An example of a level 2 intelligent controller would be an adaptive critic system in which the critic is updated (improvement of performance measure) as well as the controller.

The level 2 autonomous control architecture is shown in Figure 1. The idea behind this architecture is best understood by thinking of the flight path generator block as providing continuous optimized flight path information to the level 1 controller. In fact, the flight path generator is an immunized adaptive critic that optimizes a performance index in order to use sparse, predefined data points to generate continuous flight path information.

# 4 Immunized Computational Systems

Immunized computational systems (ICS) use the immune system metaphor along with computational (both hard and soft computing) techniques to attempt to reproduce the robustness and adaptability of a biological immune system. Any attempt to mimic the building block process of the immune system in a computational technique should contain a definition of the proposed structure along with a definition of the subspaces or building blocks. Figure 2 presents a general block diagram of the proposed immunized computational system. The proposed system has the following attributes:

- **The Constant Meso-Structure:** The solid lines in figure 2 represent the base-line computational system (BCS). This system is designed to represent an average behavior of the uncertain system. Since this design is carried out off-line, any standard technique can be used for its synthesis. The base-line system is analogous to static portion of the antibodies.
- **The Changeable Meso-Structure:** The dashed lines in figure 2 represent the changeable computational system (CCS). This represents the variable region of the antibody and epitope equivalents. This structure must be adapted on-line. To include the innate immunity equivalence, the changeable computational systems that are known a priori can be stored in look-up tables and can be used to produce the right antibody and CCS models. Similar to the variable region of the antibodies, the changeable computational systems provide diversity to the immunized computational system.
- **Computational Building Blocks:** The computational building blocks, defined later, are used to arrive at the changeable computational systems.
- **Exploratory System:** The exploratory system is basically an evolutionary algorithm variant that uses recombination, selection, and mutation to arrive at a suitable CCS.
- **Learning System:** The learning system consists of a suit of learning paradigms to learn and store important computational building blocks that are not available a priori.
- **Uncertain System:** A system that is either being emulated or being controlled. This system is constantly changing.

## 4.1 Computational Building Blocks

In this paper, computational building blocks are defined as segments of a computational system topology (for example, a neural network connection, or family of connections, along with its associated weights) that contributes in establishing a good mapping for a class of input-output characteristics. Building blocks can be of different order. The order of a building block specifies the number of specific connections defined in the building block. Examples

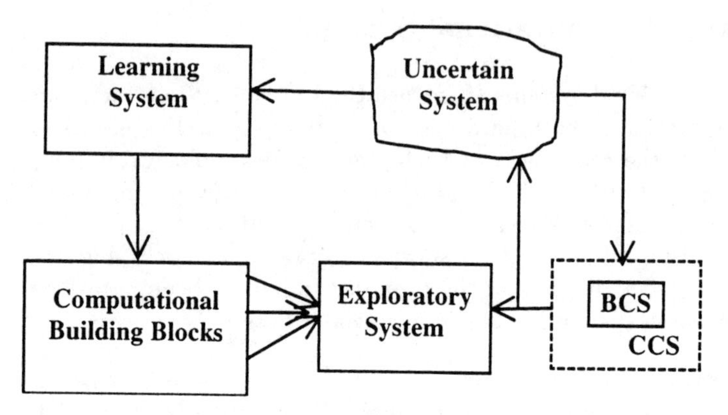


**Fig. 2.** Immunized Computational System

of building blocks using neural connections are shown in Figure 3. The building blocks are specified using a universal representation scheme that uses a neuron as the basic processing element. Thus the order 1 building block consists of two neurons and the relationship between them. In the case of Neural Networks, the relationship is the connection strength and the neurons are characterized by their type (input, hidden, output), the type of aggregation, and activation functions. In the case of a FS, the relationship is AND, OR, or THEN, and the neurons represent the input or output variables with their associated parameters (such as the *fuzzy* membership function). Determining important building blocks is problem dependent and any *a priori* knowledge will be useful here.

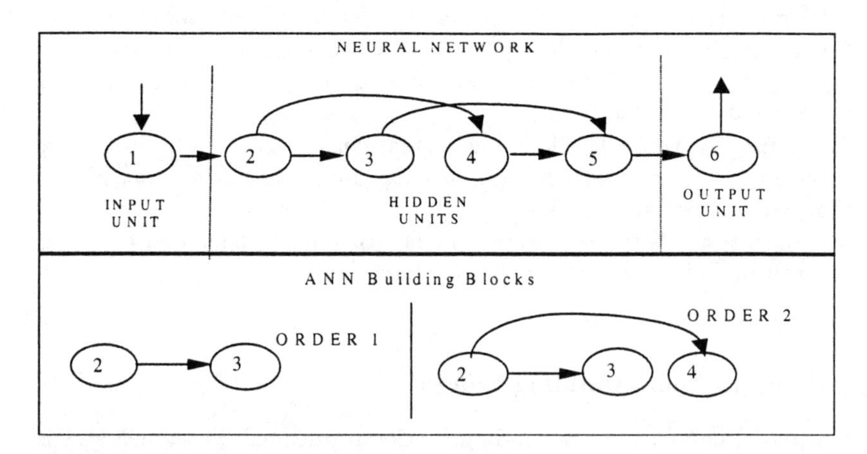


**Fig. 3.** Neural Network Building Blocks

## 4.2 The Role of Evolutionary Algorithms

Similar to the immune system, the computational building blocks need to be coded as a string of building blocks. This will represent the analogous DNA structure for the given system. For on-line processing, a population of CCS is randomly constructed using juxtapositioning of the building blocks, forming a population of messy strings (See figure 4). Next we find the best string that will represent the CCS through recombination, selection, and hyper-mutation of these strings.

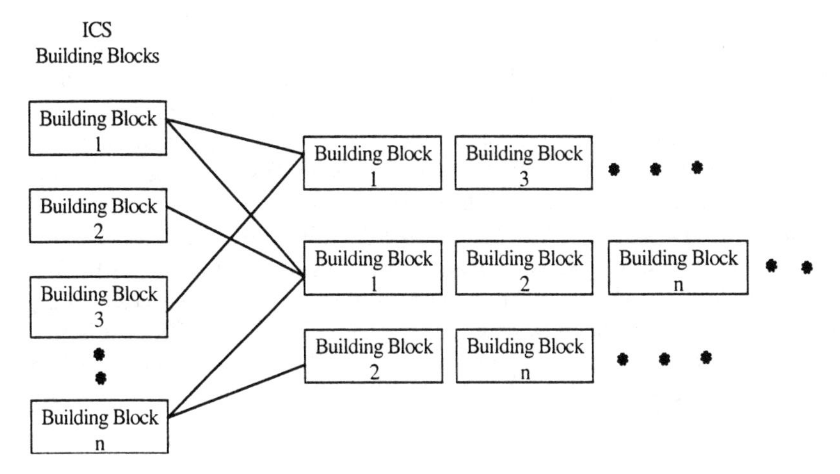


**Fig. 4.** Creation of Messy Strings from a Library of Building Blocks

Typical steps are as follows:

- From a population of N strings, arrive at a near-optimal CCS using recombination, mutation, and selection. An on-line error measure that can provide a fitness value for each candidate solution will decide optimality. Mutation takes place only on the parameters representing the topology (for example, weights for a NN) assuming a certain probability distribution of these parameters derived from the building blocks.
- Ideally, it will be desirable to have a population of all the possible CCS synthesized from the building blocks. Since this is not possible, we select a finite population of N messy strings and to ensure diversity, in every generation we introduce N/2 new messy strings drawn randomly from the available building blocks.
- The CCS chain is then decoded and the resulting computational system is superimposed with that of the BCS. The resulting computational system is evaluated for its optimality. The BCS can also be one of few possibilities. Once a near-optimal system has been found, hyper-mutation (or another preferred local learning scheme) is applied to the parameters. In

this step, no recombination is conducted, and no new strings are introduced. The selection operator is retained as it increases the number of high-affinity (or highly fit) CCS in the population.

The actual on-line processing is conducted using an evolutionary algorithm variant. Unlike any other technique, the evolutionary algorithm (EA) achieves its objective through a mix of random swapping and copying guided by a Darwinistic "survival of the fittest" strategy. EA possess great similarities to biological evolution and are guided by the notion of building blocks. The operators used for the recombination phase are similar to those used by Goldberg et al. [4]–cut, splice, and mutation. The cut operation is conducted with a specified gene-wise cut probability, $p_k$, such that the actual probability is $p_c = min\{p_k(L-1), 1\}$, where L is the current string length. The splice operator concatenates two strings at random with specified probability, $p_s$. Mutation is conducted only on the connection strengths (weights or association) using a small mutation rate. Figure 5 presents a sample sequence of operators for a computational system. After each cut and splice operation, the strings can grow longer or shorter. Selection is carried out using a binary tournament selection scheme. In the hyper-mutation phase, the connection parameters are mutated using a probability of mutation $p_{hm}$. The probability distribution for the mutation operator is assumed to be Gaussian and is derived using building block data gathered off-line.

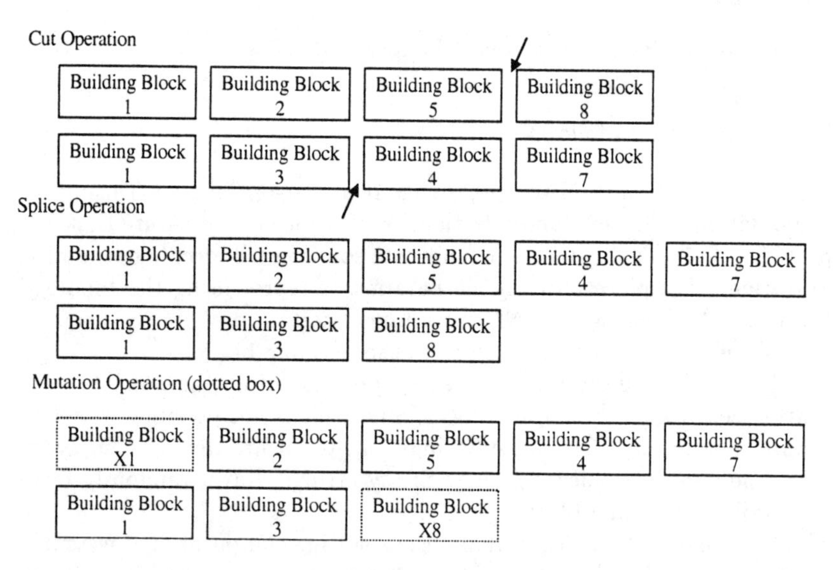


**Fig. 5.** Genetic Algorithm Operators

# 5 Immunized Adaptive Critics

## 5.1 Adaptive Critic Background

The concept of adaptive critics is a juxtaposition of neural networks, dynamic programming, and reinforcement learning ideas. Critics, both adaptive and non-adaptive have been proposed in the literature as systems that can model future performance. There are a number of ways to adapt critic networks. The simplest implementation is the heuristic dynamic programming (HDP) technique discussed by Werbos [9]. Howard's [9] formulation of the dynamic programming is the inspiration behind the Heuristic Dynamic Programming (HDP) critic. HDP is based on an attempt to approximate Howard's form of the Bellman equation.

Essentially, the critic, in addition to predicting the cost to go (future error), adapts itself with the help of the recursive relationship derived from approximate dynamic programming. Typically, backpropagation of error is used to update the weights of the critic.

## 5.2 How Adaptive Critics Work

An adaptive critic network adapts itself (see Figure 6) and at the same time it outputs a performance measure which can be used to update another system (usually a controller network). Howard's formulation of dynamic programming is the inspiration behind the simplest version of adaptive critics, namely, Heuristic Dynamic Programming (HDP) critics. HDP is based on an attempt to approximate Howard's form of the Bellman equation:

$$J(x_i) = Min_{u_i} \{U_{PM}(x_i) + \gamma J(x_{t+1}) | x_{t+1} = f(x_i, u_i, noise)\} \quad (1)$$

where $x_t$ is the state vector, $u_t$ is the control vector, $U_{PM}(.)$ is the one stage Performance Measure function, $f(.,.,.)$ is the model of the system, and $\gamma (0 < \gamma \leq 1)$ is the discount factor.

## 5.3 Immunized critics

Some of the desired features of critic adaptation will be speed, robustness, and the ability to make discontinuous jumps from one parametric space to another which is very important for handling drastically changing operating environments. We claim that adaptive critics will be useful only if they can handle fast changing operating environments. In this study, we propose to use the Immunized Computational Systems learning paradigm for achieving this objective. Here we apply the immunized Intelligent Control ideas to improve the performance estimates of the critic. In this implementation methodology, linear building blocks are used. Next, we discuss the implementation details of this application. The objective is to implement a level 2 intelligent controller

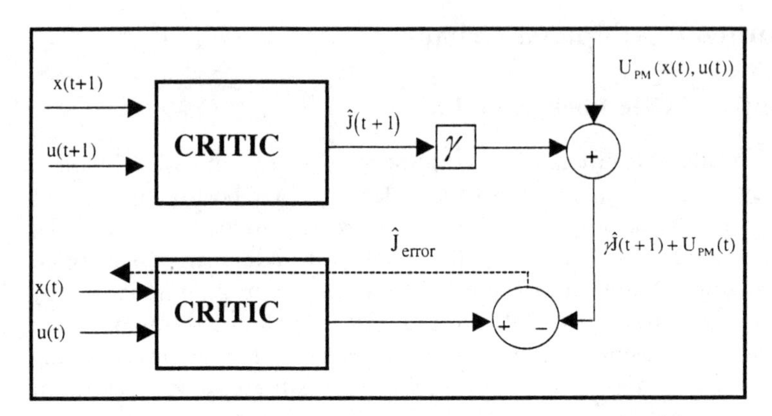


**Fig. 6.** Heuristic Dynamic Programming Adaptive Critic

using immunized critics. The implementation is carried out in an off-line Phase, which is basically the generation and organization of *a-priori* building blocks, and an on-line Phase that involves the on-line manipulation of the building blocks for uncertainty management.

**Off-Line Phase.** Step 1: To arrive at the computational building blocks, one must first define the hypersphere of uncertainties for the system. In other words, one must specify which uncertainties the system may encounter, and which of these are to be negated by the controller. It is important that the control system designer differentiates between the types of uncertainties (i.e. parametric, initial condition, environmental, etc.) and organizes *a-priori* information accordingly. *This is important because this method will be impractical for specific problems in which uncertainty measurements, estimations, or approximations are unobtainable.*

Step 2: Next, we use LQR theory to generate pre-learnt information on the critic formulation. Basically, given a linear system and a quadratic cost function as:

$$\dot{x} = Ax + Bu \tag{2}$$

$$J = \frac{1}{2}\int_0^\infty (x^T Qx + u^T Ru)dt \tag{3}$$

we have a closed form dynamic programming solution for the feedback control as:

$$u(t) = -R^{-1}B^T Sx(t) \tag{4}$$

where S is the solution of the steady state Riccati equation:

$$SA + A^T S - SBR^{-1}B^T S + Q = 0 \tag{5}$$

and the cost to go in the Bellman equation is:

$$J^o = \frac{1}{2} x^T S x \tag{6}$$

For off-line learning, simulate many different uncertainties from the definition of uncertainties presented earlier, and generate S matrices using the LQR theory (solution of the Riccati equation). The elements of the S matrix will become the pre-learnt computational building blocks.

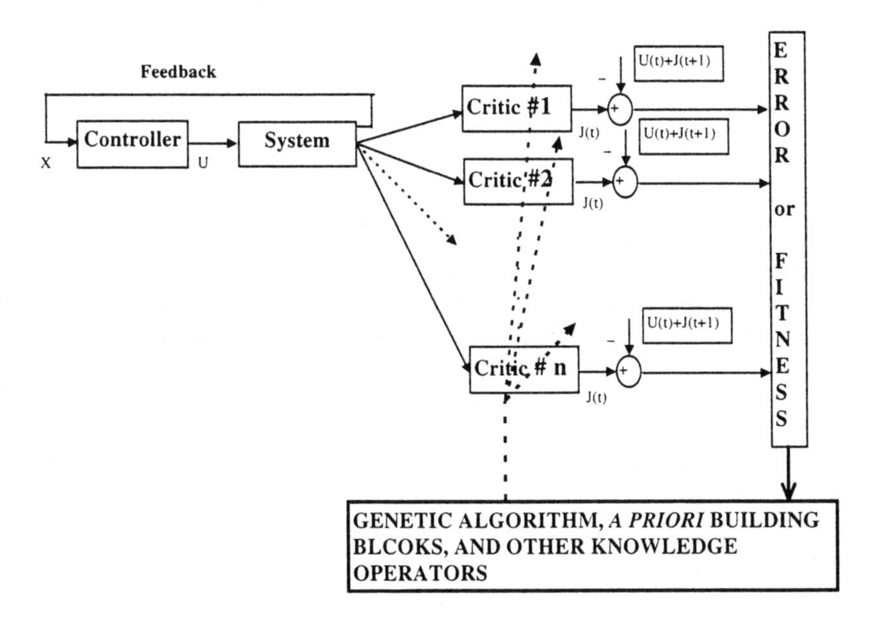


**Fig. 7.** Immunized Adaptive Critic

**On-Line Phase.** For on-line adaptation, this implementation uses a modified genetic algorithm technique to evolve the critic (elements of S). The overall concept is shown in Figure 7. The steps involved are:

Step 1: Start with a base-line S matrix and a corresponding controller (Equations 4 and 5).

Step 2: Create many different critics from the pre-learnt adaptive critic building blocks (elements of the $S$ matrix).

Step 3: Adapt the critic using a modified genetic algorithm. The parameters of the GA represent the critic building blocks ($S11, S12, ...$).

Step 4: The fitness function is defined as,

$$E = \sum_{t=T}^{T-10*dt} [J(t) - (U_{PM}(t)dt + J(t+1)]^2 \tag{7}$$

where:

$$U_{PM} = x^T Qx + u^T Ru$$

$$J(t) = \frac{1}{2} x(t)^T S(t) x(t)$$

$$J(t+1) = \frac{1}{2} x(t+1)^T S(t+1) x(t+1)$$

NOTE: The error as defined above comes from the HDP approximation to Bellman's dynamic programming equation (Equation 1).

Step 5: Every $n$-time steps, the controller is updated using the best critic estimate as follows:

$K(t) = -R^{-1} B^T S_{best}, u(t) = K(t)x(t)$. No update on the B matrix is conducted.

### 5.4 IAC Application to the Aircraft Problem

This section addresses the use of IAC as applied to an autonomous aircraft control problem. IAC can be used effectively to provide the control paradigm with an adaptive "near optimal" desired flight path. Used in conjunction with the Neural Approximator (NA) based "Level 0" and "Level 1" intelligent controllers previously defined by the authors (See Figure 1), a powerful "near autonomous" control system architecture is formed.

At the simplest level, we want to develop a path generator whose inputs are the state of the aircraft ($X_{A/C}$), and a prespecified fixed path in space ($X_{fixed}$), and whose output is a smooth, optimal, and realizable desired aircraft path (See Figure 8).

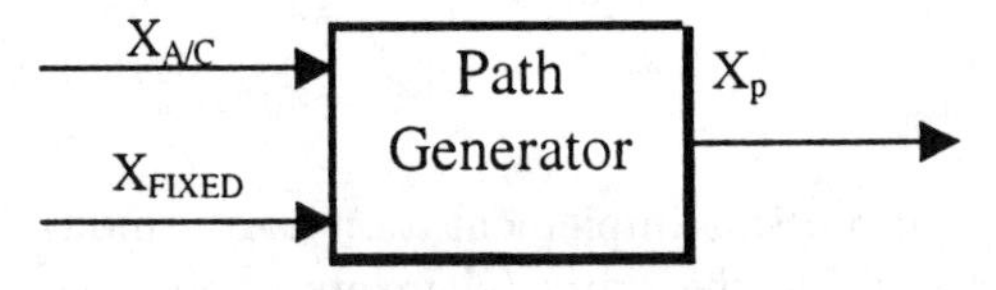


**Fig. 8.** Simplified Path Generator

The open loop path generator can be represented by the equation:

$$\delta \dot{X} = A_p \delta X_p + B_p \delta U_p \tag{8}$$

where

$$\delta X_p = X_p - X_{FIXED}$$

$$\delta U_p = X_{FIXED} - X_{A/C}$$

Additionally, $A_p$ and $B_p$ represent the dynamics of the path generator, and $X_p(t), X_{A/C}(t)$, and $X_{FIXED}(t)$ are defined as:

$X_p(t) = [V_P(t), H_P(t), \Psi_p(t)]$,
$X_{FIXED}(t) = [V_{FIXED}(t), H_{FIXED}(t), \Psi_{FIXED}(t)]$,
$X_{A/C}(t) = [V_{A/C}(t), H_{A/C}(t), \Psi_{A/C}(t)]$,
where
V = Airspeed, ft/sec
H = Altitude, feet
$\Psi$ = Heading Angle, Rad

and are defined in "earth-fixed coordinates". Note that in the open loop, $(X_{FIXED} - X_{A/C})$ is the forcing function (or the control). The open loop path generator, however, is insufficient as there is nothing to drive the path $(X_p)$ to $X_{FIXED}$. To accomplish this, we use feedback. The architecture of the closed loop path generator can be seen in Figure 9. Note that the closed loop architecture can be represented by the equation:

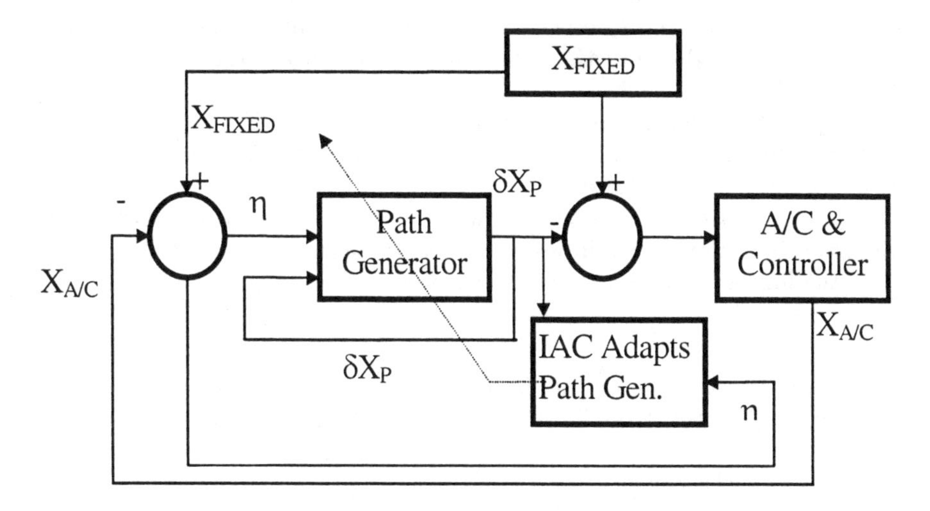


**Fig. 9.** IAC Path Generator as a Feedback System

$$\delta = A_{pCL}\delta X_p + \eta(t) \tag{9}$$

where

$$\eta = \delta U_p = X_{FIXED} - X_{A/C}(open\ loop\ control)$$

$A_{pCL}$ is the closed loop system $= A_p - B_p K_p$ with $K_p$ found from the LQR solution, and $\eta$ is viewed as a disturbance.

### 5.5 Implementation of the IAC Path Generator

The implementation of the IAC Path Generator, involves both an off-line phase, and an on-line phase.

**Off-line Phase.** The steps carried out off-line were in general for the creation of the building block pool, and the pool statistics.

Step 1: Four $A_p$ (path state) matrices were specified by modeling the system with first order dynamics. The state space B matrix for the path dynamics was held constant (identity matrix), also specified were 5 Q matrices, and R was held constant (Equation 3). Each of the four $A_p$ matrices corresponded to general maneuvers performed with different time constants. Thus, the four matrices, $A_p$ were 3x3 diagonal matrices defined by the choice of the time constants $\tau_V, \tau_H, \tau_\Psi$. The R matrix was chosen as the identity, and the Q matrices were chosen as .001R, .01R, .1R, R, and 10R. Next, the $A_p, B_p, Q$, and $R$ matrices were used to calculate 20 different S (Equation 5) matrices. The individual elements of the S matrices were specified as the IAC building blocks.

Step 2: Next the S matrices were broken into building blocks, since the S matrices were 3x3, and symmetrical, there were 6 building blocks ($S_{11}$, $S_{12}$, $S_{13}$, $S_{22}$, $S_{32}$, $S_{33}$) from each of the 20 matrices for a total of 120 *a-priori* building blocks.

Step 3: Next, the 1st and 2nd order statistics for each S matrix position were calculated, in other words, the mean $\mu$ and standard deviation $\sigma$ of $S_{11}, S_{12}$ etc. were calculated.

Step 4: Next the building blocks were ranked in order of standard deviation, and mutation probabilities were specified such that the building block with the highest standard deviation has the highest probability of mutation etc.

**On-Line Phase.** The on-line implementation was carried out inside the main aircraft control loop. For this implementation, the path generator was updated once every (simulated) second or once every 50 integration time steps (dt = 0.02 seconds).

Step 1: First the mean value of the S matrices created off-line was calculated using the means of the building blocks. The fitness of the mean S matrix was then determined.

Step 2: Next, N new S matrices were generated using a variant of the standard GA "selection" operator, by selecting building blocks from the building block (or gene) pool. N was the genetic algorithm population size.

Step 3: Next, hypermutation was applied to each new S matrix, and the fitness of each S matrix was calculated using Bellman's equation from dynamic programming (HDP).

Step 4: Now, if the best fitness of the new S matrices was better than the fitness of the previous best S matrix, replace the "best" S matrix with the S matrix corresponding to the best fitness. The "best" S matrix is then carried over into the new population, and, after a stopping criteria check, the process returns to on-line step 1.

Step 5: Continue until some stopping criteria is reached. (for this example a set number of iterations).

The implementation of the Level 2 intelligent controller was used to perform various maneuvers. The results obtained showed that the IAC methodology performed consistently well. Also, the IAC converged quickly to a desirable solution. Figure 10 presents a typical plot of the IAC evolution and Figures 11 and 12 document the performance of the overall intelligent control architecture for a 3-dimensional maneuver (only altitude and heading responses are shown) at 600 ft/sec and 800 ft/sec airspeed conditions. It is evident from these plots that the concept of immunized critics does function as desired and that the evolution of the critic happens in fewer iterations than in a typical genetic algorithm evolution.

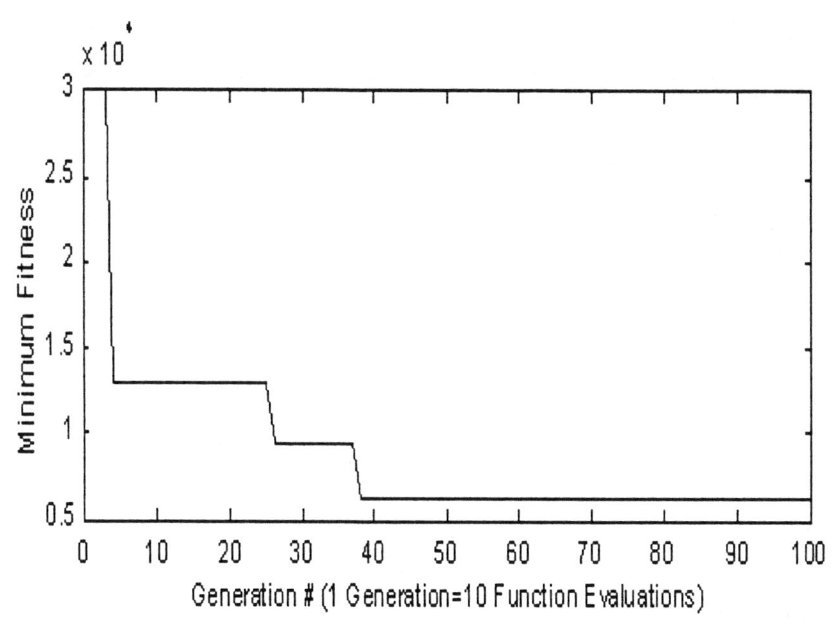


**Fig. 10.** Immunized System Evolution

## 6 Conclusion

It was found that immunized artificial systems function well as adaptive critics, and that immunized adaptive critics (IAC) can be used effectively in on-line control problems. When using IAC for path generation, modeling the

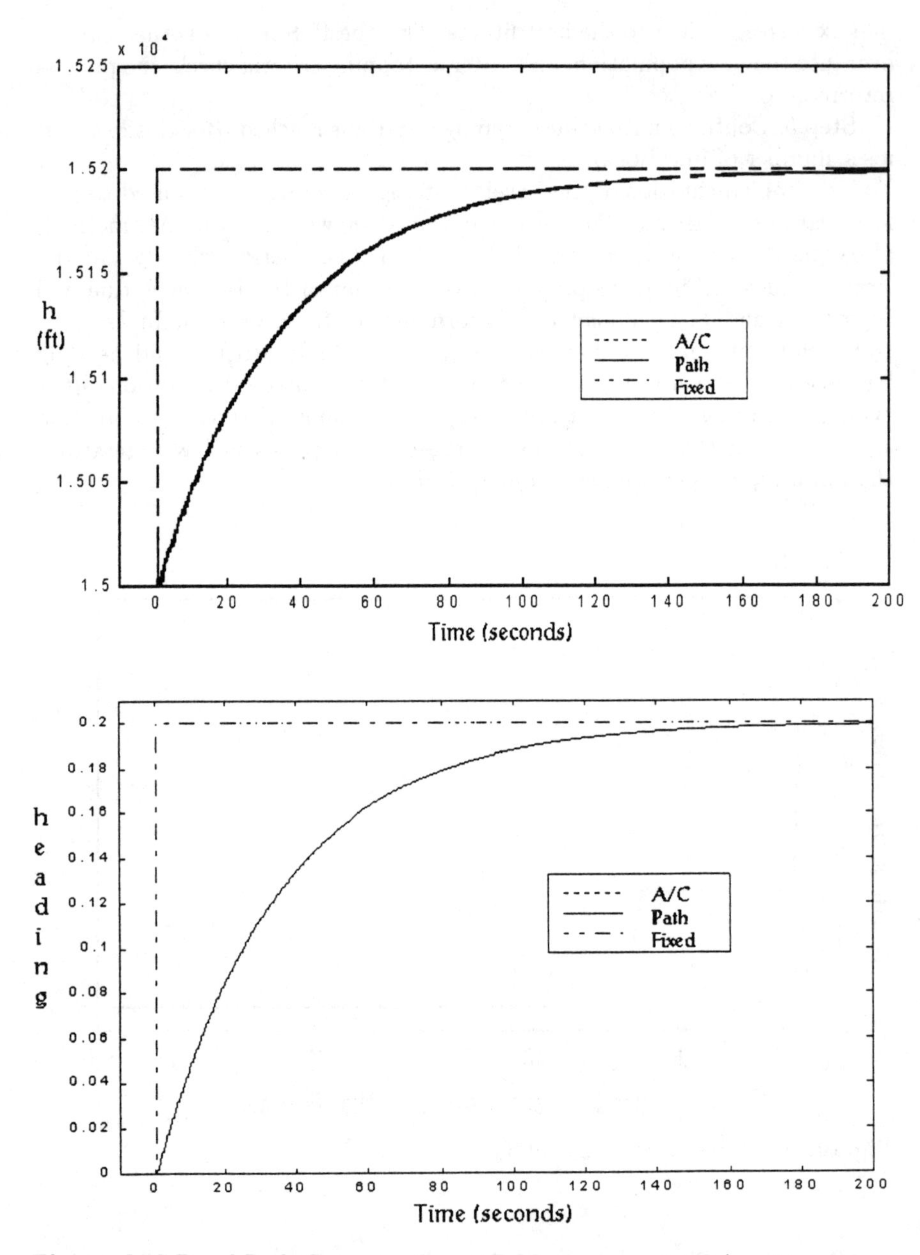


**Fig. 11.** IAC Based Path Generator for a 3-D Maneuver at 600 ft/sec Airspeed

path generator dynamics as a first order system was the simplest option. A second order system might be more appropriate as some of the dominant aircraft modes are of second order. It was also found that when using IAC

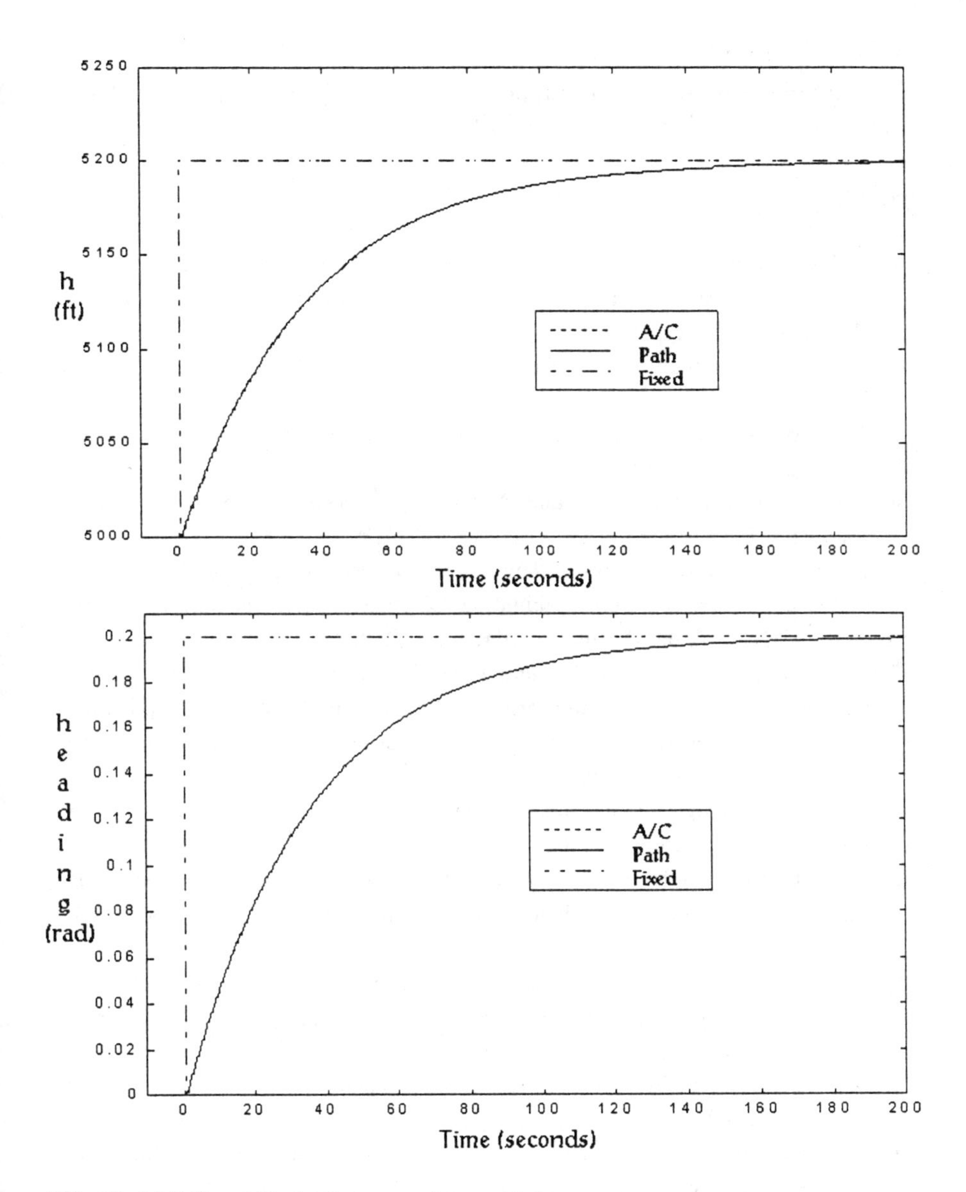


**Fig. 12.** IAC Based Path Generator for a 3-D Maneuver at 800 ft/sec Airspeed

for path generation, the IAC converges to a desired solution very quickly (see Figure 10).

**Acknowledgment**

This material is based on work supported by the National Science Foundation under Grants No. ECS-9415351 and ECS-9113283.

## References

1. A. Barto, Reinforcement Learning and Adaptive Critic Methods. Handbook of Intelligent Control: Neural, Fuzzy, and Adaptive Approaches. Van Nosttrand Reinhold, Kentucky, 1992.
2. E. Benjamin, Immunology, A Short Course, Wiley-Liss Publications, New York, NY., 1992.
3. A. E. Bryson and Y. Ho, Applied Optimal Control. Hemisphere Publishing Corporation, New York., 1965.
4. D. E. Goldberg, K. Deb, K., and B. Korb, An Investigation of Messy Genetic Algorithm (TCGA Report No. 90005), U. of Alabama, 1990.
5. K. KrishnaKumar, Immunized Neurocontrol: Concepts and Initial Results, Presented at the workshop on combinations of genetic algorithms and neural networks, COGANN'92, Baltimore, MD, June, 1992.
6. K. Krishnakumar, A. Satyadas, and J. Neidhoefer, An Immune System Framework For Integrating Computational Intelligence Paradigms With Applications To Adaptive Control, in Computational Intelligence (A Dynamic System Perspective), IEEE Press, 1995.
7. K. KrishnaKumar, Immunized artificial neural systems, World Congress on Neural Networks, Portland, July 11-15, 1993.
8. J. Neidhoefer and K. Krishnakumar, Neuro Gain Approximation, Intelligent Engineering Systems Through Artificial Neural Networks, Vol. 6, 1996, ASME Press. pp. 543-550.
9. P. J. Werbos. Approximate Dynamic Programming for Real-time Control and Neural Modeling. Handbook of Intelligent Control: Neural, Fuzzy, and Adaptive Approaches. Van Nosttrand Reinhold, Kentucky, 1993.
10. B. Wie and D. S. Bernstein, Benchmark Problems in robust control design. Journal of Guidance, Control, and Dynamics. Vol. 15, pp. 1057 - 1059, 1992.
11. J. Neidhoefer, and K. KrishnaKumar (1997), Non-linear Control Using Neural Approximators with Linear Control Theory, AIAA 97-3536, AIAA Conference on Guidance, Navigation, and Control, New Orleans, LA, August, 1997.
12. R. Brumbaugh, Aircraft Model for the AIAA Controls Design Challenge, Journal of Guidance Control and Dynamics, Vol. 17, No. 4, July-August 1994.

**Dr. Kalmanje KrishnaKumar** is an Associate Professor of Aerospace Engineering at the University of Alabama and co-founder of Flexible Intelligence Group, Tuscaloosa, Alabama. He is currently responsible for teaching and coordinating Intelligent Control, Flight Dynamics and Control, and neural networks. His research interests include immunized artificial systems, soft computing methods and their application to adaptive control, structural control, optimal control, optimal estimation, flight simulation, and training. His externally funded research includes immunized neuro-control; neural networks applications to OPAD, automated training, and large space structures; evolutionary fuzzy modeling and application to F-18 stability augmentation systems; genetic algorithms applications to flight control, adaptive control, and partitioned controllers; synthesis and experimental verification of a new concept in helicopter hover training; and flight reconstruction of recorded flight using robust estimators. He has organized several tutorial workshops on genetic algorithms: theory and control applications and evolutionary fuzzy modeling and its application to control; intelligent control; computational intelligence; and adaptive critics. He is the chairman of the AIAA intelligent systems technical committee, SAE information sciences technologies committee, the AIAA Journal of Aircraft editorial board, and the AIAA journal of guidance control and dynamics.

**Mr. James Neifhoefer** will soon complete his Ph.D. in the department of Aerospace Engineering and Mechanics at the University of Alabama in Tuscaloosa. He has recently joined the R & D team at Accurate Automation Corporation in Chattanooga, TN. His area of expertise is Intelligent Control, which is an emerging field involving the juxtaposition of ideas from Artificial Intelligence (AI) with ideas from Traditional and Modern Control Theory.

# Blueprint for a Computer Immune System*

Jeffrey O. Kephart, Gregory B. Sorkin, Morton Swimmer, and
Steve R. White

IBM Thomas J. Watson Research Center
P.O. Box 704, Yorktown Heights, NY 10598

**Abstract.** There is legitimate concern that, within the next few years, the Internet will provide a fertile medium for new breeds of computer viruses capable of spreading orders of magnitude faster than today's viruses. To counter this threat, we have developed an immune system for computers that senses the presence of a previously unknown pathogen, and within minutes automatically derives and deploys a prescription for detecting and removing it. The system is being integrated with a commercial anti-virus product, IBM AntiVirus, and will be available as a pilot in 1997.

## 1 Introduction

During the last decade, computer virus authors and anti-virus technologists have been engaged in an escalating arms race. Today, these forces are roughly in balance: computer viruses are a nuisance, but a manageable one. When a new virus appears, prescriptions for detecting and removing it are developed by human experts. This information is incorporated into the data files of anti-virus products, and is eventually distributed to end users. The time scale on which viruses spread globally is generally several months, commensurate with the time scale on which users typically receive updates.

However, the explosive growth of the Internet and the rapid emergence of applications that disregard the traditional boundaries between computers threaten to increase the global spread rate of computer viruses by several orders of magnitude. Traditionally, a PC virus has had to rely on (unwitting) human intermediaries to help it spread within a PC or from one PC to another: a human has had to execute an infected program, and to copy it from one machine to another, e.g. via diskette or ftp. But the tasks of executing and copying are becoming automated to an ever greater extent. The problem is exacerbated further by the fact that objects like documents and spreadsheets, which tend to be transferred between computers at a much greater rate than executable programs, are now increasingly likely to harbor code themselves in the form of macros, and these macros may contain viruses.

---

* This article was orginally appeared in *Proceedings of the Seventh International Virus Bulletin Conference*. Virus Bulletin Ltd., 1997.

For example, modern-day mail programs permit text documents or spreadsheets to be sent very simply as e-mail attachments. When opened by the recipient, the type of the attachment can be recognized, and an application capable of interpreting and displaying it can be launched automatically. When the application loads the attachment, any macros contained therein may be executed, giving any viral macros the opportunity to spread. Note that, in this scenario, the virus' dependence upon human intervention has been reduced substantially from what it has been traditionally. The sender can now (unwittingly) transmit an infected object by attaching it to e-mail with a few mouse clicks, one last mouse click sending it on its way. Execution is even easier: unsophisticated recipients may not even realize that, simply by opening their mail, they are automatically executing applications that may in turn automatically execute macros.

Complete automation of the cycle of transmitting a virus from computer A to computer B and then executing it on computer B cannot be far off. No great technological breakthroughs are required. Already, a number of mail programs permit the user to create agents that automatically send or process mail on behalf of the user. One can expect that, soon, viruses will exploit these capabilities, and once they do they will no longer be held back by the stumblings and bumblings of humans. Other vehicles for fully automated replication will be available soon. A few years from now, the Internet may seethe with millions or billions of mobile agents, which could serve as a fertile medium for a new type of virus that could direct its host to quickly visit a large number of sites and infect other agents there. Viruses such as these will be in control of their own destiny, replicating at rates that may be checked only by network latency and processing speed.

In short, the nature of computer viruses and their ability to propagate is on the cusp of a fundamental, qualitative change — one that demands an equally fundamental change in the way we must defend against them. Epidemiological modeling and common sense both dictate that eliminating a virus requires killing it off at a rate faster than it can spread. With humans completely removed from the replication loop, the only way to respond quickly enough to new viruses will be to remove humans from the response loop as well.

But how? Fortunately, nature supplies us with a ready answer. Higher organisms' immune systems are effective mechanisms for protecting against rapidly spreading, rapidly evolving pathogens such as bacteria and viruses. Inspired by the analogy between computer viruses and biological ones, we have designed and prototyped an "immune system for cyberspace" that is capable of automatically deriving and distributing anti-virus data within minutes of a new virus's first detection.

An exploration of the connections between our system and biological immune systems can be found in [1,2]. This paper emphasizes issues pertaining to the design and implementation of a robust, practical, industrial-strength immune system. Section 2 discusses the minimal criteria that ought to be satisfied by such a system. Then, section 3 elaborates some implementation details that illustrate how we have met these criteria in the IBM immune system design and prototype.

## 2 Requirements for a Computer Immune System

In order to describe what we mean by a computer immune system, we shall first describe briefly some of the salient features of biological immune systems, using this as a basis for a broad outline of the function of a computer immune system. Then, we shall define some minimal practical requirements that must be satisfied by any commercially viable computer immune system.

When first exposed to a pathogen, the immune system of vertebrates and many non-vertebrates reacts in a non-adaptive, non-specific way. This "innate" immune system provides a first line of defense, and, in vertebrates, also triggers a more adaptive, specific immune response. To discriminate pathogens from benign entities, the innate immune system combines knowledge of the self (e.g. proteins that are present on self-cells, but usually not on foreign cells [3]) with general knowledge of broad classes of harmful entities (signaled by double-strand RNA, which occurs in much greater concentrations in certain classes of viruses than in mammalian cells, or by the presence of a peptide produced copiously by bacteria but only in minute amounts by mammals [4]). The innate immune system can also produce a generic response to pathogens which disables or kills them.

In addition to the innate immune system, vertebrates also possess a more sophisticated, adaptive immune system whose components include antibodies, B-cells, and T-cells. When a pathogen is first encountered, only a few antibodies or immune cell receptors may bind weakly to the pathogen or fragments of it, but over the course of a few days an adaptive process produces numerous immune cells and antibodies that bind strongly enough to detect and disable the pathogen in a very precise way. Henceforth, the immune system will retain a memory of the pathogen, and be armed against repeat attacks by it [5].

A computer immune system must include components patterned on both the innate and the adaptive immune systems. Like the innate immune system it must sense pathogenic anomalies in a generic way, but by itself this is not enough. A computer immune system must also, like the adaptive immune system, develop ways of identifying pathogens very specifically, and then it must use this precise identification to purge them.

Combining these very broad statements with a number of practical considerations, we set forth some criteria that must be met to provide real-world, functional protection from rapidly spreading viruses:

- **Innate immunity.** The system must be capable of detecting the presence of a high proportion of viruses that are unknown to it specifically.

The system should recognize previously unknown viruses of all types; currently, this would include file infectors, boot-sector infectors, and macro viruses. It is particularly important that the system be geared towards detecting viruses that are found in real incidents. For example, less emphasis need be placed on detecting overwriting viruses, since these are never prevalent.

- **Adaptive immunity.** The system must be capable of automatically deriving from a single sample a "prescription" for detecting and, if possible, removing all instances of the virus.
- **Delivery and dissemination.** The system must deliver the prescription to the afflicted computer, and must also facilitate dissemination of the prescription to other machines both in its neighborhood and around the world.
- **Speed.** The system must be capable of deriving and disseminating prescriptions on a time scale faster than the virus can spread. Currently, a reasonable goal is to derive and deliver a prescription to the originally afflicted machine in less than ten minutes from when an anomaly is first detected, and to permit dissemination of the prescription to neighboring machines within less than half an hour. The system should be capable of protecting anyone from any newly discovered virus within a day at most. These requirements will become even stricter as technology permits computer viruses to spread faster.
- **Scalability.**
  1. **Analysis.** If a new, particular virulent virus begins to spread quickly, many machines at one site and/or at different sites may experience the virus simultaneously. The system must be capable of very high throughput, handling at least thousands of simultaneous requests for virus analysis.
  2. **Updates.** The system must be able to update tens of millions of PCs on at least a daily basis.
- **Safety and reliability.** The prescription produced by the immune system must be sufficiently reliable that it can be deployed worldwide without being checked by humans. Preferably the false positive rate should be at least as low and the removal information at least as accurate as is typically achieved by expert humans.
- **Security.** Virus samples must be protected in such a way that they cannot be intercepted and read by a third party while in transit. Even more importantly, appropriate measures must be taken to ensure that any prescriptions employed by a client machine are uncorrupted, genuine copies of those produced by the immune system.
- **Customer control.** Customers must be able to control the conditions under which virus samples and other information are sent out of their enterprise. They must likewise be able to control the conditions under which prescriptions are received and disseminated to the originally infected client and possibly other machines. Some customers may want

manual control in one or both directions, others may want the speed given by completely automated response.

Most of today's major anti-virus products possess a few bits and pieces from among these ingredients. Most use heuristics of various sorts to recognize previously unknown viruses. Some anti-virus vendors even use automated procedures to assist with analyzing viruses. However, designing and implementing a robust defense against rapidly-spreading viruses is a serious undertaking, and requires meeting all of the above criteria. No commercial anti-virus offering comes anywhere close to offering this level of defense today.

The remainder of this paper describes our efforts in this direction: the design and prototype of the IBM immune system for cyberspace, which is intended to defend millions of real customers against real viruses.

# 3 Implementing an Immune System for Cyberspace

In broad terms, our implementation of the immune system consists of the steps of:

1. Discovering a previously unknown virus on a user's computer.
2. Capturing a sample of the virus and sending it to a central computer.
3. Analyzing the virus automatically to derive a prescription for detecting and removing it from any host object.
4. Delivering the prescription to the user's computer, incorporating it into the anti-virus data files, and running the anti-virus product to detect and remove all occurrences of the virus.
5. Disseminating the prescription to other computers in the user's locale and to the rest of the world.

We shall now describe each of these steps in further detail, illustrating along the way how the criteria set forth in the previous section are met.

## 3.1 Discovering previously unknown viruses: the innate immune system

To be effective, an immune system must do a very good job of sensing previously unknown viruses that are present in the computer system that it is protecting. Like the "innate" immune system, the computer immune system can combine self-knowledge (embodied for example in change detection and change analysis) with generic knowledge of broad classes of potential pathogens (embodied for example in static analysis based on viral machine-code features). These and other heuristics, some based on dynamic, behavior-based analysis, can be incorporated in a very natural way into an existing anti-virus product running on user's PCs. Here we mention some of the main heuristics used to discover previously unknown file infectors, boot-sector infectors, and macro viruses, all of which are either already integrated into IBM AntiVirus, or will be shortly.

**File infectors** To catch previously unknown file-infecting viruses, we use two main heuristics. The first is based on a "generic disinfection" technique [6]; the second on a classifier that recognizes potential viruses based on characteristic machine-code features [2,7].

*Generic disinfection heuristic* The underlying principle of the generic disinfection heuristic is that a program $\mathcal{F}'$ infected with a virus can generally be restored to its original, uninfected version $\mathcal{F}$. The reason for this is simple. After a virus has carried out its own function, the best way for it to avoid immediate detection is to allow its host program to continue normally. This generally means that the virus must be able to reconstruct the host in its original form, which in turn requires that none of the original host bytes be destroyed. In other words, for non-overwriting viruses, $\mathcal{F}'$ can be regarded as a reversible transformation of $\mathcal{F}$, i.e. the original host $\mathcal{F}$ is in principle reconstructible from $\mathcal{F}'$. On the other hand, legitimate changes such as updating a program to a new version are unlikely to be similarly reversible: too much will change, and some bytes that were contained in $\mathcal{F}$ will no longer be present in $\mathcal{F}'$.

Therefore, if a program has been modified from $\mathcal{F}$ to $\mathcal{F}'$ and the generic disinfection algorithm could recover $\mathcal{F}$ from $\mathcal{F}'$, it may be concluded with a high degree of confidence that $\mathcal{F}'$ contains a virus. If so, the user is given the option to carry out the disinfection, and a sample of the program is captured.

*Generic disinfection algorithm* As employed in IBM AntiVirus, the generic disinfection algorithm works as follows. When the product is first installed, a fingerprint of each executable file is computed and stored in a database. The fingerprint consists of less than 100 bytes of information about each program $\mathcal{F}$, including its size, date, and various checksums. On subsequent scans of the system, the fingerprint is recomputed and compared with the stored one. If it has changed, the new version of the program, $\mathcal{F}'$, will be scanned for known viruses. If the change cannot be attributed to any known virus, the generic disinfection algorithm tries to reconstruct the original program $\mathcal{F}$ from the new version $\mathcal{F}'$ plus the fingerprint.

The reconstruction is attempted roughly as follows. First, some of the fingerprint data are used to locate the beginning and end of $\mathcal{F}$ within $\mathcal{F}'$, say at offsets $b$ and $e$ respectively. Then, if $e - b = |\mathcal{F}|$, the length of $\mathcal{F}$, the checksum of the bytes between $b$ and $e$ is computed. If the checksum matches the original checksum contained in the fingerprint, the block of bytes between $b$ and $e$ is taken to be an exact reconstruction of $\mathcal{F}$. If $e - b > |\mathcal{F}|$ or $e < b$, then a series of trial reconstructions is attempted, in which a block $\mathcal{F}_1$ beginning at $b$ is concatenated with a block $\mathcal{F}_2$ ending at $e$, with $|\mathcal{F}_1| + |\mathcal{F}_2| = |\mathcal{F}|$. If the checksum of a reconstruction matches the original checksum, the reconstruction is assumed to be correct.

*Generic disinfection implementation* The number of candidate reconstructions of $\mathcal{F}$ can be of the same order as its length. Since computing a single checksum requires an amount of computation proportional to $|\mathcal{F}|$, a naive implementation of the generic disinfection algorithm would require running time quadratic in the file length. In practical terms, it would take several days to reconstruct an average executable on an average PC. Fortunately, for CRC checksums (cyclic redundancy check [8]), there is a very efficient implementation (modeled on the Karp-Rabin hash for string matching [9]) allowing all the checksums together to be computed in linear time, and in a fraction of a second on a PC.

To see how this it works, suppose $e - b > |\mathcal{F}|$. In this case, our working assumption is that the original file has been split at an unknown point into blocks $\mathcal{F}_1$ and $\mathcal{F}_2$, with a block of virus bytes introduced between them. A first candidate reconstruction hypothesizes that the split occurred as close before $e$ as is consistent with our recognition of $e$ as the endpoint of the original file $\mathcal{F}$; this is checked by computing the checksum in the standard way. Then, successive candidates are generated by extending the beginning of the block $\mathcal{F}_2$ backwards one byte at a time, with a corresponding backwards shrinkage from the end of block $\mathcal{F}_1$.

The key point is that the checksum of each candidate need not be computed from scratch, but can be calculated very quickly from that of its predecessor. Suppose that the bytes between offsets $b$ and $e$ in $\mathcal{F}'$ have the form $G_1\alpha \ldots \beta G_2$, where the combined length of blocks $G_1$ and $G_2$ is $|\mathcal{F}| - 1$, and $\alpha$ and $\beta$ are single bytes. Then the candidate reconstruction $\mathcal{G}_1\alpha\mathcal{G}_2$ will be followed by $\mathcal{G}_1\beta\mathcal{G}_2$, with a change in just one byte.

The CRC checksum of a *bit* string $b_{n-1}, \ldots, b_0$ is by definition the coefficient bit string of the remainder of the polynomial $\sum_{i=0}^{n-1} b_i x^{i+d}$ on division by a fixed irreducible degree-$d$ polynomial $P(x)$ over the integers modulo 2. Returning to *bytes*, linearity of the checksum implies that the exclusive-OR difference $\gamma$ between successive candidates is:

$$\gamma \triangleq \mathrm{CRC}[\mathcal{G}_1\alpha\mathcal{G}_2] \oplus \mathrm{CRC}[\mathcal{G}_1\beta\mathcal{G}_2] = \mathrm{CRC}[(\alpha\oplus\beta), 0^{|\mathcal{G}_2|}]$$

where $0^n$ represents a sequence of $n$ bytes, each of value 0. Expressed as a polynomial (once more over *bits*), this difference is:

$$\gamma(x) = \sum_{j=0}^{7} \left[(\alpha_j \oplus \beta_j) x^{8|\mathcal{G}_2|+j+d} \bmod P(x)\right] \bmod P(x).$$

Note that $\delta_k(x) \triangleq x^{k+d} \bmod P(x)$ can be computed from its predecessor, as $(x\delta_{k-1}(x)) \bmod P(x)$. This turns out to be a trivial computation in the bit-string representation:

$$\delta_k = \mathrm{LeftShift}[\delta_{k-1}] \oplus \mathrm{CRC}\,[\mathrm{MSB}(\delta_{k-1})]$$

where MSB represents the most significant bit, and the LeftShift operation shifts the bit string one position to the left, dropping the MSB from the left and bringing in a zero bit on the right. Since $|G_2|$ increases by one at each successive trial, $\gamma$ can be computed quickly, and in turn so can $\mathrm{CRC}[\mathcal{G}_1\beta\mathcal{G}_2] = \mathrm{CRC}[\mathcal{G}_1\alpha\mathcal{G}_2]\oplus\gamma$. The computation of $\gamma$ may also be performed efficiently on bytes rather than bits, using shifts, exclusive-ORs, and a 256-element table of the CRC's of all byte values.

Rather remarkably, the generic disinfection algorithm can use a related trick to reconstruct programs infected with a limited class of *overwriting* viruses: viruses that replace some of the host with the virus to keep the host's length unchanged [6].

*Generic disinfection performance* The generic disinfection heuristic has an extremely low false positive rate. Since its incorporation into IBM AntiVirus in 1994, there have been no confirmed reports of a false positive. The false negative rate is also extremely low. In laboratory experiments, it caught over 99% of all non-overwriting virus infections. The proportion of viruses that overwrite their hosts is about 15%, but none of these are known to spread successfully because they are too harmful to go undetected for long. Thus in practice generic disinfection is extraordinarily effective. Of course, there is one important drawback: generic disinfection can only catch viruses in programs that have been seen in their uninfected state. But if a file-infecting virus spreads appreciably on a machine, the generic disinfection algorithm will almost certainly catch it.

*Classifier* A second method for detecting previously unknown viruses, the virus classifier, does not require prior knowledge of an uninfected version of a program. A classifier's function is to identify an object as either viral or non-viral; a classifier is constructed through a *training* procedure that takes as input a collection of known viruses and a collection of known non-viruses. The classification learning problem is hard in general and in this particular application; here the classification also needs to be accurate and robust.

Classifiers base their decisions on the presence or absence of various *features*, in this case short byte sequences common to several viruses. Candidate features are found using suffix arrays, a standard data structure for text algorithms [10]. The classifier itself is a simple hyperplane separator: the number of times each feature string occurs in a sample is tallied; the tallies are multiplied by weights and added together; and the sample is considered likely to be viral if the sum exceeds a threshold. The selection of features from the thousands of strings that occur repeatedly, and the determination of the feature weights, are particularly knotty problems: standard methods result in hopeless overtraining and abyssmal performance on non-training data. The techniques we used to overcome these obstacles will be described in a future publication, and have two patents pending.

The file-infector classifier contains roughly 1000 5-byte features. To elude virus scanners, some viruses use a simple form of encryption, taking the exclusive-OR of their own machine code with a repeated one- or two-byte key.

To catch them, the features we use are not direct machine-code fragments, but transformations that are invariant with respect to such encryption. In particular, the 5-byte feature derived from the 7-byte fragment $\langle b_1\, b_2\, b_3\, b_4\, b_5\, b_6\, b_7\rangle$ is its second-order exclusive-OR difference, $\langle b_1 \oplus b_3, b_2 \oplus b_4, b_3 \oplus b_5, b_4 \oplus b_6, b_5 \oplus b_7\rangle$. A file is classified by computing its invariant, tallying the number of times each feature occurs in the invariant, and computing a thresholded, weighted sum of the feature tallies.

Initial tests indicate that the classifier can detect roughly 85% of viruses on which it was not trained. However, with comprehensive false-positive tests still pending, we expect that to eliminate some false positives we will also have to reduce the detection rate somewhat. Still, by combining the generic disinfection and virus classification techniques, we believe that IBM AntiVirus will be able to detect approximately 99% of all new file infectors that actually spread in the wild.

**Boot-sector infectors.** A classifier for boot-sector infectors has also been implemented; in fact it came first. The boot-sector classifier [2] was trained separately on a corpus of several hundred legitimate and viral boot sectors.

This classifier uses roughly 30 three- and four-byte plaintext fragments. Although they were derived purely mechanically, the fragments turn out to be semantically meaningful bits of code. Many of them appear among a set of generic boot-sector signatures that had been hand-crafted by a human expert.

The boot-sector classifier's false-positive rate is quite low, but a few false positives have occurred. All have ultimately been attributed to special boot sectors that offer enhanced security for PC's, and that do several things that are virus-like. Since the "neural net" boot virus detector was first deployed in IBM AntiVirus in 1994, it has caught roughly 75% of all new boot sector viruses. Recent improvements include using an emulator to identify any additional relevant sectors, and decrypt them if necessary, prior to examination by the classifier. The improvements already made are believed to have increased the detection rate to roughly 90%, and further gains are expected.

**Macro viruses.** Currently, many new macro viruses are just simple variants of known ones. Consequently, fuzzy detection using simple signatures is sufficient to catch roughly two thirds of all new macro viruses. We are developing other techniques, including a classifier trained specifically on macro viruses, that are expected to bring the detection rate up to the high levels attained for file-infectors and boot-infectors. Rigorous false-positive testing is still required before the trade-off between minimizing false negatives and minimizing false positives can be tuned appropriately.

### 3.2 Capturing and transmitting virus samples

Whenever a heuristic identifies a potential virus, a sample is captured and compressed. Information about the type of virus, the version of the anti-virus program, etc., are included with the sample data, and the result is encrypted. The infected client PC then sends the encrypted sample to an administrative PC via a secure protocol that authenticates that the sample was generated by a legitimate version of IBM AntiVirus.

The administrator is given the opportunity to review the sample to ensure that it does not contain proprietary or sensitive data or code. Alternatively, the administrator may choose to configure the system to send samples outside the corporate firewall automatically. In either case, in the planned commercial version of the immune system, the sample is sent over the Internet to a concentrator located outside both the corporate and IBM firewalls, where other such samples from other administrative domains are collected. Another computer pulls the samples through the IBM firewall, and yet another through a final firewall and into the immune system laboratory.

There the sample is analyzed by the adaptive immune system, which is faced with the task of developing a specific response: means for detecting, verifying and removing all instances of the virus.

### 3.3 Deriving a prescription: the adaptive immune system

The adaptive component of the computer immune system can be viewed as an analog to the antibodies, B-cells, T-cells, and other elements of the adaptive biological immune system. In the current implementation, it does *not* reside on the client PC, for reasons of performance (the algorithms are CPU- and memory-intensive), convenience (we can focus development efforts on a single platform) and security (the algorithms require a database of infected files).[1]

When a sample is received, the address of the sender is recorded, and the sample and information pertaining to it and the environment in which it was found are uncompressed and decrypted. The sample is checked against the most current copy of the signature file because it is possible that the PC on which the virus was captured had a slightly out-of-date signature file. This step is particularly important for a rapidly spreading virus, about which many independent reports could be sent to the virus analyzer at nearly the same time. If the virus is known, the relevant anti-virus data can be sent back to the originally infected PC immediately. Otherwise, information about the type

[1] Eventually, it could be advantageous to decentralize virus analysis, even to the point of having the innate and adaptive immune systems together on each PC. This would be truer to the biological analogy, but more importantly it could be helpful for different computers to use different signatures to detect the same virus. For an interesting treatment of the virtues of diversity in computer systems, see Forrest et al. [11].

of virus is used to set up an appropriate environment for creating samples, or to route the sample to a machine where the appropriate environment can be found. So, file and boot virus samples are sent to an emulator (or to a real machine running the appropriate platform), Microsoft Word macro viruses to a WindowsNT environment running both Office 95 and Office 97,[2] etc.

Once the sample has been placed in an appropriate environment, it is encouraged to create additional samples of itself. If this succeeds, further analysis isolates code portions of the virus, which are useful for signature extraction and other purposes. Then, an "autosequence" procedure uses pattern matching to extract the virus's method of attachment and its basic structure. From this, a prescription for verifying and removing the virus is derived, and a virus signature is extracted. Finally, the virus data are tested, and integrated with data files that contain complete information for all known viruses. The resultant update is sent to the afflicted PC.

For the majority of viruses, the entire procedure takes less than two minutes from beginning to end on a dual 200MHz Pentium Pro PC running the Windows NT operating system. The remainder of this section treats its steps in greater detail.

**Replication.** The virus sample is placed in the appropriate environment and it is lured to infect a diverse suite of "decoy" or "goat" programs. For binary file infectors, there are several dozen .COM and .EXE-format decoys; for boot infectors, a few floppy and hard disk images; and for macro viruses, several documents or spreadsheets. Some viruses infect an object only when it is used, so the immune system executes, reads, writes to, copies, opens, and otherwise manipulates them.

Other viruses actively seek objects to infect, so decoys are placed where the most commonly used programs are typically located. For binary file infectors, this includes the root directory, the current directory, and other directories in the path. The next time the infected file is run, it is likely to select one of the decoys as its victim.

Periodically, each of the decoys is examined to see if it has been modified. If so, it is almost certain that an unknown virus is loose in the system, and that each of the modified decoys contains a sample. These virus samples are stored in such a way that they will not be executed accidentally.

Since viruses can be particular about the conditions under which they replicate, the decoys are run under several different environmental settings if necessary. The date may be changed a few times, as may the operating system version and other parameters. This helps to increase the chances of replication, and also helps expose differences in viral progeny that depend upon such parameters.

---

[2] Microsoft changed the underlying macro language used in their Office application suite between these versions. However, the new language (VBA5) is backwards compatible and the viruses must be replicated on both platforms.

**Behavioral analysis.** For file and boot infectors, sample creation occurs in an emulated environment. The emulator produces a detailed log of system behavior. After the sample creation phase, the log is analyzed by an expert system that has been programmed with rules allowing it to determine various aspects of the virus's behavior [12,13]. For example, for file infectors the expert system is able to produce information about the types of executables the virus can infect, whether or not the virus "goes resident", and the conditions under which it infects its victims (e.g. the victim was just opened, closed, executed, etc.). Ultimately this information will be automatically incorporated into a "help" file describing the virus to customers and virus experts.

Replicating the virus in an emulated environment has the advantage of giving us data on the virus's behaviour, allowing us to automate the task, and keeping the virus isolated from the rest of the system while it is active. The disadvantage is the near-impossibility of performing high-quality PC emulation. Currently our emulator only runs code compatible with an 80386 in real mode. As a backup, we have another, hardware-based solution, but it is slower and has not yet been integrated into the automated system.

Macro viruses are replicated in an analogous manner. In the case of Word for Windows macro viruses, Word is placed in an armoured Windows NT environment. Word is driven by a script that loads the virus and attempts to infect various "decoy" or "goat" documents. After the virus has run, results are collected and the environment is restored.

**Code/data segregation.** Both the autosequencing and automatic signature extraction steps, to follow, need to know which portions of the virus are code and which are data. For file and boot infectors, we use an 80386 chip emulator that has been modified so that, when a conditional branch is encountered, *all* paths are taken. When the emulation is complete, portions of the virus that were executed as code are so identified, and the rest is tagged as data.

**Autosequencing.** Given several pairs of uninfected and infected decoy programs — generated in the sample creation phase — we use pattern-matching algorithms to extract a description of the virus's structure and of how it attaches itself to any host [14,15].

Pattern matching is first done within each ⟨uninfected, infected⟩ file pair to determine the viral portions (strings occurring only in the infected file) and their locations. Then, the viral portions extracted from all the pairs are compared to identify patterns that are constant across all instances. (The comparison takes into account simple forms of encryption, as before.) Finally, an effort is made to locate portions of the original file that may have been sequestered within one of the variable regions of the virus. A simple example of the output from this stage is depicted in figure 1.

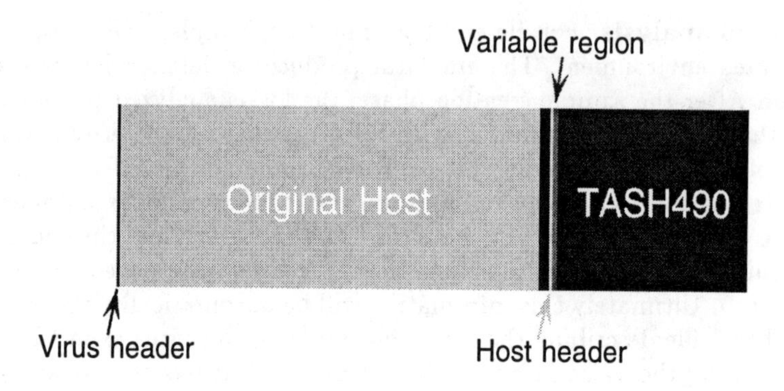


**Fig. 1.** Pictorial representation of attachment pattern and structure of the TASH490 virus, derived completely automatically

This "autosequencing" analysis provides several useful items of information:

1. The locations of all the pieces of the original host within an infected file, independent of the content and length of the host. This information is automatically converted into the repair language used by IBM AntiVirus.
2. The locations and structures of all components of the virus. Structural information includes the contents of regions of the virus that are observed to be invariant across different samples, and which have been classified as code in the code/data segregation step. This information has two purposes:
   (a) It is automatically converted into the verification language used by IBM AntiVirus.
   (b) It is passed to the automatic signature extraction component for further processing.

**Automatic signature extraction.** From among the byte sequences produced by the autosequencing step, the signature extractor must select a virus signature carefully to avoid both false negatives and false positives. That is, the signature must be found in every instance of the virus, and must almost never occur in uninfected programs.

First, consider the false negative problem. The samples captured by the decoys may not represent the full range of variable appearance of which the virus is capable. As a general rule, non-executable "data" portions of programs, which can include representations of numerical constants, character strings, and work areas for computations, are inherently more variable than are "code" portions, which represent machine instructions. To be conservative, "data" areas are excluded from consideration as possible signatures. Byte sequences that are both "invariant" according to the autosequencer, and "code" according to the code/data segregator, are the ideal input to the signature extractor.

The signature extractor is thus left with the problem of minimizing false positives. In the biological immune system, false positives that accidentally recognize self cause auto-immune diseases. In both traditional anti-virus software and the computer immune system, false positives are annoying to customers, and so infuriating to vendors of falsely-accused software that at least one lawsuit against a major anti-virus software vendor has resulted.

Briefly, the automatic signature extractor examines each subsequence of $S$ contiguous bytes (referred to as "candidate signatures") within its input. and estimates the probability for that $S$-byte sequence to be found among normal, uninfected "self" programs. Typically, $S$ is chosen to be between 16 and 24. The probability estimate is made by forming a list of all sequences of $\leq 5$ bytes in the input data; tallying their frequencies in a corpus of roughly 20,000 ordinary, uninfected programs comprising a gigabyte of data; and using simple formulas based on a Markov model to combine the frequencies into a probability estimate that each candidate signature will be found in a set of programs statistically similar to the corpus. The signature with the lowest estimated false-positive probability is selected.

Characterizations of this method show that the probability estimates are poor on an absolute scale because code tends to be correlated on a scale longer than 5 bytes. However, the relative ordering of candidate signatures is good, so the method generally selects one of the best possible signatures [16]. The signature extractor has been used for several years now to generate signatures used by IBM AntiVirus. Judging from the relatively low false-positive rate of the signatures (compared with those of other anti-virus software), the algorithm's ability to select good signatures is *better* than can be achieved by typical human experts.

**Testing and integration.** The extracted signature is tested by verifying that it detects all the samples of the virus (including the original sample), and that it generates no false positives on the corpus of uninfected programs. The removal prescription is tested on each infected decoy to ensure that it produces a functionally equivalent version of the corresponding original decoy. Optionally, the sample creation step can be re-done with a fresh set of decoys, and both the signature and the removal information can be tested on them as well. If the anti-virus data pass the test, they are automatically integrated with the complete data file containing information for all known viruses.

### 3.4 Delivering the prescription

Finally, the data file update is sent back to the client from which the virus sample was received. In the current prototype, the update is sent directly to the client machine. In the commercial version, it will retrace the path by which it received: it will be pushed through the immune system laboratory firewall, pushed through the IBM firewall to the concentrator, pulled through the client company's firewall to its administrative machine, and finally delivered to the afflicted PC.

### 3.5 Disseminating the prescription

Having received the prescription, the administrator will (automatically) disseminate the cure to all machines that might need it, including the one on which the virus was originally found.

In the current prototype and in the planned commercial release, each PC runs IBM AntiVirus in the background upon receiving the update. All copies of the virus lurking in the system are detected, and the user is given the option to disinfect.

In the commercial version, the master virus data files in the immune system laboratory would also be mirrored at the "antivirus online" web site, `www.av.ibm.com`. Thus subscribers all over the world would be protected against new viruses soon after their discovery, provided that they download the updates frequently.

## 4 Evaluation and Final Remarks

Now we return to the criteria set forth in section 2, reproduced here in italics, and discuss the extent to which the immune system described in section 3 meets each of them.

- **Innate immunity.** *The system must be capable of detecting the presence of a high proportion of viruses that are unknown to it specifically. The system should recognize previously unknown viruses of all types; currently, this would include file infectors, boot-sector infectors, and macro viruses. It is particularly important that the system be geared towards detecting viruses that are found in real incidents. For example, less emphasis need be placed on detecting overwriting viruses, since these are never prevalent.*
  The discovery rate is roughly 99% for file infectors and 90% for boot-sector infectors. The figure for file infectors is averaged over non-overwriting viruses, which we feel is legitimate because overwriters have never successfully spread in the wild. Currently, the discovery rate is an unacceptably low 65% for macro viruses, but several techniques under development are expected to boost the discovery rate to at least 90% by the time the pilot is launched later this year.

- **Adaptive immunity.** *The system must be capable of automatically deriving from a single sample a "prescription" for detecting and, if possible, removing all instances of the virus.*
The adaptive immune system prototype can usually produce an adequate supply of samples from a single sample of a file infector or a macro virus. (Less emphasis has been placed on boot-sector replication since such viruses are much less likely to take advantage of the Internet to spread quickly; still, this is not ideal.) In cases where samples are produced, a signature can be extracted in almost every case, even for encrypted viruses. For file infectors, automatic extraction of repair information can be tricky, and the success rate is lower than for signature extraction. For macro viruses, the success rate for extraction of both signatures and repair information is extremely high.
- **Delivery and dissemination.** *The system must deliver the prescription to the afflicted computer, and must also facilitate dissemination of the prescription to other machines both in its neighborhood and around the world.*
In the prototype, the prescription is delivered directly from the adaptive immune system to the afflicted PC. In the commercial version still being imlemented, the prescription is delivered to the afflicted PC and disseminated in its locale by the administrative component of IBM AntiVirus, and made available to the rest of the world via updates downloadable from `www.av.ibm.com`.
- **Speed.** *The system must be capable of deriving and disseminating prescriptions on a time scale faster than the virus can spread. Currently, a reasonable goal is to derive and deliver a prescription to the originally afflicted machine in less than ten minutes from when an anomaly is first detected, and to permit dissemination of the prescription to neighboring machines within less than half an hour. The system should be capable of protecting anyone from any newly discovered virus within a day at most. These requirements will become even stricter as technology permits computer viruses to spread faster.*
The immune system prototype easily satisfies the speed requirements. Once the sample is received, it typically takes less than two minutes to derive a full prescription for detecting and removing a file infecting virus, and roughly five minutes for a macro virus. Even if one allows a few minutes for the sample to be delivered via the network to IBM and for the prescription to be delivered over the network from IBM, the criterion for rapid delivery should be met comfortably. Dissemination of the prescription to other machines in the vicinity of the one that discovered the virus will be achieved by simple extensions to the existing IBM AntiVirus administrative software, which permits administrators to update hundreds or thousands of IBM AntiVirus clients within an administrative domain. Even by conservative estimates, it would take less than half an hour to send updates to, say, 1000 clients. Finally, by incorporating the prescrip-

tion into the IBM AntiVirus data files and making them available from the web, a very large number of customers can be protected from the new virus within hours of its first discovery.

- **Scalability.**
  - **Analysis.** *If a new, particular virulent virus begins to spread quickly, many machines at one site and/or at different sites may experience the virus simultaneously. The system must be capable of very high throughput, handling at least thousands of simultaneous requests for virus analysis.*
    The commercial pilot will be able to handle a limited number of multiple requests simultaneously. A proprietary design, slated for incorporation into the full commercial version of the immune system next year, will be able to handle a high volume of simultaneous requests.
  - **Updates.** *The system must be able to update tens of millions of PCs on at least a daily basis.*
    A large number of customers may download up-to-the-minute updates from the Web, enabling them to be protected very soon after a new virus is discovered.
- **Safety and reliability.** *The prescription produced by the immune system must be sufficiently reliable that it can be deployed worldwide without being checked by humans. Preferably the false positive rate should be at least as low and the removal information at least as accurate as is typically achieved by expert humans.*
  Tests suggest that the automatic signature extraction algorithm selects signatures that are less prone to false positives than those chosen by human experts [16]. The removal information extracted by the autosequence algorithm tends to be of high quality. This, coupled with the fact that IBM AntiVirus verifies the exact identity of a virus prior to removing it from a host program, means that botched repairs based an automatically generated prescription are very rare. Certainly, the rate is very much lower than the figure of 10% we have measured for a competing anti-virus product that presumably uses prescriptions derived by human experts!
- **Security.** *Virus samples must be protected in such a way that they cannot be intercepted and read by a third party while in transit. Even more importantly, appropriate measures must be taken to ensure that any prescriptions employed by a client machine are uncorrupted, genuine copies of those produced by the immune system.*
  Standard secure protocols are included in the design of the immune system. Encryption is used to ensure that virus samples cannot be intercepted by a third party, and digital signatures used to verify the origin of virus samples, anti-virus prescriptions, and updates.
- **Customer control.** *Customers must be able to control the conditions under which virus samples and other information are sent out of their enterprise. They must likewise be able to control the conditions under*

*which prescriptions are received and disseminated to the originally infected client and possibly other machines. Some customers may want manual control in one or both directions, others may want the speed given by completely automated response.*
Especially when the immune system is first made available commercially, administrators may wish to review the virus samples that are sent to IBM for automatic analysis to ensure that confidential material is not inadvertently included. Manual throttling of the flow of samples to IBM will always be an option, but as mechanisms that reduce such concerns are developed and implemented, administrators may permit the samples to be sent automatically. Likewise, manual control over the delivery of the prescription to the afflicted PC and other machines on the network must always remain an option, but we anticipate that with time it will become increasingly common to let updates occur automatically with no intervention from the administrator.

In summary, the existing prototype meets many but not all of the criteria. As we ready ourselves for the first commercial pilot in 1997, our primary emphases include implementing and testing our algorithms for boosting the detection rate of new macro viruses, finishing the implementation of the communication protocols between the IBM AntiVirus administrative and client components, and completing implementation of the network software that transfers virus samples and anti-virus prescriptions between IBM and the IBM AntiVirus Administrator program.

The IBM immune system is the product of several years of automation efforts. So far, six U.S. patents relating to it and its components have been granted [17,18,15,6,7,19].

**Acknowledgments**

The authors thank their many colleagues at IBM's High Integrity Computing Laboratory, particularly Bill Arnold, Dave Chess, and Ed Pring, for numerous discussions about automatic virus analysis and the design of the immune system. Bill Arnold and Dave Chess invented the idea of using decoy programs. John Evanson, Riad Souissi, Bill Schneider, Frederic Perriot, Jean-Michel Boulay, Hooman Vassef, and August Petrillo contributed to the development of the adaptive immune system, and Alexandre Morin and Gerald Tesauro made major contributions to the virus classifier.

## References

1. J.O. Kephart. A biologically inspired immune system for computers, in R. A. Brooks and P. Maes, eds., *Artificial Life IV. Proc. of the 4th International Workshop on the Synthesis and Simulation of Living Systems,* 130–139. MIT Press 1994.

2. J.O. Kephart et al. Biologically inspired defenses against computer viruses, *Proceedings of IJCAI '95*, 985–996, Montreal, August 19–25, 1995.
3. C.A. Janeway, Jr. How the immune system recognizes invaders. *Scientific American*, 269(3):72–79, September 1993.
4. P. Marrack and J.W. Kappler. How the immune system recognizes the body. *Scientific American*, 269(3):81–89, September 1993.
5. Paul, William E., ed. *Immunology: Recognition and Response... Readings from Scientific American.* New York: W.H. Freeman and Company, 1991.
6. J.O. Kephart and G.B. Sorkin. Generic disinfection of programs infected with a computer virus. U.S. Patent 5,613,002; March 1997.
7. J.O. Kephart, G.B. Sorkin and G.J. Tesauro. Adaptive statistical regression and classification of computational bit strings ... U.S. Patent (to be issued); allowed March 1997.
8. D. Bertsekas and R. Gallager. Data Networks, Prentice-Hall, Inc., Englewood Cliffs, New Jersey, 1987.
9. R.M. Karp and M.O. Rabin. Efficient randomized pattern-matching algorithms. *IBM Journal of Research and Development*, 31:249–260, 1987.
10. M. Crochemore and W. Rytter. Text Algorithms, Oxford University Press, New York, 1994.
11. S. Forrest, A. Somayaji, and D.H. Ackley. Building Diverse Computer Systems. In *Proceedings of 6th Workshop on Hot Topics in Operating Systems*, 67–72, IEEE Computer Society Press, Los Alamitos, CA, 1997.
12. M. Swimmer. Dynamic detection and classification of computer viruses using general behavior patterns. In *Proceedings of the Fifth International Virus Bulletin Conference*, 75–88. Virus Bulletin Ltd., 1995.
13. M. Swimmer. Fortschrittliche Virus–Analyse — Die Benutzung von statischer und dynamischer Programm–Analyse zur Bestimmung von Virus–Charakteristika. Master's Thesis, Fachbereich Informatik, Universitaet Hamburg, May 1995.
14. W.C. Arnold and G.B. Sorkin. Automated analysis of computer viruses. In *Proceedings of the Sixth International Virus Bulletin Conference*, 149–159. Virus Bulletin Ltd., 1996.
15. D.M. Chess, J.O. Kephart and G.B. Sorkin. Automatic analysis of a computer virus's structure and means of attachment to its hosts. U.S. Patent 5,485,575; September 1995.
16. J.O. Kephart and W.C. Arnold. Automatic extraction of computer virus signatures. In *Proceedings of the Fourth International Virus Bulletin Conference*, 179–194. Virus Bulletin Ltd., 1994.
17. W.C. Arnold, D.M. Chess, J.O. Kephart, and S.R. White. Automatic immune system for computers and computer networks. U.S. Patent 5,440,723, August 1995.

18. J.O. Kephart. Method and apparatus for evaluating and extracting signatures of computer viruses and other undesirable software entities. U.S. Patent 5,452,442; September 1995.
19. W.C. Arnold, D.M. Chess, J.O. Kephart, G.B. Sorkin and S.R. White. Searching for patterns in encrypted data. U.S. Patent 5,442,699. August 1995.

# An Anomaly Detection Algorithm Inspired by the Immune System

Dipankar Dasgupta[1] and Stephanie Forrest[2]

[1] Department of Mathematical Sciences
The University of Memphis
Memphis, TN 38152, USA.
[2] Department of Computer Science
The University of New Mexico
Albuquerque, NM 87131.

**Abstract.** Detecting anomaly in a system or a process behavior is very important in many real-world applications such as manufacturing, monitoring, signal processing etc. This chapter presents an anomaly detection algorithm inspired by the negative-selection mechanism of the immune system, which discriminates between *self* and *other*. Here self is defined to be *normal data patterns* and non-self is any deviation exceeding an allowable variation. Experiments with this anomaly detection algorithm are reported for two data sets - time series data, generated using the Mackey-Glass equation and a simulated signal. Compared to existing methods, this method has the advantage of not requiring prior knowledge about all possible failure modes of the monitored system. Results are reported to display the performance of the detection algorithm.

## 1 Introduction

The normal behavior of a system is often characterized by a series of observations indexed in time. The problem of detecting anomalies can be viewed as finding non permitted deviations of a characteristic property in the system of interest. The detection of anomaly is an important task in many diagnostic or dynamical systems. In safety-critical applications, it is essential to detect the occurrence of unnatural events as quickly as possible before any significant performance degradation results. This can be done by continuous monitoring of the system for changes from the normal behavior patterns. For example, drilling or high speed milling processes require continuous monitoring to assure quality production; machines such as jet engines require continuous monitoring to assure safe operation.

There have been several techniques suggested in the literature for detecting anomalies and faults in monitored systems. These include control charts [21], model-based methods [15], knowledge-based expert systems [13], pattern recognition and clustering [25], hidden markov models [23], and neural networks [16]. Recently, neural network-based methods have been increasingly used for anomaly detection [2,18]. Two different neural network approaches have received the most attention - Multi-Layer Perceptrons (MLP)[20] and Adaptive Resonance Theory (ART) [14][22].

However, most existing methods require either prior knowledge about various anomaly conditions [16] or precise theoretical models of the monitored system. But a robust method should detect any unacceptable (unseen) change rather than looking for specific known novel activity patterns. This chapter investigates a new anomaly detection method that addresses some of these deficiencies. In the next section, the basic detection algorithm based on an immune system model is described. The application of the model for anomaly detection is discussed in section 3, which include the data preprocessing and the implementation details of generating a detector set for monitoring. Section 4 reports the experimental results and the performance of the proposed detection algorithm with different control parameters. Conclusions are given in section 5.

## 2 A Negative Selection Algorithm

This approach is inspired by the information-processing properties of natural immune system. Animal immune systems are capable of distinguishing virtually any foreign cell or molecule from the body's own cells - this is known as the self-nonself discrimination problem [19]. In the immune system, T cells have receptors on their surface that can detect foreign proteins (antigens). During the generation of T cells, receptors are made by a pseudo-random genetic rearrangement process. Then they undergo a censoring process, called negative selection, in the *thymus* where T cells that react against self-proteins are destroyed, so only those that do not bind to self-proteins are allowed to leave the thymus. This complex censoring process is very important in self-nonself discrimination. The artificial immune system [12] is an abstract of the complex chemistry of antibody/antigen recognition in natural immune systems. The basic principle of the negative selection algorithm is as follows:

- Define *Self* as a normal pattern of activity or stable behavior of a system/process which needs to be monitored. In particular, we build up a database of normal behavior of each process of interest, then logically split the pattern sequence to represent as a multiset $S$ of equal-size strings of length $l$ over a finite alphabet.
- Generate a set $R$ of *detectors*, each of which fails to match any string in $S$. We use a partial matching rule, in which two strings match if and only if they are identical at at least $r$ contiguous positions, where $r$ is a suitably chosen parameter (as described in [12]).

- Monitor new observations (of $S$) for changes by continually matching the detectors against the representative of $S$. If any detector ever matches, a change (or deviation) must have occurred in system behavior .

In the original description of the algorithm [12], candidate detectors are generated *randomly* and then tested (censored) to see if they match any of the self string. If a match is found, the candidate is rejected. This process is repeated until a desired number of detectors are generated. A probabilistic analysis is used to estimate the number of detectors that are required to provide a given level of reliability. The major limitation of the random generation approach appears to be computational difficulty of generating valid detectors, which grows exponentially with the size of self. Also for many choices of $l$ and $r$, and compositions of self, the random generation of strings for detectors may be prohibitive.

In this work, detector sets are generated using an improved algorithm which runs in linear time with respect to the size of self [10]. The algorithm has two phases. First it employs a dynamic programming technique to count recurrences in order to define an enumeration of all unmatched strings (i.e. all feasible detectors). Second, a random subset of this enumeration is chosen to generate a detector set. In other words, given a collection of self strings $S$ and matching threshold $r$, the first phase of the algorithm determines the total number of unmatched strings that exists for the defined self ($S$); then in the second phase, some of them are selected to generate a diverse set of detectors for monitoring data patterns (representative of the *self*).

## 3 Anomaly Detection

In this implementation, the anomaly detection problem is reduced to the problem of detecting whether or not a string has changed (actually matched using negative selection), where a change (or match) implies a shift in the normal behavior patterns.

### 3.1 Data Preprocessing

Preprocessing can be viewed as constructing an alternative representation in an attempt to capture the semantics of the data while preserving the information content. Furthermore, any change that exceeds allowable variation in the data pattern should ideally be reflected in the representation space . This can be a problem when perhaps very small changes in real-valued data need to be monitored. To handle this, an encoding method is used that maps close real-valued data into a discrete form. An analog value is first normalized with respect to a defined fixed range to determine the interval in which it belongs, and then the interval is encoded into binary form. However, if the value falls outside range ($MIN, MAX$), it will encode to all 0's or all 1's depending on which side of the range it crossed. Accordingly, if each datum item is encoded by $m$ binary digits (which may be chosen according to the desired precision), then there would be $2^m - 2$ different intervals between the maximum ($MAX$) and minimum ($MIN$) ranges of data. Each interval size, $d$ is then quantized as $(MAX - MIN)/(2^m - 2)$. Thus, an analog value $x$, $MIN \leq x \leq MAX$, where $MAX = MIN + (2^m - 2).d$ in magnitude can be quantized (within an absolute error of magnitude $d$) to an interval and encoded to the binary form according to the interval number it belongs to. For example, if the magnitude of $x$ is such that $MIN + n_a.d \leq x \leq MIN + (n_a + 1).d$, then it encodes to binary string corresponding to the interval number, $n_a$ (where $n_a$ can vary from 1 to $2^m - 2$).

### 3.2 Implementation Details

In our current implementation, analog data is sampled from a moving time window and each data value in the window is encoded in binary using the above mentioned coding scheme. Each window, therefore, is a sequence of data items. A historical database is then constructed from a succession of windows sliding along the time series to capture the semantics (regularities) of the normal behavior of the system. The number of such windows needed for the normal database will depend on how much inherent variability there is in the monitored process. So, as long as the time series data pattern maintains similar behavior, collected strings should be sufficient to define normal behavior of the system. This collection of strings for windows is the self ($S$). Then strings are generated that do not match any of the strings in $S$ to become member of the detector set using the negative selection algorithm discussed above. The generation of detectors in this detection algorithm is time-consuming and therefore, usually performed off-line, as in the case of neural networks training for anomaly detection or developing rules for anomaly-detecting expert-systems. Overall, the approach can be summarized as follows:

1. Collect time series (sensor) data sufficient to exhibit the normal behavior of a system (these may be raw data at each time step, or average values over a longer time interval).
2. Examine the database to determine the range of variation ($MAX, MIN$ values) of data and choose the data encoding parameter ($m$) according to the desired precision.
3. Encode each value in binary form using the above coding scheme.
4. Consider a suitable window size to capture the semantics in data pattern.
5. Slide the window along the time series and store the encoded string for each window as "self" for processing by the negative selection algorithm.
6. Generate a set of detectors that do not match any of the self strings according to the partial matching rule with suitably chosen $r$. It is desirable

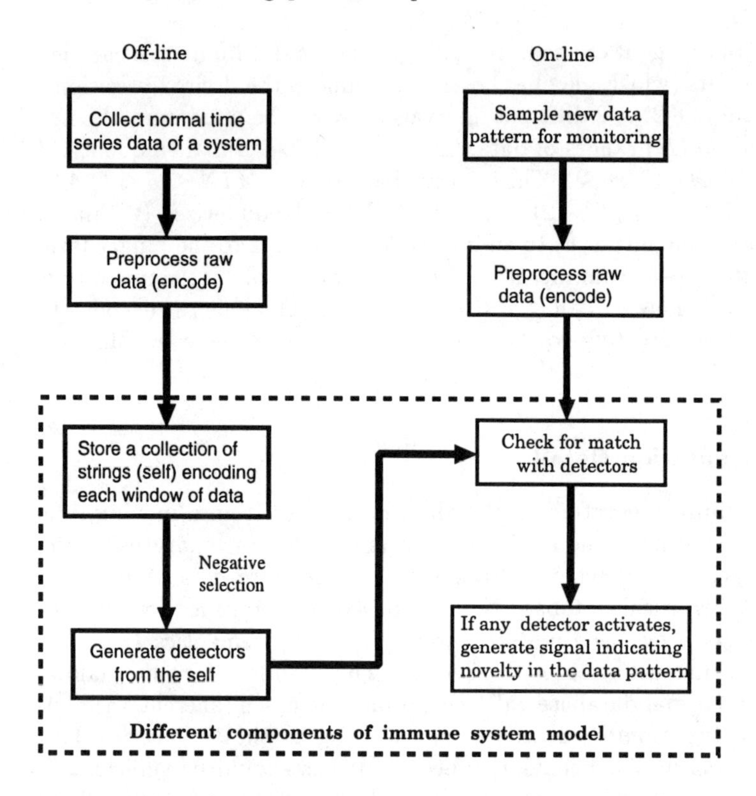


**Fig. 1.** Schematic diagram showing the processing stages of the immunity-based anomaly detection system

that the detectors are spread enough to cover the unmatched string (non-self) space. Also an estimate for the size of the detector set is needed to ensure a certain level of reliability in detecting changes [12].

7. Once a unique set of detectors is generated from the normal database , it can detect (probabilistically) any change (or abnormality) in patterns of unseen time series data.
8. When monitoring the system, we used the same preprocessing parameters as before to encode new data patterns. If a detector is ever activated (matched with current pattern), a change in behavior pattern is known to have occurred and an alarm signal is generated regarding the abnormality. The same matching rule is adopted (for monitoring the system) as was used in generating detectors.

Basic parameters controlling preprocessing are:

BITS_PER_DATA ($m$) — this will dictate the degree of numerical precision with which real numbers are represented in binary form. For example, 5-bit data encoding gives 30 intervals into which the range [MIN, MAX] of data is divided.

WINDOW_SIZE ($w$) — the number of samples encoded in a single pattern (each string in self).

SHIFT — the number of samples by which one pattern is shifted from the previous one in a moving window. For example, if SHIFT = 1 with a window size $w$, the patterns will be $\{x_1, x_2, ..., x_w\}$, $\{x_2, x_3, ..., x_{(w+1)}\}$ .... etc.

# 4 Experiments

Dasgupta and Forrest [7,9] experimented with several data sets to investigate the performance of the negative selection algorithm for detecting anomaly. These include Mackey Glass series, simulated cutting tool dynamics in a milling process, and some sensory data. In this chapter, two of these examples are reported — Mackey-Glass series and a simulated data series (figure 5), where signals of varying amplitude are observed under normal behavior .

In the first example, time series is generated using the Mackey-Glass series [11][17], and perform some experiments to monitor the dynamics of the series in varying conditions. Two examples of the series are studied, one in which the change is relatively slight and supposedly harder to detect, and another in which a rather substantial change occurs.

The *Mackey-Glass equation* is a nonlinear delay-differential equation with dynamics that have been studied in many fields [17]. The equation is

$$\frac{dx}{dt} = \frac{ax(t-\tau)}{[1 + x^c(t-\tau)]} - bx(t)$$

The constants are generally taken [5] to be a = 0.2, b = 0.1 and c =10, and the delay parameter $\tau$ determines the complexity of the dynamic behavior displayed by the time series. In some cases, the equation was used as a task for short-term prediction based on previous samples presented [24]. In other cases, it has been used to detect changes in the value of $\tau$ [5][22], and that is the task we adapt.

The normal series is generated using $\tau = 30$, the slight anomaly is $\tau = 27$, and the substantial anomaly using $\tau$ =17 (as used in [5]). The series is generated by solving the differential equation numerically using a fourth-order Runga-Kutta method and considering a sample interval of 6 for each integration step. To eliminate the initial value effect of the series, 1000 observations starting from an initial value vector of 1.1 was run before considering the data for experiments. In these experiments, 2000 samples are taken for generating the self and different test databases (see figure 2).

In all experiments, we set $m = 5$ for binary encoding of data (i.e. the interval number it belongs to). Results of the experiments are shown in Tables 1 and 2. Two different window sizes were considered with various parameter settings in each case. In first set of experiments, self strings were generated using non-overlapping sliding windows, and in the second set, overlapping

**Table 1.** Detection of *slight changes* in Mackey-Glass series (figure 3) using the immune system model. Here $r$ is the matching threshold and $N_r$ is the number of detectors generated. Results are averaged over 50 runs, where the number of detections in successful runs (mean and standard deviation) and reliability of detection are shown in columns 4 and 5 respectively.

| Encoding parameters | $r$ | $N_r$ | Anomaly Detection Mean(Std. dev) | Anomaly Detection Success_rate |
|---|---|---|---|---|
| Win_size =4, Win_shift=4, Self_length, $l = 20$, Self_size, $N_s = 500$ | 9 | 30 | 11.34 (3.52) | 100% |
| | | 40 | 14.96 (3.78) | 100% |
| | | 50 | 16.99 (4.20) | 100% |
| | 10 | 30 | 4.78 (2.77) | 98% |
| | | 50 | 7.82 (3.16) | 100% |
| | | 70 | 11.48 (3.51) | 100% |
| Win_size =6, Win_shift=2, Self_length, $l = 30$, Self_size, $N_s = 998$ | 10 | 20 | 8.08 (3.30) | 100% |
| | | 30 | 12.12 (4.08) | 100% |
| | | 40 | 14.58 (4.82) | 100% |
| | 12 | 30 | 5.80 (2.70) | 96% |
| | | 50 | 9.38 (2.99) | 100% |
| | | 70 | 14.80 (4.82) | 100% |

**Table 2.** Results for *substantial* anomaly detection of Mackey-Glass time series (as in figure 4). Here $r$ is the matching threshold and $N_r$ is the number of detectors generated for monitoring novel patterns. Columns 4 and 5 give the success rate of detections in two different set of experiments (averaged over 50 runs). Column 4 shows the average detection of novel patterns in successful runs.

| Encoding parameters | $r$ | $N_r$ | Anomaly Detection Mean(Std. dev) | Anomaly Detection Success |
|---|---|---|---|---|
| Win_size =4, Win_shift=4, Self_length, $l = 20$, Self_size, $N_s = 500$ | 9 | 30 | 13.24 (2.86) | 100% |
| | | 40 | 18.35 (3.91) | 100% |
| | | 50 | 20.65 (4.36) | 100% |
| | 10 | 30 | 6.10 (2.83) | 98% |
| | | 50 | 9.62 (2.93) | 100% |
| | | 70 | 13.66 (3.87) | 100% |
| Win_size =6, Win_shift=2, Self_length, $l = 30$, Self_size, $N_s = 998$ | 10 | 20 | 8.34 (3.12) | 100% |
| | | 30 | 11.22 (4.10) | 100% |
| | | 40 | 15.98 (5.09) | 100% |
| | 12 | 30 | 6.84 (2.66) | 98% |
| | | 50 | 9.34 (4.65) | 100% |
| | | 70 | 15.24 (5.11) | 100% |

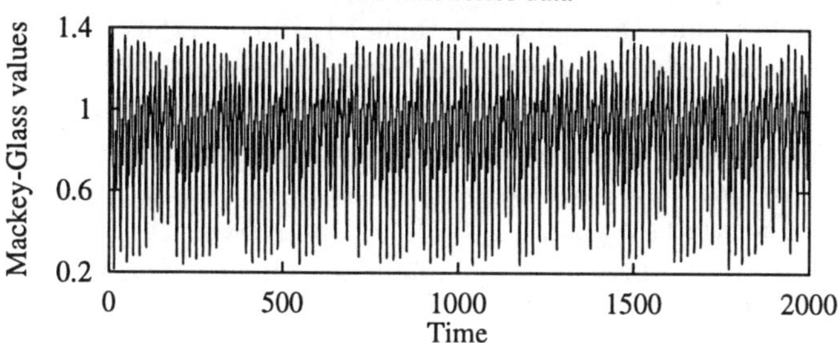


**Fig. 2.** Mackey-Glass time series data considered as normal pattern

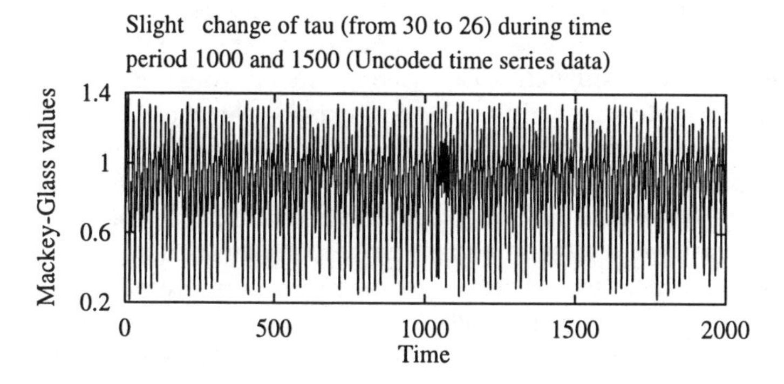


**Fig. 3.** Above example with slight changes in data pattern in a particular region

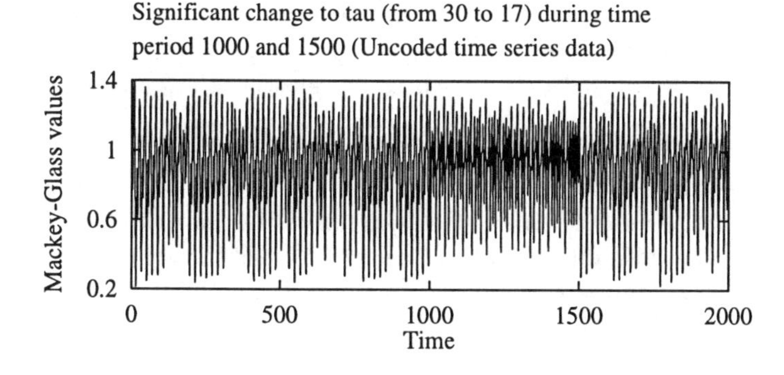


**Fig. 4.** Shows significant changes in data pattern

windows were used. A diverse set of detectors were generated in such a way that they do not match each other by $r$-contiguous bit rule.

It is observed that the algorithm could detect the anomalies in both cases. It noticed slight changes (Table 1) almost as efficiently as substantial changes (Table 2) in the data, since the number of changed strings in the encoded form are almost same in two cases (between time period 1000 and 1500). Strangely, the detection rates in the two cases are similar even though there are much more wide spread changes in the data in the latter case. This is because of the limitation of binary encoding, which does not map small and large changes proportionately (known as a Hamming cliff) in the representation space. To alleviate this limitation other encoding techniques such as gray, scatter code etc. need to be explored.

We next considered the second data series - a typical example found in many signal processing applications (figure 5), where signals of varying amplitude are observed under normal behavior. The data patterns, however, show regularities over a period of time. Detecting unknown changes (noise) in this signal pattern is a very difficult task, although monitoring such changes is essential in some applications. However, most existing threshold-based methods fail to detect small changes because of varying boundary conditions . We conducted experiments with similar parameter settings as in the previous example. Figure 6 shows a typical result demonstrating that the proposed algorithm can easily detect noisy signals by monitoring with a small set of detectors. In particular, we generated 20 detectors from initial data (data during 0 to 50 time steps are assumed as the normal pattern of signals). The detector set was then used to monitor future signal patterns (test signals), and it could detect changes during the time period 75 and 85. This suggests that the detection of gradual change can be monitored with a suitable detector set.

We observed that the performance of the algorithm varies with the choice of the matching threshold ($r$) for a defined string length ($l$) and encoding. With larger $r$, the generated detectors become sensitive to any anomaly in the data patterns, so more detectors are necessary to achieve a desired level of overall reliability. On the other hand, if $r$ is too small, it may not be possible to generate a reasonable size detector set from the available self, since there may not exist any unmatched strings (non-self) at that value of $r$. The choice of a suitable value is desirable for optimal performance of the algorithm. This suggests that the value of $r$ can be used to tune the reliability of detection against the risk of false positives.

### 4.1 Comparison with a Neural Network Approach

Further experiments were carried out for comparing the results with a neural network (in particular, ART1 [3,5]) using the same data set. An ART [4] is a self-organizing competitive learning ANN which can develop stable recognition codes in response to arbitrary sequences of input patterns.

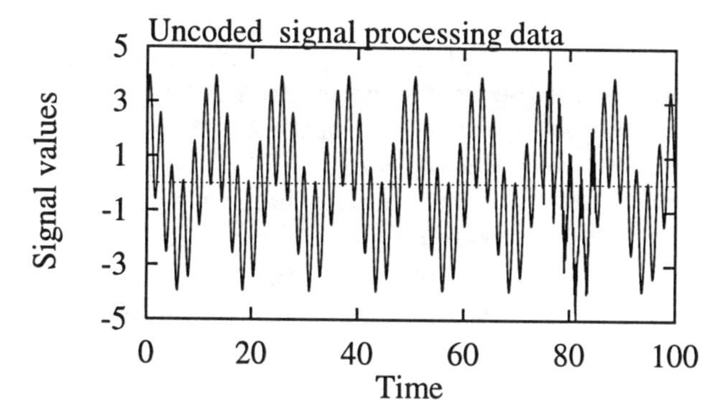


**Fig. 5.** An example of signal processing data series. Here the signals are noisy during the time period 75 and 85.

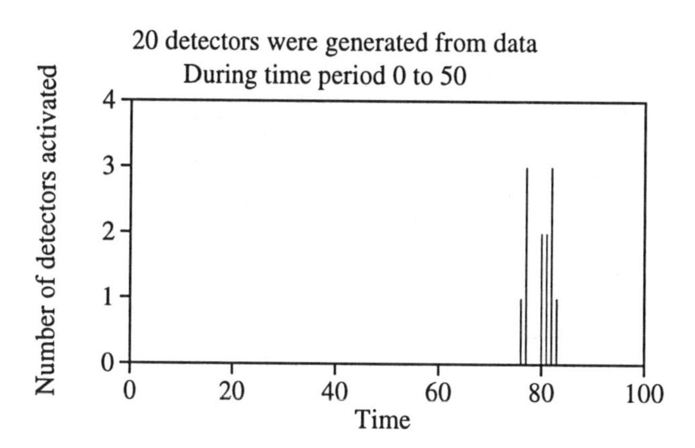


**Fig. 6.** The vertical lines indicate the activation of detectors indicating the changes in signal pattern. The detectors are only activated during the time period when signals get distorted as in figure 5.

The ART1 is the binary version of the family of ART networks. The ART architecture has two layers: the comparison layer and the recognition layer. The neurons in these layers interact with each other through bottom-up and top-down connections, which are modified to store binary information during the on-line learning phase. When an input pattern is presented, the ART network tries to classify it into one of the existing categories based on its similarity to the stored template of each category. A number of stable pattern templates or categories are created as the network completely learns the system behavior. However, when a totally different (or novel) pattern is presented, the network either updates one of the existing category or generate a new category according to the degree of novelity.

Figure 7 shows a sample result of these experiments which indicates the formation of templates and subsequent updating (recoding) of existing templates during the unsupervised learning phase of the ART network. The graph leveled off well within 40 time steps which exhibits that the network settles into a steady resonance state. However, during the time period between 75 and 85 there are generation of new templates and recoding of existing templates which indicate the anomaly in the signal pattern. Though the results qualitatively agree in both cases (ANN and AIS), further detail study and a careful quantitative comparison of two approaches is an important area of further research.

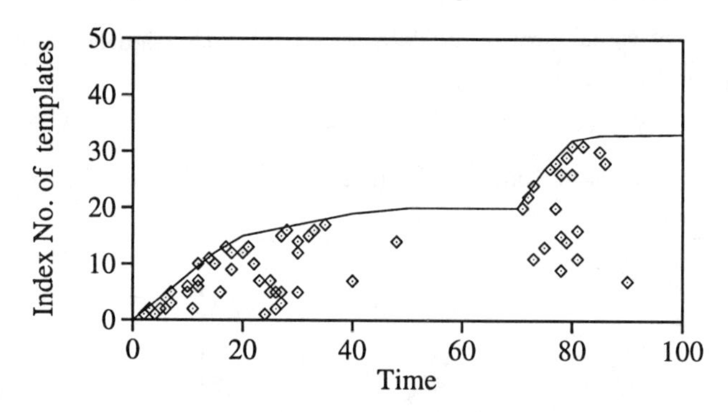


**Fig. 7.** The generation of new and recoding of existing templates (after the training phase) indicate anomaly in signal patterns

However, based on our initial experiments, the following similarities and differences between the negative selection algorithm [12] and the ART network have been observed on anomaly detection in time series data [6,7]:

- An ART network detects novel patterns deterministically, whereas in the immunological approach detection is probabilistic (particularly, the generation of detectors).
- The ART network tries to recognize/classify an input pattern in the space defined by the training data set (actual encoded space of data or signals), but on the contrary the anomaly detection algorithm based on the negative selection, recognizes patterns in the complement space as novel.
- ART network's (binary version, ART1) pattern recognition mechanism deals with Hamming space, but the current implementation of the negative selection approach uses an $r$-contiguous space matching rule.
- ART's vigilance threshold ($\rho$) provides a degree of sensitivity in discriminating input patterns, and forming clusters (or classes). A $\rho$ value near zero gives a network with low discrimination, and a value near one gives a network with high discrimination (forming many clusters). An optimal

vigilance value creates a reasonable number of clusters with minimum error. A similar effect is also noticed while choosing a matching threshold, $r$, in the negative selection algorithm.

- In an ART network, a cluster (or class) is represented in its neural memory as a template. A template is an abstraction of the patterns in a cluster which are formed and modified during the learning (training) process. So the number of templates increases (for a fixed parameter setting) according to the diversity in input patterns. In the negative selection algorithm, the effect of such diversity in data is opposite; also there is an indication that for an independent self (a training data set), the size of a detector set remains almost unchanged for a fixed probability of success (or failure) [12].
- An ART network learns the semantics of the time series on-line, and in principle, the rate of template formation reduces to zero when the learning is complete; but the negative selection algorithm detector generation is off-line, and largely depends on the normal time series (training) data and other parameters of the algorithm. However, it may be possible to produce detectors on-line using a different algorithm for generating detectors.
- During testing (or monitoring) new data patterns in an ART network, the existence of novel patterns is determined by examining the frequency and the degree of template formation and recoding. Activation of any detector (or a threshold number) determines the change in the behavior pattern of data in the implementation of the negative selection algorithm.
- Recognizing an input pattern is a global decision over the ART network (while determining the class memberships of object represented by the input patterns), whereas the recognition of a novel pattern by detectors in the negative selection algorithm is a decentralized local decision, which appears to be an important advantage over the ART methodology. This property results in generating a quick response to any changes, and may be very useful in monitoring safety-critical systems.

## 5 Conclusions

This chapter discussed a new approach for anomaly detection based on a negative selection algorithm inspired by the natural immune system. The objective of this work is to develop an efficient detection algorithm that can be used to alert an operator to any changes in steady-state characteristics of a monitored system. This approach collects knowledge about the normal behavior of a system from a historical data set, and generates a set of detectors that probabilistically notice any deviation from the normal behavior of the system. The detection system can be updated by generating a new set of detectors as the normal system behavior shifts due to aging, system modifications etc. Forrest et. al [12] showed that a small set of detectors can have a very high probability of noticing changes to the original data set. However, it is observed that generating an optimal set of detectors is critical to the success of this method.

The empirical results of this anomaly detection method are encouraging and the method appears to have significant advantages over other approaches. Since it does not look for any particular (or known) anomaly, it can detect any shift from the normal. In other words, this method does not examine new data patterns to look for an anomaly (fault) class, but indicates that these patterns are novel with respect to the normal data pattern. So this algorithm can be incorporated into other diagnostic tools for further classification. In most monitoring systems, the detection of a spurious change in data is not as important as the gradual change in the data pattern over a period of time, so our probabilistic detection algorithm appears to be a feasible alternative approach to such problems. Also it may be may be needed to choose a anomaly detection threshold in order to allow some instantaneous variations in new patterns from the established normal patterns while monitoring real sensor data.

There are a number of parameters which are tunable in both the preprocessing and the detector generation stage. In preprocessing stage, desired precision can be achieved while encoding similar analog data, and the window size may be suitably chosen to capture the semantic of the data patterns. Note that the system can be monitored using different time-scales simultaneously. Also instead of directly encoding the time series data, it may be necessary to transform data (e.g. by Fourier transform) depending on the properties of (sensor) data. In cases of multi-variate data series, the system can be monitored by a single set of detectors, constructing self string by concatenation of patterns of data (window) for each variable. A desired level of reliability can be achieved by changing the window size, matching threshold, and the number of detectors. Other matching rules and generation algorithms are the topics of further investigation.

The Mackey-Glass equation considered here as an example of time series data; other methodologies (in particular, ART networks) in anomaly detection also used similar example [5]. However, nonperiodic nature of the Mackey-Glass dynamics restricts its use for continuous monitoring test. There are many potential application areas in which this method may be useful. For example, in milling process, the tool breakage can be detected by monitoring the pattern characteristics of cutting forces [1] [8]. The remarkable detection abilities of animal immune systems suggest that the immunity-based systems are worth exploring in real-world applications. Future research will investigate various computational properties of the immune system, improvements to the existing detection algorithm, and exploring new application areas.

## Acknowledgements

This research was partly carried out by the first author at the University of New Mexico, Department of Computer Science, Albuquerque, NM 87131. The authors acknowledges many suggestions and comments from Patrik D'haeseleer, Derek Smith and Ron Hightower. The author also express his appreciation to Tom Caudell, and David Ackley. The second author received a grant from National Science Foundation (grant IRI-9157644).

## References

1. Y. Altintas and I. Yellowley. In-Process Detection of Tool Failure in Milling using Cutting Force Models. *Journal of Engineering for Industry*, 111, pp. 149–157, May 1989.
2. C. M. Bishop. Novelty detection and neural network validation. *IEE Proceedings - Vision, Image and Signal processing*, 141(4), pp. 217–222, August 1994.
3. G. A. Carpenter and S. Grossberg. A massively parallel architecture for a self-organizing neural pattern recognition machine. *Computer Vision, Graphics, and Image Processing*, 37, pp. 54–115, 1987.
4. G. A. Carpenter and S. Grossberg. *Competitive Learning: From Interactive Activation to Adaptive Resonance*, chapter 5, pages 213–250. MIT Press, Cambridge, 1987.
5. Thomas P. Caudell and David S. Newman. An Adaptive Resonance Architecture to Define Normality and Detect Novelties in Time Series and Databases. In *IEEE World Congress on Neural Networks*, pages IV166–176, Portland, Oregon, 3-7 July 1993.
6. Dipankar Dasgupta, Artificial Neural Networks and Artificial Immune Systems: Similarities and Differences. In the proceedings of the *IEEE International Conference on Systems, Man and Cybernetics*, Orlando, October 12-15, 1997.
7. Dipankar Dasgupta. Using Immunological Principles in Anomaly Detection. In *Proceedings of the Artificial Neural Networks in Engineering (ANNIE'96)*, St. Louis, USA, November 10-13 1996.
8. Dipankar Dasgupta and Stephanie Forrest. Tool breakage detection in milling operations using a negative-selection algorithm. Technical Report Technical Report No. CS95-5, Department of Computer Science, University of New Mexico, 1995.
9. Dipankar Dasgupta and Stephanie Forrest. Novelty detection in time series data using ideas from immunology. In *ISCA 5th International Conference on Intelligent Systems*, Reno, Nevada, June 19-21, 1996.

10. P. D'haeseleer, S. Forrest, and P. Helman. An immunological approach to change detection: algorithms, analysis, and implications. In *Proceedings of IEEE Symposium on Research in Security and Privacy*, Oakland, CA, May 1996.
11. J. Doyne Farmer. Chaotic Attractors of an Infinite-Dimensional Dynamical System. *Physica 4D*, pp. 366–393, 1982.
12. S. Forrest, A. S. Perelson, L. Allen, and R. Cherukuri. Self-Nonself Discrimination in a Computer. In *Proceedings of IEEE Symposium on Research in Security and Privacy*, pp. 202–212, Oakland, CA, 16-18 May, 1994.
13. Paul M. Frank. Fault Diagnosis in Dynamic Systems using Analytical and Knowledge-based Redundancy - A survey and some new results. *Automatica*, 26(3), pp. 459–474, 1990.
14. H. B. Hwarng and C. W. Chong. A Fast-Learning identification system for SPC: An Adaptive Resonance Theory approach. *Intelligent Engineering Systems Through Artificial Neural Networks*, 4, pp. 1097–1102, 13-16 November, 1994.
15. Rolf Isermann. Process Fault Detection based on Modeling and Estimation Method - A survey. *Automatica*, 20, pp. 387–404, 1984.
16. R. Kozma, M. Kitamura, M. Sakuma, and Y. Yokoyama. Anomaly Detection by neural network models and statistical time series analysis. In *Proceedings of IEEE International Conference on Neural Networks*, Orlando, Florida, June 27-29, 1994.
17. M. C. Mackey and L. Glass. Oscillation and Chaos in Physiological Control Sysyems. *Science*, 197, pp. 287–289, July 1977.
18. G. Martinelli and R. Perfetti. Generalized Cellular Neural Networks for Novelty Detection. *IEEE Transactions on circuits and systems-I: Fundamental theory and applications*, 41(2), pp. 187–190, February 1994.
19. J. K Percus, O. Percus, and A. S. Person. Predicting the size of the antibody combining region from consideration of efficient self/non-self discrimination. *Proceedings of the National Academy of Science*, 60, pp. 1691–1695, 1993.
20. S. Roberts and L. Tarassenko. A Probabilistic Resource Allocating Network for Novelty Detection. *Neural Computation*, 6, pp. 270–284, 1994.
21. W. A. Shewhart. *Economic Control of Quality of Manufactured Product*. 1931. Reprinted in 1980 by the American Society for Quality Control, pp. 304-318.
22. Scott D. G. Smith and Richard A. Escobedo. Engineering and Manufacturing Applications of ART-1 Neural Networks. In *Proceedings of IEEE International Conference on Neural Networks*, Orlando, Florida, June 27-29, 1994.
23. Padhraic Smyth. Hidden Markov Model for fault detection in dynamic system. *Pattern Recognition*, 27(1), pp. 149–164, 1994.
24. M. F. Tenorio and W. T. Lee. Self-Organizing Networks for Optimum Supervised Learning. *IEEE Transactions on Neural Networks*, 1(1), pp. 100–110, March 1990.

25. S. G. Tzafestas. *Fault Detection in Dynamic Systems, Theory and Applications*, chapter :System Fault Diagnosis Using the Knowledge-Based Methodology. Prentice Hall, 1989.

# Immunity-Based Management System for a Semiconductor Production Line*

Toyoo Fukuda[1], Kazuyuki Mori[2], and Makoto Tsukiyama[2]

[1] School of Policy Studies
Kwansei Gakuin University
2-1 Gakuen, Sanda, Hyogo 669-13
JAPAN

[2] Industrial Electronics & Systems Laboratory
Mitsubishi Electric Corporation
Amagasaki, Hyogo 661
JAPAN

**Abstract.** A production line of semiconductor is large scale and complex system. A control system of the line is considered to be difficult to control because there exist lots of malfunctions such as maintenance of equipment, equipment break down and unbalance of WIP to disturb production of wafers in the semiconductor production system.

We have been exploited some methods and systems using simulations or expert systems approach to solve these disturbances [2],[3],[4]. However, the semiconductor production systems had been large and complex and the environments of the systems have been changing dynamically, so that we could not exploit a perfect control system of semiconductor production by using only these methods.

This paper presents a method applying an artificial immunity based system described by multi agent nets to adapt itself to dynamical environment.

## 1 Introduction

A production line of semiconductor is large scale and complex system. It takes time and costs to fabricate the ultra high density LSI in a great amount of volume. A semiconductor line has the following characteristics; varieties of specification of products, changes of products in time, changes of fabricating machines, changes of demands of market and malfunctions of machines. It means that the production line is changing dynamically, so that the constant

* A short version of this paper was first published in the Proceedings of the IEEE International Conference on Systems, Man, and Cybernetics, pp 363-368, October 1997, Orlando, Florida.

operation is not expected. Conventional operation management of production is neither optimal nor realistic[2],[3].

The artificial immunity based system is an information processing model of the natural immune systems which play an important role to detect abnormality and protect themselves observed widely in the animals and human body. The key abilities found in the immune system which are beneficial to the engineering field are detecting self/non self, adaptation to the environmental changes, memory and distributed information processing[4].

By applying artificial immunity system, the dynamic adaptability for the operation management of semiconductor production line to many varieties of changes can be realized as follows. A virtual immune agent is defined on the operations management system. The roles of immune agent consist of three steps.

1. Sensing mode: The immune agent always monitors the status of system such as malfunction of machines, changes of demands, changes of process.
2. Decision mode: The agent decides whether the changes induces the operational change to be done or not with referring to the experienced changes by using genetic recombination.
3. Controlling mode: The agent produces the best solution against the systems changes.

The paper describes the information processing framework of the artificial immunity based system for the complex and large scale semiconductor production line with illustrative examples.

## 2 Problem of Semiconductor Production System

### 2.1 Characteristics of semiconductor production system

A semiconductor production system discussed here are very large and complex. The production of the LSI (memories, ASIC and MPU) is characterized by the repeated resorting to some process classes: cleaning, diffusion, photolithograph, etching, implantation and measuring process classes as shown in figure 1.

There are more than 200 of these operations to fabricate a wafer. WIP (Work In Process) including a lot of variety of products in the production line are over 1000 lots of wafer products[5].

### 2.2 Objectives of the semiconductor production

In the semiconductor production system, it is needed to keep to be high utilization of equipments and to minimize the cycle time of products and to meet the due date of all products. And also processing priorities and

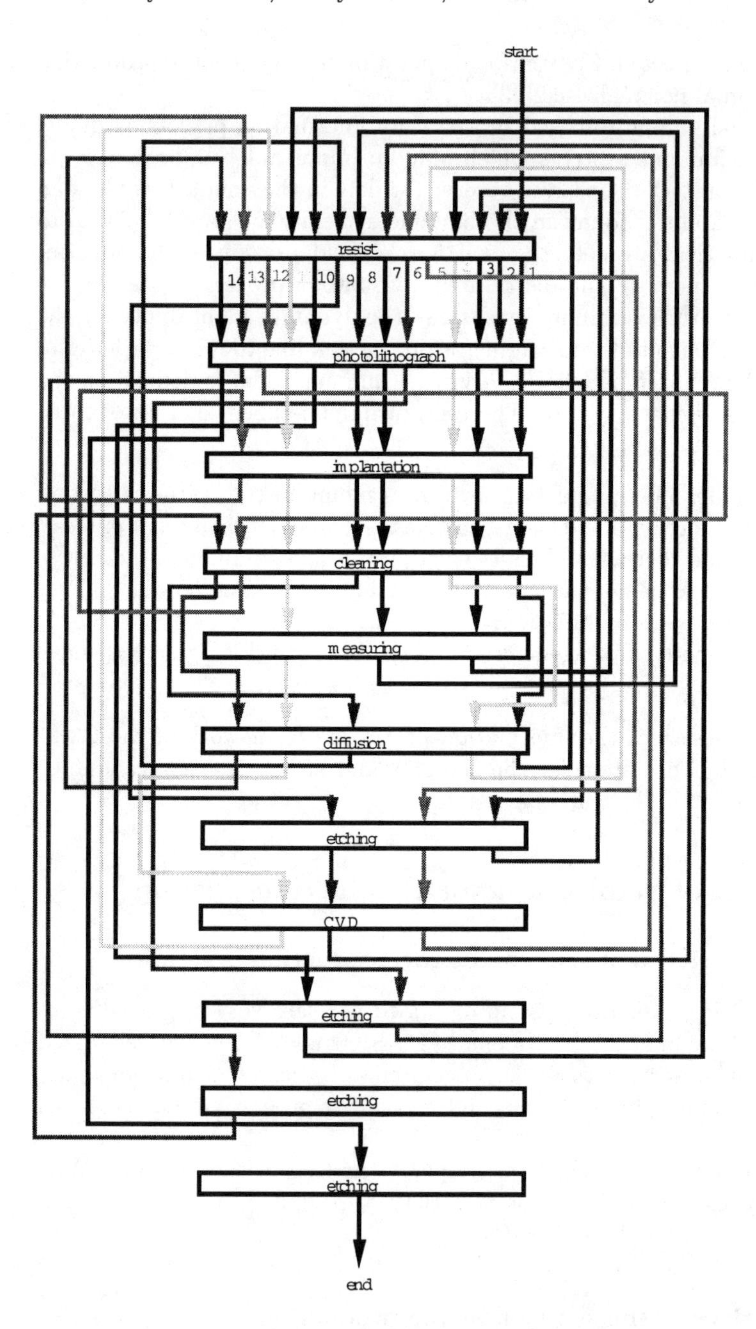


**Fig. 1.** A process flow of a semiconductor production

dispatching policies should be changed to adapt unanticipated events such as machine break down, adding engineering lots and low yields.

These objectives have trade-off relation each other. For example, though keeping high WIP become to be high utilization, the cycle time of the products becomes longer.

### 2.3 Problem

It is a difficult problem to make decision of optimal product mix size in the semiconductor production system and dispatching products under a unexpected situation. Because there exist lots of malfunctions such as maintenance of equipment, equipment break down and unbalance of WIP to disturb production of wafers in the semiconductor production system as mentioned before.

We have been exploited some methods and systems using simulations or expert systems approach to solve these disturbances [2],[3],[4]. However, the semiconductor production systems had been large and complex and the environments of the systems have been changing dynamically, so that we could not exploit a perfect control system of semiconductor production by using only these methods.

This paper proposes a method that dispatching agents which consist of some agents make dispatch to adjust the WIP or to minimize the product cycle time by agent interaction among a detector agent which indicates the malfunctions of the line, a specific mediator agent which identifies the detector agent and a specific inhibitor agent, and a restoration agent.

## 3 Immunity-Based System and Multi-Agent Nets

### 3.1 Definition of multi agent nets

We define some classes in the multi agent nets to represent immunity based agent systems. The multi agent net is of the colored petri net [6] extended by Kumagai [7] to represent an autonomous distributed system.

An agent net is an instance of its agent class. Each agent net represents an agent of the autonomous distributed systems. The autonomous distributed system is represented by a set of the agent nets.

Characteristics of the multi agent nets are as following below.

- Agent nets of the same class have the same structure and different identifier.
- The class of the agent net is identified by a color set.
- Tokens and agents are identified by a color set.
- Tokens have states and their state transition is specified by an agent net, except when a token indicates a simple or a combination of data.

It is easy to represent and analyze the autonomous distributed systems such as immunity based systems on account of above characteristics.

### 3.2 Implementation of the immunity based autonomous distributed systems by the multi agent nets

A production component of a semiconductor production line can be modeled by the petri nets.

Figure 2 shows a petri net model of an example line which is very simple, and consists of 3 processing operations and 3 equipments.

In this model, each place of $p7$, $p8$ and $p9$ corresponds to each buffer of processing operation represented by the transition $t5$, $t6$ and $t7$ respectively. Each token in place $p18$, $p19$ and $p20$ corresponds to each resource of equipment. For examples, the transition $t5$ can fire because each input place $p7$ and $p18$ of transition $t5$ has a token in figure 2.

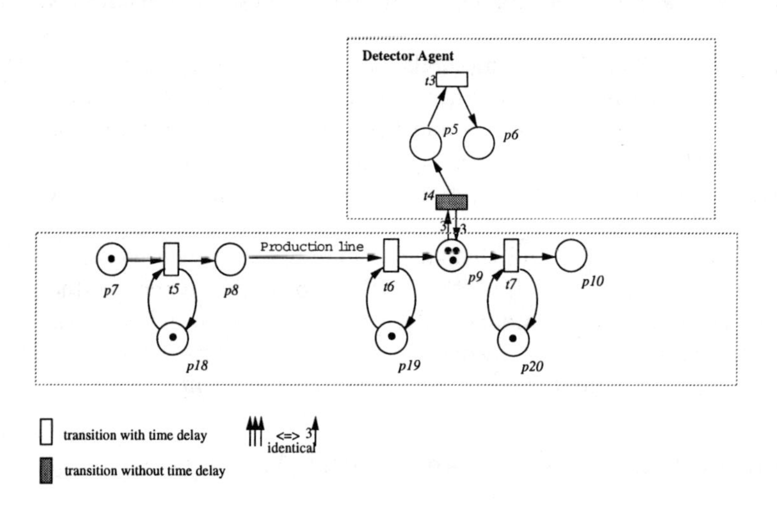


**Fig. 2.** An example of agents

The token in place $p7$ has specific color set. If the transition $t5$ can fire, then each token in input place $p7$ and $p18$ of the transition $t5$ is removed and new token occurs in output place $p8$ and $p18$ of the transition $t5$. The new token inherits the color of token removed in place $p7$, and is added new information which rule was applied. Figure 3 shows examples of color set of token.

For example the token 1 in this figure represents that rule r18, r19 and r20 was applied in firing transition $t5$, $t6$ and $t7$ respectively.

Overall of the semiconductor production line can be constructed in combination with the production components. Moreover, this basic model can extend an autonomous distributed system by adding detector agents, mediator agents, inhibitor agents and restoration agents as follows.

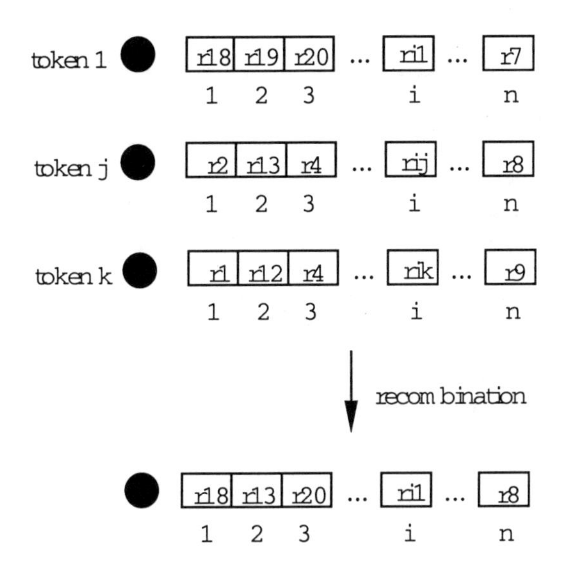


**Fig. 3.** An example of color set of tokens

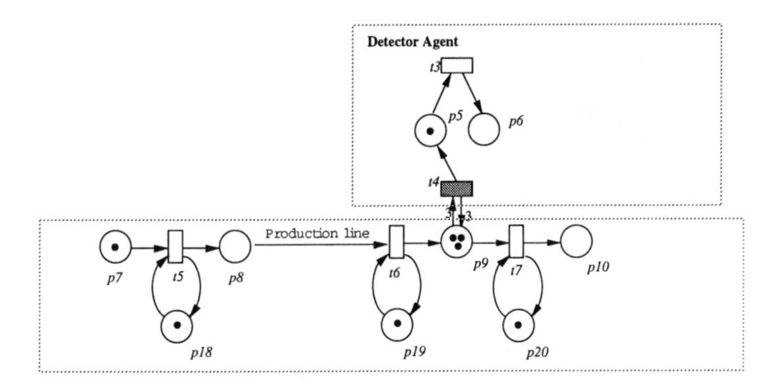


**Fig. 4.** An example of agents

**(1) Detector agent.** The detector agent corresponds to B cells having receptor for a specific antigen. The detector agents detect a specific malfunction which corresponds to the specific antigen. In figure 2, transition $t4$ can fire when sum of tokens in buffer place $p9$ is over 3. After firing the $t4$, a token which can indicate a malfunction, is added new color set generated by genetic recombination with color sets of three tokens and occurs in the place p5 in figure 4.

If there exists any mediator agent having a receptor place like $p15$ which can rendezvous with the place $p5$ indicating the malfunction as shown in figure 5, then the place $p15$ of the mediator agent rendezvous with the place $p5$ of the detector agent.

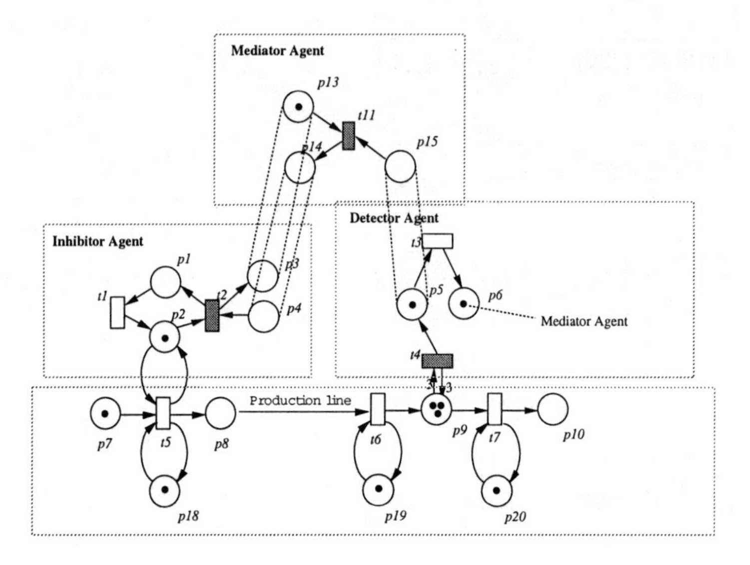


**Fig. 5.** An example of agents

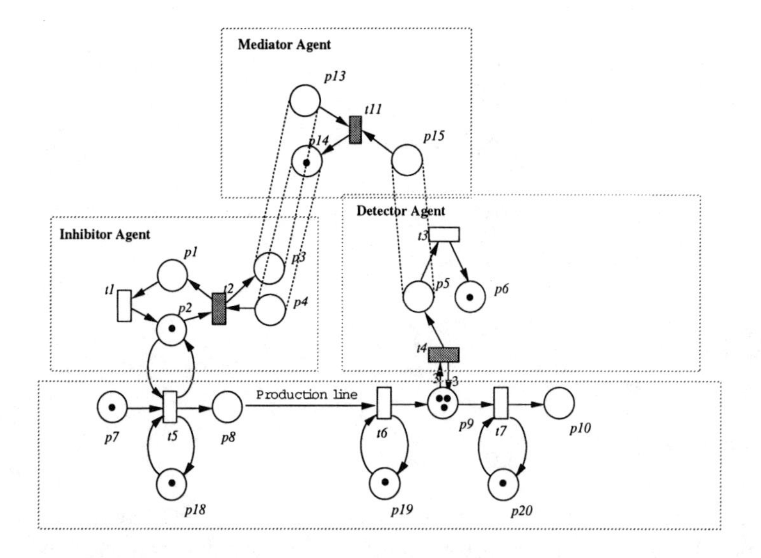


**Fig. 6.** An example of agents

If there exists no mediator agent having the specific place which can rendezvous with the place indicating the malfunction, new mediator agent can be created by firing transition $t3$.

**(2) Mediator agent.** The mediator agent corresponds to lymphokines secreted from T cells to activate B cells. The mediator agent can activate the

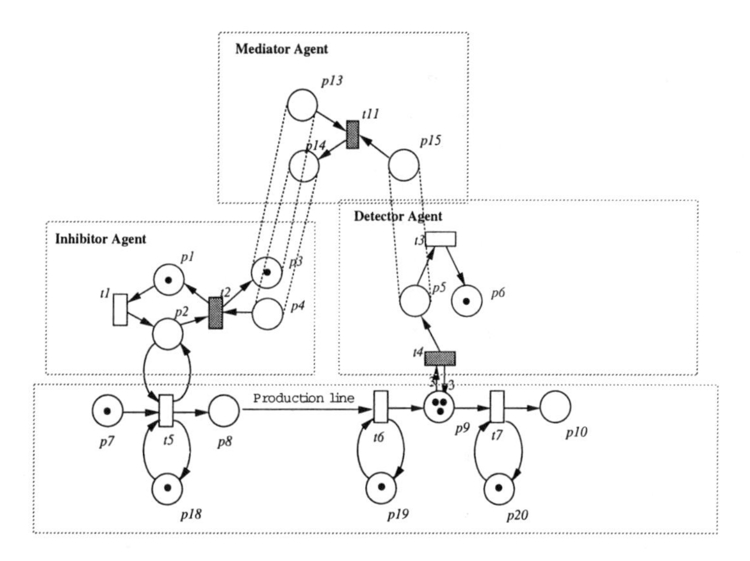


**Fig. 7.** An example of agents

inhibitor agent to inhibit firing specific transition. A mediator agent in the figure 5 can mediate the inhibitor agent and detector agent by fusion of place $p3$ and $p13$, fusion of the place $p4$ and $p14$, and fusion of place $p5$ and $p15$. Another type of mediator agent can restore the inhibition by inhibitor agent.

**(3) Inhibitor agent.** The inhibitor agent corresponds to B cell killing specific antigen. In figure 5, transition $t5$ can fire only when each place of $p2$, $p7$ and $p18$ has over one token. If there exists no token in the place $p2$, transition $t5$ cannot fire. The inhibitor agent can inhibit firing transition $t5$ by removing all tokens from place $p2$.

In an inhibitor agent as shown in figure 6, transition $t2$ can fire after fusion the place $p4$ and $p5$. By firing $t2$, each token in the place $p2$ and $p4$ removes form the place $p2$ and $p4$, then new token occurs to place $p1$ and $p3$ respectively as shown in figure 7.

In this condition, transition $t6$ which represents processing can not fire until tokens occur in the place $p2$ by firing transition $t1$.

**(4) Restoration agent.** The restoration agent corresponds to helper T cells. There is similarity between restoration agents and the detector agents to the effect that indicates the condition. The restoration agents indicate a malfunction which represents that there exists no lot processed in the related equipment. If there exists a token in the place $p1$ and $p11$ when there exists no token in place $p2$ as shown in figure 8, transition $t5$ can fire after following steps.

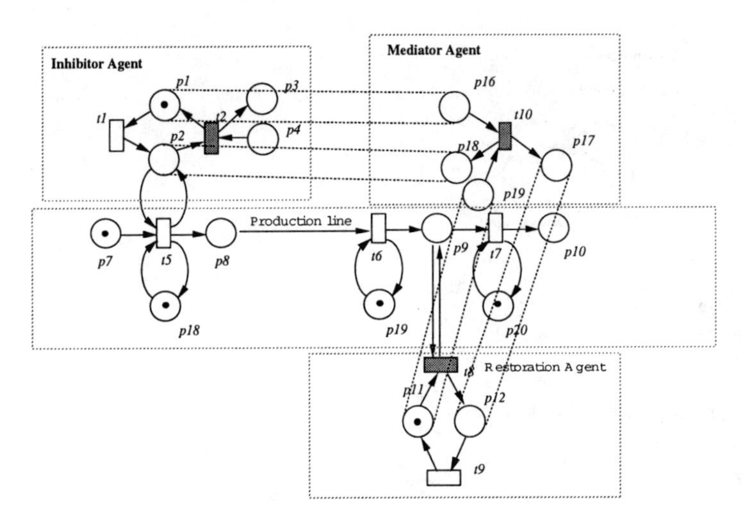


**Fig. 8.** An example of agents

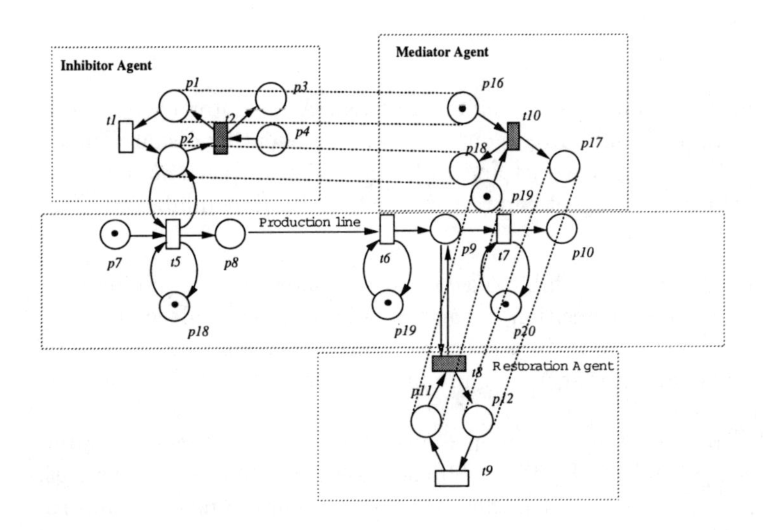


**Fig. 9.** An example of agents

First step is fusion of the place $p1$ and $p16$ and fusion of the place $p11$ and $p19$. After first step, the marking of the nets is shown in figure 9.

Second step is to fire transition $t10$. After firing the transition $t10$, each token in place $p16$ and $p19$ is removed, then new tokens occur in place $p17$ and $p18$ as shown in figure 10.

Third step is fusion of place $p18$ and $p2$ and fusion of place $p17$ and $p12$. After third step, the marking of the nets is shown in figure 11. In this marking, the transition $t5$ can fire.

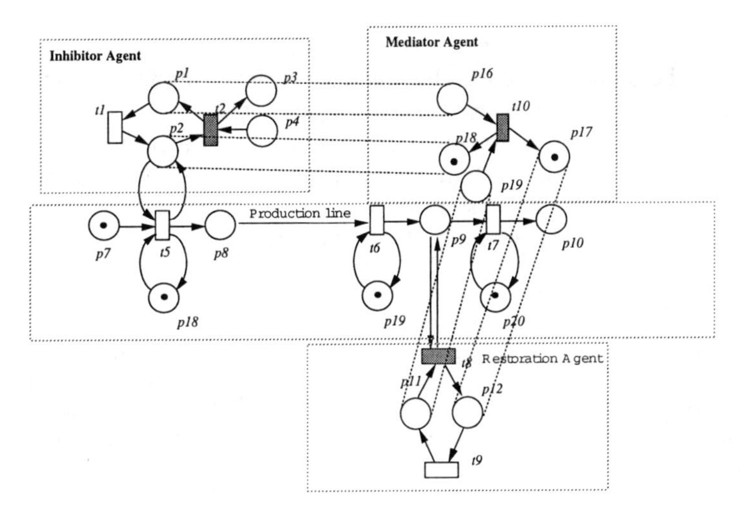


**Fig. 10.** An example of agents

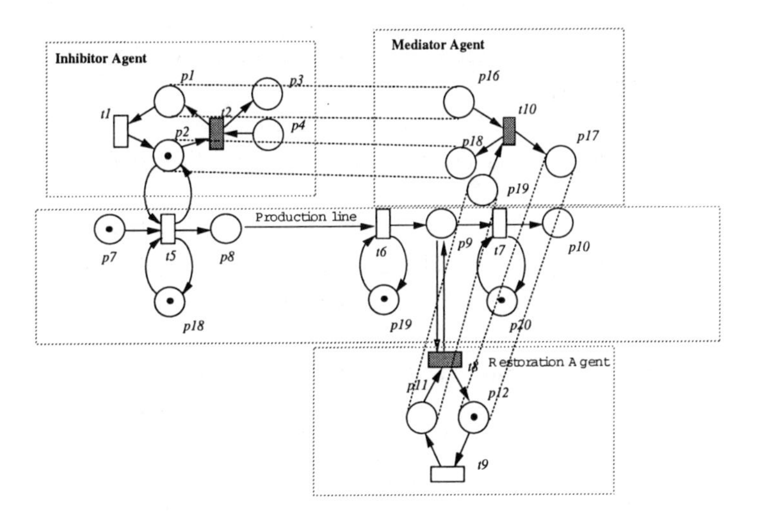


**Fig. 11.** An example of agents

# 4 Conclusion

The production line of semiconductor is large scale and complex system. The control system of the line is considered to be difficult to control, because there exist lots of malfunctions such as maintenance of equipment, equipment break down and unbalance of WIP to disturb production of wafers.

This paper proposed a framework of an autonomous distributed system for a semiconductor production control system, and defined some agents to represent the control system. The framework is an immunity based system which consists of the detector agents, the mediator agents, inhibitor agents and the restoration agents defined by the multi-agent nets.

The detector agents, the mediator agents, inhibitor agents and the restoration agents correspond to receptors, lymphokines, B cells killing specific antigen and helper T cells in immune system respectively.

Characteristics and advantages using the framework are as follows:

- decision making in real time
- tolerant to changing environment
- analysis of the autonomous distributed system using petri nets tools

However we have not made sure the effectiveness of the framework in practical systems. Future researches are to apply the framework to practical systems and verify the effectiveness.

## References

1. Tonegawa, S. (1983); Somatic generation of antibody diversity; *Nature*,Vol. 302 14 APRIL (pp.575-581).
2. D. V. Savell, R. A. Aerez and S. W. Koh (1989); Scheduling Semiconductor Wafer Production: An Expert System Implementation; *IEEE EXPERT*, FALL (pp.9-15).
3. M. Tsukiyama, K. Mori and T. Fukuda (1993); Strategic Level Interactive Scheduling and Operational Level Real-time Scheduling for Flexible Manufacturing Systems; *Applications of Artificial Intelligence in Engineering VIII*, Vol.2, Elsevier Applied Science (pp.615-625).
4. K. Mori, M. Tsukiyama and T. Fukuda (1994); Immune Algorithm and its Application to Factory Load Dispatching Planning; *1994 JAPAN-U.S.A. Symposium on Flexible Automation* (pp.1343-1346).
5. P. Castrucci (1995); The future fab: Changing the paradigm; *Solid State Technology*, January (pp.49-56).
6. K. Jensen (1992); *Coloured Petri Nets*, Vol.1, Springer-Verlag.
7. S. Kumagai and T. Miyamoto (1996); An Agent Net Approach To Autonomous Distributed Systems; *1996 IEEE Int. Conf. on Systems, Man, and Cybernetics* (pp.3204-3209).

# Appendix
# Indexed Bibliography

# An Indexed Bibliography of Artificial Immune Systems

(Books, Proceedings, Journal Articles, Ph.D Theses, and Technical Reports)

**Important Note**: The field of Artificial Immune Systems is too young to be well defined, and its scope and limitations sre unknown. So this bibliographic collection is neither complete nor very accurate. Some references are of synthetic approaches to understand and simulate the immune system, and others that develop computational methodologies inspired by the immune system to solve real-world problems. While this bibliography has been compiled with the utmost care, the editor takes no responsibility for any errors, missing information, the contents and quality of the references, nor for the usefulness and/or the consequences of applying the models or methodologies.

## References


1. F. Abbattista, G. Di Danto, G. Di Gioia and M. Fanelli. An associative memory based on the immune networks. In *Proceedings of the International Conference on Neural Networks*, 1996.
2. Hideyuki Aisu and Hiroyuki Mizutani. Immunity-based learning - Integration of distributed search and constraint relaxation. *Presented at ICMAS Workshop on Immunity-Based Systems*, December 10, 1996.
3. Pascal Ballet, Jacques Tisseau, and F. Harrouet A Multi-agent system to model an human humoral response. In the proceedings of *the 1997 IEEE International Conference on Systems, Man, and Cybernetics*, Orlando, Florida, October 13, 1997.
4. H. Bersini and V. Calenbuhr. Frustrated Chaos in Biological Networks. In *Journal of Theoretical Biology*, Vol. 188, No 2, pp. 187-200, 1996.
5. H. Bersini and V. Calenbuhr. Frustration Induced Chaos in a System of Coupled ODE's. In *Chaos, Soliton and Fractals*, Vol. 5, No 8, pp. 1533-1549, 1995.
6. H. Bersini and F. Varela. The Immune Learning Mechanisms: Recruitment Reinforcement and their applications. *In Computing with Biological Metaphors*, Chapman and Hall - R. Patton (Ed.), 1993.
7. H. Bersini and F. Varela. The Immune Recruitment Mechanism: A Selective Evolutionary Strategy. In *Proceedings of the 4th International Conference on Genetic Algorithms* - R. Belew and L. Booker (Eds.) - Morgan Kaufman - pp. 520-526, 1991.
8. H. Bersini and F. Varela. Hints for Adaptive Problem Solving Gleaned from Immune Network. In *Parallel Problem Solving from Nature*, H.P. Schwefel and H. M'hlenbein (Eds.), Publisher - Springer-Verlag, pp. 343 - 354, 1990.

9. V. Calenbuhr, F. Varela, and H. Bersini. Immune Idiotypic Network. In *International Journal of Bifurcation and Chaos*, Vol. 6 No 9, pp. 1691-1702, 1996.
10. V. Calenbuhr, H. Bersini, J. Stewart and F. Varela. Natural Tolerance in a Simple Immune Network. In *Journal of Theoretical Biology*, 177, pp. 199-213, 1995.
11. V. Calenbuhr, H. Bersini, F. J. Varela, and J. Stewart. The Impact of the Structure of the Connectivity Matrix on the Dynamics of a Simple Model for the Immune Network. In *Proceedings of the 1st Copenhagen Symposium on Computer Simulation in Biology*, Ecology and Medicine - Mosekilde, E. (Ed.), pp. 41 - 45, 1993.
12. J. Carneiro, J. Faro, A. Coutinho, and J. Stewart. A model of the immune network with B-T cell co-operation. I-Prototypical Structures and Dynamics. *J. Theor. Biol.* 182, 513, 1996.
13. J. Carneiro, A. Coutinho, and J. Stewart. A model of the immune network with B-T cell co-operation. II-The simulation of ontogenesis. *J. Theor. Biol.* 182, 531, 1996.
14. J. Carneiro. Towards a comprehensive view of the immune system. PhD Thesis. University of Porto. Portugal, 1997.
15. F. Celada and P. E. Seiden. Affinity maturation and hypermutation in a simulation of the humoral immune response. *Eur. J. Immunol.*, 26:1350–1358, 1996.
16. F. Celada and P. E. Seiden. Modeling Immune Cognition. In *proceedings of the IEEE International Conference on Systems, Man, and Cybernetics*, October 11-14, 1998.
17. Franco Celada and Philip E. Seiden. A computer model of cellular interactions in the immune system. *Immunology Today*, 13(2):56–62, 1992.
18. D. Chowdhury and D. Stauffer. Systamatics of the Models of Immune Response and Auto-Immune Disease. Journal of Statistical Physics (*Plenum*), vol.59, 1019, 1990.
19. D. Chowdhury, D. Stauffer and P.V. Choudary. A Unified Discrete Model of Immune Response. Journal of Theoretical Biology (*Academic Press*), vol.145, 207, 1990.
20. D. Chowdhury and B.K. Chakrabarti. Robustness of the Network Models of Immune Response. *Physica A* (*Elsevier*), vol.167, 635, 1990.
21. D. Chowdhury, M. Sahimi and D. Stauffer. A Discrete Model for Immune Surveillance, Tumor Immunity and Cancer. *Journal of Theoretical Biology* (*Academic Press*), vol.152, 263, 1991.
22. D. Chowdhury and D. Stauffer. Statistical Physics of Immune Networks. Physica A (*Elsevier*), vol.186, 61-81, 1992.
23. D. Chowdhury and D. Stauffer. Bursting of soap films. *Physica A* (*Elsevier*), vol.186, 237-249, 1992.

24. D. Chowdhury. A unified model of immune response II: continumm approach. *Journal of Theoretical Biology (Academic Press)*, vol.165, 135, 1993.
25. D. Chowdhury, J.K. Bhattacharjee and A. Bhattacharya. Dynamics of crumpling of fluid-like amphiphilic membranes. *Journal of Physics A (IOP, U.K.)*, vol.27, 257, 1994.
26. D. Chowdhury, V. Deshpande and D. Stauffer. Modelling immune network through cellular automata: a unified mechanism of immunological memory. *International Journal of Modern Physics C (World Sc.)*, vol. 5, 1049, 1994.
27. D. Chowdhury and D. Stauffer. Zellularautomaten in der Immunologie. (in German), *Magazin Fuer Computer Technik*, February 1991, page 204.
28. D. Chowdhury. Roles of intra-clonal and inter-clonal interactions in immunological memory: illustration with a toy model. Ind. J. Phys. 69B, 539, 1995.
29. Irun R. Cohen. The cognitive paradigm and the immunological homunculus. *Immunology Today*, 13(12):490–494, 1992.
30. I.R. Cohen. The cognitive principle challenges clonal selection. *Immunol. Today*, Vol. 13, pp. 441-444, 1992.
31. I.R. Cohen. A cognitive paradigm of the immune system. *Immunol. Today*, Vol. 13, pp. 490–494, 1992.
32. D. E. Cooke and J. E. Hunt. Recognising Promoter Sequences Using an Artificial Immune System. in Proc. Intelligent Systems in Molecular Biology (ISMB'95), Pub AAAI Press, pp 89-97, (1995).
33. J. Coutinho. Beyond clonal selection and network. Immunol. Rev. 110, 63, 1989.
34. Dipankar Dasgupta. An Artificial Immune System as a Multiagent Decision Support System. In *IEEE Int. Conf. on Systems, Man, and Cybernetics*, San Diego, 1998.
35. Dipankar Dasgupta. Artificial Neural Networks and Artificial Immune Systems: Similarities and Differences. In the proceedings of the *IEEE International Conference on Systems, Man and Cybernetics*, Orlando, October 12-15, 1997.
36. Dipankar Dasgupta and Nii Attoh-Okine. Immunity-based systems: A survey. In *Proceedings of the IEEE International Conference on Systems, Man, and Cybernetics*, pages 363–374, Orlando, Florida, October 12-15 1997.
37. Dipankar Dasgupta. Artificial Neural Networks Vs. Artificial Immune Systems. In the proceedings of the *Sixth International Conference on Intelligent Systems*, Boston, June 11-13, 1997.
38. Dipankar Dasgupta. A new Algorithm for Anomaly Detection in Time series Data. In *International Conference on Knowledge based Computer Systems* (KBCS-96), Bombay, India, December 16-18, 1996.
39. Dipankar Dasgupta. Using Immunological Principles in Anomaly Detection. In *Proceedings of the Artificial Neural Networks in Engineering* (ANNIE'96), St. Louis, USA, November 10-13 1996.

40. Dipankar Dasgupta and Stephanie Forrest. Novelty Detection in Time Series Data using Ideas from Immunology. In *ISCA 5th International Conference on Intelligent Systems*, Reno, Nevada, June 19- 21 1996.
41. Dipankar Dasgupta and Stephanie Forrest. Tool Breakage Detection in Milling Operations using a Negative-Selection Algorithm. Technical Report CS95-5, Department of Computer Science, University of New Mexico, 1995.
42. R. Deaton, M. Garzon, J. A. Rose, R. C. Murphy, S. E. Stevens, Jr and D. R. Franceschett. DNA Based Artificial Immune System for Self-Nonself Discrimination. In the proceedings of the 1997 IEEE International Conference on Systems, Man, and Cybernetics, Orlando, Florida, October 13, 1997.
43. R. J. DeBoer, P. Hogeweg, and A. S. Perelson. Growth and recruitment in the immune network. In A. S. Perelson and G. Weisbuch, editors, *Theoretical and Experimental Insights into Immunology*, pages 223–247. Springer-Verlag, Berlin, 1992.
44. R. J. DeBoer and A. S. Perelson. Size and connectivity as emergent properties of a developing immune network. *J. Theoret. Biol.*, 149:381–424, 1991.
45. R. J. DeBoer, L. A. Segel, and A. S. Perelson. Pattern formation in one and two dimensional shape space models of the immune system. *J. Theoret. Biol.*, 155:295–333, 1992.
46. J. H. B. De Monvel and O. C. Martin, Memory capacity in large idiotypic networks. Bull. Math. Biol. 57, 109, 1995.
47. V. Detours, B. Sulzer, and A. S. Perelson. Size and connectivity of the idiotypic network are independent of the discreteness of the affinity distribution. *J. Theoret. Biol.*, 183:409–416, 1996.
48. V. Detours, Modeles formels de la selection des cellules B et T. PhD Thesis, University Paris 6, France, 1996.
49. V. Detours, H. Bersini, J. Stewart and F. Varela, Development of an Idiotypic Network in Shape Space. In *Journal of Theoretical Biology* - 170, 1994.
50. P. D'haeseleer, S. Forrest, and P. Helman. An immunological approach to change detection: algorithms, analysis, and implications. In Proceedings of the 1996 *IEEE Symposium on Computer Security and Privacy*, IEEE Computer Society Press, Los Alamitos, CA, pp. 110-119, 1996.
51. P. D'haeseleer, S. Forrest, and P. Helman. A distributed approach to anomaly detection. Submitted to *ACM Transactions on Information System Security*, 1997.
52. Werner Dilger. Decentralized Autonomous Organization of the Intelligent Home According to the Principles of the Immunity System. In the proceedings of the 1997 *IEEE International Conference on Systems, Man, and Cybernetics*, Orlando, Florida, October 13, 1997.
53. J. D. Farmer. A rosetta stone for connectionism. *Physica D*, 42:153–187, 1990.
54. J. D. Farmer, N. H. Packard, and A. S. Perelson. The immune system, adaptation, and machine learning. *Physica D*, 22:187–204, 1986.

55. J. Faro and S. Velasco. Studies on a recent class of network models of the immune system. *J. Theor. Biol.* 164, 271, 1993.
56. M.A. Fishman and A.S. Perelson. Modeling T cell-antigen presenting cell interactions. *J. thoer. Biol.*, Vol. 160, pp. 311–342, 1993.
57. S. Forrest, A. Somayaji, and D. H. Ackley. Building diverse computer systems. In Proceedings of the *Sixth Workshop on Hot Topics in Operating Systems*, IEEE Computer Society Press, Los Alamitos, CA, pp. 67-72, 1997.
58. S. Forrest, S. Hofmeyr, and A. Somayaji. Computer Immunology. In *Communications of the ACM* Vol. 40, No. 10, pp. 88-96, 1997.
59. S. Forrest, B. Javornik, R. E. Smith and A. S. Perelson. Using genetic algorithms to explore pattern recognition in the immune system. In *Evolutionary Computation* 1:3, pp. 191-211, 1993.
60. S. Forrest, S. A. Hofmeyr, A. Somayaji, and T. A. Longstaff. A sense of self for Unix processes. In Proceedings of the 1996 *IEEE Symposium on Computer Security and Privacy*, IEEE Computer Society Press, Los Alamitos, CA, pp. 120-128, 1996.
61. S. Forrest, A. S. Perelson, L. Allen, and R. Cherukuri. Self-nonself discrimination in a computer. In Proceedings of the *IEEE Symposium on Research in Security and Privacy*, IEEE Computer Society Press, Los Alamitos, CA, pp. 202-212, 1994.
62. S. Forrest and A. S. Perelson. Genetic algorithms and the immune system. In H. Schwefel and R. Maenner (Eds.) *Parallel Problem Solving from Nature*, Springer-Verlag, Berlin (Lecture Notes in Computer Science), 1991.
63. Steven A. Frank. *The Design of Natural and Artificial Adaptive Systems.* Academic Press, New York, M. R. Rose and G. V. Lauder edition, 1996.
64. T. Fukuda, K. Mori and M. Tsukiyama. Immune Networks using Genetic Algorithm for Adaptive Production Scheduling. In *15th IFAC World Congress*, Vol.3, pp.57–60, 1993.
65. C. J. Gibert and T. W. Routen. Associative memory in an immune-based system. In *Proceedings of the 12th National Conference on Artificial Intelligence* (AAAI-94), pages 852–857, Seattle, July 31-August 4 1994.
66. P. Hajela and J. Lee. Constrained Genetic Search Via Schema Adaptation: An Immune Network Solution. *Structural Optimization*, Vol 12, No. 1, pp. 11-15, 1996.
67. P. Hajela, J. Yoo and J. Lee. GA Based Simulation of Immune Networks - Applications in Structural Optimization. *Journal of Engineering Optimization*, 1997.
68. E. Hart and P. Ross. Immune system for robust scheduling. *ICEC' 98.*
69. P. Helman and S. Forrest. An Efficient Algorithm for Generating Random Antibody Strings. Technical Report 94-07, University of New Mexico, Albuquerque, NM, 1994.

70. R. Hightower, S. Forrest, and A. S. Perelson. The evolution of cooperation in immune system gene libraries. Technical Report CS-92-20, University of New Mexico, Albuquerque, NM, 1992.
71. R. Hightower, S. Forrest, and A. S. Perelson. The evolution of emergent organization in immune system gene libraries. In L. J. Eshelman (Ed.) Proceedings of the Sixth International Conference on Genetic Algorithms, Morgan Kaufmann, San Francisco, CA, pp. 344–350, 1995.
72. R. Hightower, S. Forrest and A. S. Perelson. The Baldwin effect in the immune system: learning by somatic hypermutation. In R. K. Belew and M. Mitchell (Eds.) *Adaptive Individuals in Evolving Populations*, Addison-Wesley, Reading, MA, pp. 159-167, 1996.
73. Hirofumi Hirayama and Yuzo Fukuyama. Analysis of dynamical transition of immune reactions of idiotype network. Presented at ICMAS Workshop on Immunity-Based Systems held on December 10, 1996.
74. Hirofumi Hirayama and Yuzo Fukuyama. A Priority in Immune System — A Hypothetical Theoretical Study. Presented at ICMAS Workshop on Immunity-Based Systems held on December 10, 1996.
75. S. Hofmeyr, S. Forrest, and A. Somayaji. Lightweight intrusion detection for networked operating systems. In *Journal of Computer Security*, July, 1997.
76. Geoffrey W. Hoffmann. A neural network model based on the analogy with the immune system. *Journal of Theoretical Biology*, 122:33–67, 1986.
77. J. E. Hunt, C. M. King and D. E. Cooke, Immunizing against fraud. Proc. Knowledge Discovery and Data Mining, IEE Colloquium, October 1996.
78. J. E. Hunt and D. E. Cooke, Learning Using An Artificial Immune System. In *Journal of Network and Computer Applications: Special Issue on Intelligent Systems: Design and Application*, Vol. 19, pp. 189-212, 1996.
79. J. E. Hunt and A. Fellows. Introducing an Immune Response into a CBR system for Data Mining. In *BCS ESG'96 Conference and published as Research and Development in Expert Systems XIII*, 1996.
80. J. E. Hunt, D. E. Cooke and H. Holstein. Case memory and retrieval based on the Immune System. In the First International Conference on Case Based Reasoning, Published as Case-Based Reasoning Research and Development, Ed. Manuela Weloso and Agnar Aamodt, *Lecture Notes in Artificial Intelligence* 1010, pp 205 -216, October 1995.
81. J. E. Hunt and D. E. Cooke, An Adaptive. Distributed Learning System based on the Immune System. In *Proc. of the IEEE International Conference on Systems Man and Cybernetics*, pp 2494 - 2499, 1995.
82. J. Hunt and J. Timmis. Evolving and Visualizing a Case Database using an Immune Network. In *European Conference on Artificial Intelligence* (ECAI 98), 1998.

83. Mark Neal, John Hunt and Jon Timmis. Augmenting an Artificial Immune Network. In *IEEE Int. Conf. on Systems, Man, and Cybernetics*, San Diego, 1998.
84. Shingo Ichikawa, Akio Ishiguro, Yuji Watanabe, and Yoshiki Uchikawa. Moderationism in the Immune System: Gait Acquisition of a Legged Robot Using the Metadynamics Function. In *IEEE Int. Conf. on Systems, Man, and Cybernetics*, San Diego, 1998.
85. A.Ishiguro, S.Ichikawa and Y.Uchikawa. A Gait Acquisition of 6-Legged Walking Robot Using Immune Networks, In *Proc. of IROS'94*, Vol.2, pp.1034-1041, 1994.
86. A.Ishiguro, Y.Watanabe and Y.Uchikawa. An Immunological Approach to Dynamic Behavior Control for Autonomous Mobile Robots. In *Proc. of IROS'95*, Vol.1, pp.495-500, 1995.
87. A.Ishiguro, T.Kondo, Y.Watanabe and Y.Uchikawa. Dynamic Behavior Arbitration of Autonomous Mobile Robots Using Immune Networks. In *Proc. of ICEC'95*, Vol.2, pp.722-727, 1995.
88. A.Ishiguro, T.Kondo, Y.Watanabe and Y.Uchikawa. Immunoid: An Immunological Approach to Decentralized Behavior Arbitration of Autonomous Mobile Robots. In *Lecture Notes in Computer Science*, Vol. 1141, Springer, pp.666-675, 1996.
89. A.Ishiguro, S.Kuboshiki, S.Ichikawa and Y.Uchikawa. Gait Control of Hexapod Walking Robots Using Mutual-coupled Immune Networks. In *Advanced Robotics*, Vol.10, No.2, pp.179-195, 1996.
90. A.Ishiguro, T.Kondo, Y.Watanabe, Y.Shirai and Y.Uchikawa. Emergent Construction of Artificial Immune Networks for Autonomous Mobile Robots. In *Proc. of SMC'97*, pp.1222-1228, 1997.
91. Akio Ishiguro, Yuji Watanabe, Toshiyuki Kondo, Yasuhiro Shirai, Hoshiki Uchikawa. Immunoid: A Robot with a Decentralized Behavior Arbitration Mechanisms Based on the Immune System. Presented at *ICMAS Workshop on Immunity-Based Systems*, December 10, 1996.
92. C.A. Janeway, Jr. How the immune system recognizes invaders. *Scientific American*, 269(3):72–79, September 1993.
93. N. K. Jerne. The immune system. *Scientific American*, 229(1):52–60, 1973.
94. N. K. Jerne. Towards a network theory of the immune system. *Ann. Immunol. (Inst. Pasteur)*, 125C:373–389, 1974.
95. N. K. Jerne. The generative grammar of the immune system. *The EMBO Journal*, 4(4):847–852, 1985.
96. Catriona Kennedy. Evolution of Self-Definition. In *IEEE Int. Conf. on Systems, Man, and Cybernetics*, San Diego, 1998.
97. J.O. Kephart. A biologically inspired immune system for computers, in R. A. Brooks and P. Maes, eds., *Artificial Life IV. Proc. of the 4th International*

*Workshop on the Synthesis and Simulation of Living Systems,* 130–139. MIT Press 1994.

98. J.O. Kephart et al. Biologically inspired defenses against computer viruses, *Proceedings of IJCAI '95*, 985–996, Montreal, August 19–25, 1995.
99. T. B. Kepler and A. S. Perelson. Modeling and optimization of populations subject to time-dependent mutation. *Proc. Natl. Acad. Sci. USA*, 92:8219–8223, 1995.
100. K. KrishnaKumar. An immune system framework for integrating computational intelligence paradigms. In Computational Intelligence, A Dynamic Perspective, IEEE Press, 1995.
101. K. KrishnaKumar and J. C. Neidhoefer. Immunized Neurocontrol, Expert Systems with Applications, Vol. 13, No. 3, pp. 201-214, 1997.
102. K. KrishnaKumar, J. Neidhoefer. Immunized Adaptive Critics, ICNN'97, Houston, TX, June, 1997.
103. K. KrishnaKumar. Immunized Neurocontrol: Concepts and Initial Results, *International workshop on combinations of genetic algorithms and neural networks* (COGANN-92), IEEE Press, pp. 146-168, 1992.
104. P. Marrack and J.W. Kappler. How the immune system recognizes the body. *Scientific American*, 269(3):81–89, September 1993.
105. Robert E. Marmelstein, David A. Van Veldhvizen and Gary B. Lamont. A Distributed Architecture for an Adaptive Computer Virus Immune. In *the IEEE International Conference on Systems, Man, and Cybernetics*, San Diego, October, 1998.
106. David McCoy and Venkat Devarajan. Artificial Immune Systems for Aerial Image Segmentation. In the proceedings of the 1997 IEEE International Conference on Systems, Man, and Cybernetics, Orlando, Florida, October 13, 1997.
107. Ronald R. Mohler, Carlo Bruni, and Alberto Gandolfi. A System Approach to Immunology. *Proceedings of the IEEE*, 68(8):964–990, 1980.
108. D. Morawietz, D. Chowdhury, S. Vollmar and D. Stauffer. Simulation of the kinetics of the Widom model of microemulsion. Physica A (*Elsevier*), vol.187, 126, 1992.
109. K. Mori, M. Tsukiyama and T. Fukuda. Immune Algorithm with Searching Diversity and its Application to Resource Allocation Problem. *The Trans. of the Institute of Electrical Engineers of Japan*, Vol.113-C, No.10, pp.872–878 (in japanese), 1993.
110. K. Mori, M. Tsukiyama and T. Fukuda. Immune Algorithm and its Application to Factory Load Dispatching Planning. *1994 JAPAN-U.S.A. Symposium on Flexible Automation*, pp.1343–1346, 1994.
111. K. Mori, M. Tsukiyama and T. Fukuda. Load Dispatching Planning by Immune Algorithm with Diversity and Learning. *7th Int. Conf. on Systems Research, Informatics and Cybernetics*, Vol.II, pp.136–141, 1994.

112. K. Mori, M. Tsukiyama and T. Fukuda. Multi-Optimization by Immune Algorithm with Diversity and Learning. *2nd Int. Conf. on Multi-Agent Systems, Workshop Notes on Immunity-Based Systems*, pp.118–123, 1996.
113. K. Mori, M. Tsukiyama and T. Fukuda. Application of an Immune Algorithm to Multi-Optimization Problems. *The Trans. of the Institute of Electrical Engineers of Japan*, Vol.117-C, No.5, pp.593–598 (in japanese), 1997.
114. K. Mori, M. Tsukiyama and T. Fukuda. Artificial Immunity Based Management System for a Semiconductor Production Line. In *1997 IEEE Int. Conf. on Systems, Man, and Cybernetics*, Vol.1, pp.852–856, 1997.
115. K. Mori, M. Tsukiyama and T. Fukuda. Adaptive Scheduling System Inspired by Immune System. In *IEEE Int. Conf. on Systems, Man, and Cybernetics*, San Diego, 1998.
116. Mihaela Oprea and Stephanie Forrest. Simulated evolution of antibody gene libraries under pathogen selection. In *IEEE Int. Conf. on Systems, Man, and Cybernetics*, San Diego, 1998.
117. William E. Paul, (ed.) *Immunology: Recognition and Response ... Readings from Scientific American.* New York: W.H. Freeman and Company, 1991.
118. A. Perelson, R. Hightower, and S. Forrest. Evolution (and learning) of V-region genes. *Research in Immunology* Vol. 147, pp. 202–208, 1996.
119. Alan S. Perelson and Gerard Weisbuch. Immunology for physicists. *Preprint for Review of Modern Physics*, June 1995.
120. J. K Percus, O. Percus, and A. S. Person. Predicting the size of the antibody combining region from consideration of efficient self/non-self discrimination. *Proceedings of the National Academy of Science*, 60:1691–1695, 1993.
121. Alan S. Perelson. Immune network theory. *Immunological Reviews*, (10):5–36, 1989.
122. A. S. Perelson and G. F. Oster. Theoretical studies of clonal selection: Minimal antibody repertoire size and reliability of self- non-self discrimination. *J. Theoret. Biol.*, 81:645–670, 1979.
123. Calton Pu, Andrew Black, Crispin Cowan, Jonathan Walpole, A Specialization Toolkit to Increase the Diversity in Operating Systems. *Presented at ICMAS Workshop on Immunity-Based Systems*, December 10, 1996.
124. Mitchell A. Potter and Kenneth A. De Jong. The Coevolution of Antibodies for Concept Learning. In the *Proceeding of the Parallel Problem Solving from Nature (PPSN)*, Amsterdam, 1998.
125. Glenn W. Rowe. *The Theoretical Models in Biology.* Oxford University Press, first edition, 1994.
126. Rira M. Z. Santos and Américo T. Bernardes. The stable-chaotic transition on cellular automata used to model the immune repertoire. *Physica A*, 219:1–12, 1995.

127. L. A. Segel and A. S. Perelson. Computations in shape space: A new approach to immune network theory. In A. S. Perelson, editor, *Theoretical Immunology, Part Two, SFI Studies in the Sciences of Complexity*, pages 321–343. Addison-Wesley, Reading, MA, 1988.
128. P. E. Seiden and F. Celada. A model for simulating cognate recognition and response in the immune system. *J. Theoret. Biol.*, 158:329–357, 1992.
129. D. J. Smith, S. Forrest, D. H. Ackley, and A. S. Perelson Using lazy evaluation to simulate realistic-size repertoires in models of the immune system. *Bulletin of Mathematical Biology*, 1997.
130. D. J. Smith, S. Forrest, R. R. Hightower, and A. S. Perelson Deriving shape-space parameters from immunological data for a model of cross-reactive memory. *Journal of Theoretical Biology* Vol. 189: 141-150, 1997.
131. R. E. Smith, S. Forrest, and A. S. Perelson. Searching for diverse, cooperative populations with genetic algorithms. In *Evolutionary Computation* 1:2, pp. 127-149, 1993.
132. D. J. Smith, S. Forrest, and A. S. Perelson. Immunological memory is associative. In ICMAS Worshop on Immunity-based Systems, 1996.
133. R. Smith, S. Forrest, and A. S. Perelson. An immune system model for maintaining diversity in a genetic algorithm. In L. D. Whitley (Ed.) Proceedings of a Workshop on Foundations of Genetic Algorithms, Morgan Kaufmann, Los Altos, CA, 1993.
134. D. J. Smith, S. Forrest, D. H. Ackley, and A. S. Perelson. Modeling the effects of prior infection on vaccine efficacy. In Proceedings of the 1997 IEEE International Conference on Systems, Man, and Cybernetics, October 12-15, 1997, Orlando, FL, 1997.
135. A. Somayaji, S. Hofmeyr, and S. Forrest. Principles of a Computer Immune System. Presented at New Security Paradigms Workshop September, 1997.
136. D. Stauffer and M. Sahimi. High-dimensional simulation of simple immunological models. *J. Theoret. Biol.*, 166:289–297, 1994.
137. Dietrich Stauffer and Gérard Weisbuch. High-dimensional simulation of the shape-space model for the immune system. *Physica A*, 180:42–52, 1992.
138. David Tarlinton. Antigen presentation by memory b cells: The sting is in the tail. *Science*, 276:374–375, April 1997.
139. J. Timmis, J. Hunt and M. Neal, Augmenting an Artificial Immune Network using Ordering, Self-recognition and Histo-compatibility Operators, In the proceedings of the IEEE SMC Conference, 1998.
140. Franciso J. Varela and John Stewart. Dynamics of a class of immune networks I. Global Stability of idiotype interactions. *Journal of Theoretical Biology*, 144(1):93–101, 1990.
141. Frank T. Vertosick and Robert H. Kelly. Immune network theory: a role for parallel distributed processing? *Immunology*, 66:1–7, 1989.

142. Frank T. Vertosick and Robert H. Kelly. The immune system as a neural network: A multi-epitope approach. *Journal of Theoretical Biology*, 150:225–237, 1991.
143. F. Varela, A. Coutinho, B. Dupire and N.N. Vaz. Cognitive networks: immune, neural and otherwise. in *Theoretical Immunology* (A.S. Perelson, ed.), Part 2, Redwood City: Addison-Wesley, p. 359, 1988.
144. Y.Watanabe, A.Ishiguro, Y.Shirai and Y.Uchikawa. Emergent Construction of Behavior Arbitration Mechanism Based on the Immune System. Advanced Robotics, 1998.
145. Richard G. Weinand. Somatic mutation, affinity maturation and antibody repertoire: A computer model. *Journal of Theoretical Biology*, 143(3):343–382, 1990.
146. G. Weisbuch and M. Oprea. Capacity of a model immune network. *Bull. Math. Biol.*, 56:899–921, 1994.
147. Gerard Weisbuch. A shape space approach to the dynamics of the immune system. *Journal of Theoretical Biology*, 143(4):507–522, 1990.
148. Y. Ishida and F. Mizessyn. An Immune Network Approach for Sensor-Based Diagnosis with Sensor Faults: An Experimental Simulation for Cement Plant. NAIST Technical Report, NAIST-IS-TR 95027, 1995.
149. Y. Ishida. An Immune Network Approach to Sensor-Network with Self-Organization for Sensor and Process Faults. NAIST Technical Report, NAIST-IS-TR 95028, 1995.
150. Y. Ishida and Y. Tokimasa. An Immune Network Approach for Sensor-Based Diagnosis with Measurement Noise and Gross Errors. NAIST Technical Report, NAIST-IS-TR 95029, 1995.
151. Y. Ishida and N. Adachi. An Immunological Algorithm and Its Application to Disturbance Rejection. NAIST Technical Report, NAIST-IS-TR 95030, 1995.
152. Y. Ishida. Note on Immune Network and Majority Network. NAIST Technical Report, NAIST-IS-TR 95031, 1995.
153. Y. Ishida. Distributed and Autonomous Sensing based on Immune Network. Proc. of AROB 96, pp. 214-217, 1996.
154. Y. Ishida and N. Adachi. Active Noise Control by an Immune Algorithm: Adaptation in Immune System as an Evolution. Proc. ICEC 96, pp. 150-153, 1996.
155. Y. Ishida and A. Nogi. Reasoning about Structure of Interval Systems: An Approach by Sign Directed-Graph. Proc. QR 96, pp. 93-102, 1996.
156. Y. Ishida and Y. Tokimasa. Diagnosis by a Dynamic Network inspired by Immune Network. Proc. WCNN 96, San Diego, USA, pp. 508-511, 1996.
157. Y. Ishida. Active Diagnosis by Immunity-Based Agent Approach. Proc. DX 96, Val-Morin, Canada, pp. 106-114, 1996.
158. Y. Ishida. A Model of Group Choice for Artificial Society. In H. Asama Eds., Proc. DARS 96, Springer-Verlag, Tokyo, 1996.

159. Y. Ishida, and N. Adachi. An Immune Algorithm for Multiagent: Application to Adaptive Noise Neutralization. Proc. IROS 96, Osaka, pp. 1739-1746, 1996.
160. Y. Ishida and Y. Tokimasa. Data Reconcilliation Combined with Data Evaluation by Sensor Networks with Immune Net Metaphor. Proc. of the 35th IEEE Conference on Decision and Control 96, in CD-ROM, 1996.
161. Y. Ishida. The Immune System as a Self-Identification Process: a survey and a proposal. Presented at ICMAS International Workshop on Immunity-Based Systems (IMBS96), Kyoto, December 10-13, pp. 2-12, 1996.
162. Y. Ishida. Agent-Based Architecture of Selection Principle in the Immune System. Presented at ICMAS International Workshop on Immunity-Based Systems (IMBS96), Kyoto, December 10-13, pp. 92-104, 1996.
163. Y. Ishida. An Immune Network Approach to Sensor-Based Diagnosis by Self-Organization. Complex Systems, Vol. 10, No. 1, pp. 73-90, 1996.
164. Y. Ishida. The Immune System as a Prototype of Autonomous Decentralized Systems: An Overview. In Proc. of *International Symposium on Autonomous Decentralized Systems* (ISADS'97), Berlin, April 9 - 11, pp. 85-92, 1997.
165. Y. Ishida. Active Diagnosis by Self-Organization: An Approach by The Immune Network Metaphor. In Proc. of the *International Joint Conference on Artificial Intelligence*, Nagoya, pp. 1084-1089, 1997.

# Author Index


David H. Ackley 144
Ruth Lev Bar-Or 65
Hugues Bersini 22
Jorge Carneiro 47
Debashis Chowdhury 89
Denise Cooke 157
Dipankar Dasgupta 3, 262
Stephanie Forrest 105, 144, 262
Toyoo Fukuda 210, 278
John Hunt 157
Akio Ishiguro 187
Jeffrey O. Kephart 242
Clive King 157
Kalmanje Krishnakumar 221
Kazuyuki Mori 210, 278
Mark Neal 157
James Neidhoefer 221
Alan S. Perelson 105, 144
Lee A. Segel 65
Derek J. Smith 105, 144
Gregory B. Sorkin 242
John Stewart 47
Morton Swimmer 242
Wai-Yuan Tan 115
Jon Timmis 157
Makoto Tsukiyama 210, 278
Yoshiki Uchikawa 187
Yuji Watanabe 187
Steve R. White 242
Zhihua Xiang 115

# Subject Index


action selection, 203
actively infected T cells, 117
acquired immunity, 89
adaptive critics, 221
adaptive immune systems, 251
adaptive immunity, 6
adaptive resonance theory, 263
agents, 281
aircraft control, 222, 234
anomaly detection, 263, 264
anti-viral drugs, 116
anti-virus software, 255
antibody, 194, 214
antigen, 194, 214
antigen receptors, 146
antigenic challenge, 6
antigenic distance, 151
antigenic stimulation, 49
AntiVirus, 242
artificial immune algorithm, 219
artificial immune network, 199
artificial immune system, 263
artificial immunology, 65
artificial intelligence, 187
associative memory, 105, 111
associative recall, 106
autoimmune disease, 67
autonomous distributed system, 281
autonomous agents, 27
autonomous control, 222
autonomous mobile robots, 187, 188
autosequencing, 254

B-cells, 90, 251
B-lymphocytes, 189
B-T cell co-operation, 47
Boltzmann distribution, 35

cell-population dynamics, 102
cellular automata, 95
cellular immunity, 4
Central Immune System, 47
cerebellar cortex, 106
classifier, 163
classifier systems, 34
clonal selection, 5
cognitive, 83
colored petri net, 281
combinatorial optimization, 211
complex system, 278
complex adaptive systems, 27
computer simulation, 51, 145
computer viruses, 242
consensus-making, 195
control of chaos, 22, 28
cross-reactive memory, 105, 148
cross-reactive response, 108
cross-reactivity, 145, 150

data preprocessing, 264
decentralized behavior arbitration, 206
decentralized processing mechanism, 189
decoy programs, 14
decreasing peaks function, 216
delay-differential equation, 267
detection algorithm, 263
detector agents, 281
detector generation, 274
detectors, 263
diversity, 210
drug resistance, 116, 121, 124, 130
dynamic programming, 231, 232, 264

effector, 73–75

epidemic infection, 147
epidemic strains, 151
epidemiological modeling, 243
evolutionary algorithms, 4, 22
extended Kalman filter, 127

feedback, 65, 68, 80
fixed point, 93
free HIV, 115, 116
function optimization, 210
functional networks, 10

genetic algorithms, 23, 210, 233, 236

hamming distance, 109
hamming space, 272
hepatitis C virus, 144
historical database, 265
HIV-infected, 115
humoral immunity, 4

idiotope, 194
immune algorithm, 213
idiotypic networks, 10, 89
immune system, 158
immune network, 162, 163, 187, 191
immune networks, 22, 25, 30
immune response, 106
immune system, 3, 5, 65, 89, 106, 263
immunity, 50
immunized adaptive critic, 226
immunized adaptive critic, 222, 237
immunodeficiency virus, 144
immunoglobulin, 213
immunoglobulins, 49
immunologcal memory, 102
immunological computation, 4
immunological memory, 105, 108
immunology, 83
influenza, 149
informative entropy, 212
intelligent control, 221–223
internal image, 98

latently infected T cells, 116
learning algorithm, 32, 34
learning phase, 176
limit cycle, 93
lymphocyte population, 211
lymphocytes, 6, 90

machine learning, 180
Mackey-Glass series, 267
macro viruses, 252
macros, 242
matching algorithm, 159
matching threshold, 6
memory, 49
memory cell, 213
metabolism, 193
metadynamics, 190, 203
MHC-protein, 67
mortgage fraud, 172, 175
multi agent nets, 278
multi-modal function, 210
mutual recognition, 211

natural immunology, 83
nearest-neighbour, 101
negative-selection algorithm, 11, 263
neural networks, 4, 22, 34, 180
neuro-control, 222
normal behavior, 267
normal database, 266

object oriented approach, 176
objective function, 211
observation model, 127
optimize, 69
original antigenic sin, 105, 148

parallel search, 210
parametric plasticity, 35, 37
paratope, 189

partial matching rule, 263
pathogens, 66
pattern recognition, 159
Peripheral Immune System, 47
plasma cell, 66, 146
prior infection, 145

Q-learning, 28, 34, 36
quadratic Kalman filter, 131
quality production, 262

real world problem, 180
regulation, 4
reinforcement learning, 25, 27, 28, 231
repertoire, 50
representation space, 264
Runga-Kutta method, 267

Second generation immune network, 47
Self, 263
self organisation, 158
self-nonself discrimination, 5, 263
self-regulatory, 6
semiconductor production systems, 275
semiconductor production line, 278
shape space, 99
shubert function, 210
signature extractor, 255
sliding window, 267
somatic hyper-mutation, 6
somatic theory, 213
sparse distributed memory, 105, 108
spatial organization, 65, 79
spatio-temporal patterns, 93
stability augmentation, 225
state transition, 281
state space models, 115, 124, 138
stimulation threshold, 161
stochastic differential equations, 119, 123, 135
stochastic process, 6
stochastic system model, 115, 123, 135
system behavior, 264

T-cells, 91, 251
T-lymphocytes, 189
Taylor series, 124
TCR, 55
third generation network model, 60
thymus, 263
time series, 265
token, 281
trafficking, 4

unified model, 94

vaccination, 49, 106, 144, 147
vaccine efficacy, 145, 149
varying boundary conditions, 270
visualization tool, 176

window automata, 93
WIP (Work In Process), 279

Printing: Saladruck, Berlin
Binding: Buchbinderei Lüderitz & Bauer, Berlin